Atlas of
HYPERTENSION

Fourth Edition

EDITOR

Norman K. Hollenberg, MD

Professor of Radiology
Harvard Medical School;
Director, Physiologic Research
Department of Medicine
Brigham and Women's Hospital
Boston, Massachusetts

SERIES EDITOR

Eugene Braunwald, MD, MD (Hon), ScD (Hon)

Distinguished Hersey Professor of Medicine
Faculty Dean for Academic Programs at
* Brigham and Women's Hospital and Massachusetts Hospital*
Harvard Medical School;
Vice President for Academic Programs
Partners HealthCare System
Boston, Massachusetts

Developed by Current Medicine, Inc., Philadelphia

CM
CURRENT
MEDICINE

Philadelphia

CURRENT MEDICINE, INC.

400 Market Street, Suite 700 • Philadelphia, PA 19106

Developmental Editor . . . .*Elise M. Paxson*
Editorial Assistant . . . .*Annmarie D'Ortona*
Cover Design . . . .*John McCullough*
Design and Layout . . . .*William C. Whitman, Jr.*
Illustrators . . . .*John McCullough, Marie Dean, Wieslawa Langenfeld, Maureen Looney*
Assistant Production Manager . . . .*Margaret La Mare*
Indexing . . . .*Holly Lukens*

Printed in Singapore by Imago Productions (FE) Pte. Ltd.

Library of Congress Cataloging-in-Publication Data

Atlas of hypertension / editor, Norman K. Hollenberg.--4th ed.
    p. ; cm.
    Rev. ed. of: Hypertension, c2001.
    Includes bibliographical references and index.
    ISBN 1-57340-196-X
    1. Hypertension--Atlases. I. Hollenberg, Norman K. II. Hypertension.
    [DNLM: 1. Hypertension--physiopathology. 2. Hypertension--therapy. 3. Medical
Illustration. WG 17 A884374 2003]
    RC685.H8 H825 2003
    616.1'32--dc21

                                          2002036836

ISBN 1-57340-196-X

www.current-science-group.com

PREFACE

In the preface to the third edition of the *Atlas of Hypertension*, I expressed surprise and delight that there was to be such a third edition. The many thousands of copies purchased and distributed, and I hope read and used, could not have been anticipated. As it turned out, the third edition was as popular as the first and second, and so we have a fourth edition.

In the preface to the third edition, I pointed out that the goal was to have a single chapter on pathogenesis, which would reflect the fact that pathogenesis was well worked out— rather than the multiple chapters that are necessary in our current state of ignorance. Although we have made major advances in our understanding of pathogenesis, largely through the study of genes in animal models, in fact we are very little closer to under-standing pathogenesis than we were when this series began. On the other hand, as will be evident in the chapters dealing with pathogenesis, we have made advances, and these are nicely covered in the individual chapters.

In the area of clinical trials, we have made substantial advances since the last edition. Our sole new contributor, Dr. Kenneth A. Jamerson, provides a superb overview of our advance in understanding therapeutics and epidemiology based on clinical trials. His chapter and that of Matthew Weir, which focuses on renal aspects, summarize quite an extraordinary array of trials completed in the past several years.

In the area of therapeutics based on individual therapeutic agents, there have been fewer advances. The angiotensin-receptor blockers, which were the "new kids on the block" at the time of the third edition, are now firmly established. Eplerenone, the new aldosterone antagonist, has not yet found approval by a regulatory agency at the time of the publica-tion of this fourth edition, but is likely to do so before the fifth edition, and is likely to be a singular advance. The same might have been said of omapatrilat, the vasopeptidase inhibitor, in the preface to the third edition. At the moment, the future of omapatrilat lies somewhat under a cloud at the regulatory agency and in the community. Given our poor track record in achieving goal blood pressure in high-risk patients, especially the patient with type 2 diabetes mellitus, it is my hope that omapatrilat will be made available to physicians for such patients and for detailed review in the fifth edition.

All chapters have been revised, adding new material where appropriate and modifying material in the text where new information is provided in new context.

Writing these prefaces has created an opportunity for me to take a global view to address the issue of which advances over the past several years are sufficiently important that they merit review in an edition of this sort. I am pleased that the advances made have been frequent and substantial.

Norman K. Hollenberg, MD, PhD

CONTRIBUTORS

R. WAYNE ALEXANDER, MD, PHD
R. Bruce Logue Professor and Chair
Director of Cardiology
Emory University
Atlanta, Georgia

JOHN AMERENA, MBBS, FRACP
Senior Lecturer
Department of Clinical and Biomedical Science
University of Melbourne School of Medicine;
Geelong Hospital
Geelong, Australia

RICHARD B. ANDERSON, EdD
President
CoMMensa, Inc.
Arlington, Massachusetts

HENRY R. BLACK, MD
Charles J. and Margaret Roberts Professor
  of Preventive Medicine
Rush Medical College;
Associate Vice President for Research
Rush-Presbyterian–St. Luke's Medical Center
Chicago, Illinois

EMMANUEL L. BRAVO, MD
Department of Nephrology and Hypertension
The Cleveland Clinic Foundation
Cleveland, Ohio

HANS R. BRUNNER, MD
Professor of Medicine
Division of Hypertension
Lausanne University
University Hospital
Lausanne, Switzerland

ROBERT M. CAREY, MD
Professor of Medicine
Dean, School of Medicine
University of Virginia Health Sciences Center
Charlottesville, Virginia

WILLIAM J. ELLIOTT, MD, PHD
Professor
Department of Preventive Medicine, Internal
  Medicine and Pharmacology
Rush Medical College;
Attending Physician
Rush-Presbyterian–St. Luke's Medical Center
Chicago, Illinois

KATHY K. GRIENDLING, PHD
Professor of Medicine
Department of Medicine
Emory University
Atlanta, Georgia

CARLENE MINKS GRIM, MD
Shared Care Research and Education
Torrance, California

CLARENCE E. GRIM, RN, MSN
Professor
Department of Cardiovascular Medicine
Medical College of Wisconsin
Milwaukee, Wisconsin

RANDOLPH A. HENNIGAR, PHD, MD
Associate Professor of Pathology
Department of Pathology
Emory University
Atlanta, Georgia

NORMAN K. HOLLENBERG, MD
Professor of Radiology
Harvard Medical School;
Director, Physiologic Research
Department of Medicine
Brigham and Women's Hospital
Boston, Massachusetts

KENNETH A. JAMERSON, MD
Associate Professor of Internal Medicine
Division of Hypertension
University of Michigan Medical Center
Ann Arbor, Michigan

STEVO JULIUS, MD
Professor of Internal Medicine and Physiology
Frederick G.L. Huetwell Professor of Hypertension
Department of Internal Medicine
University of Michigan
Ann Arbor, Michigan

WILLIAM B. KANNEL, MD, MPH, FACC
Professor of Medicine and Public Health
Department of Preventive Medicine
Boston University School of Medicine
Boston, Massachusetts

BARRY J. MATERSON, MD, MBA
Professor of Medicine
Department of Medicine
University of Miami
Miami, Florida

DOMENIC A. SICA, MD
Professor of Medicine and Pharmacology
Chairman, Section of Clinical Pharmacology
  and Hypertension
Division of Nephrology
Medical College of Virginia
Campus of Virginia Commonwealth University
Richmond, Virginia

HELMY M. SIRAGY, MD, FACP, FAHA
Professor of Medicine
Department of Medicine
University of Virginia Health System
Charlottesville, Virginia

BERNARD WAEBER, MD
Professor of Medicine
Division of Pathophysiology
Lausanne University
University Hospital
Lausanne, Switzerland

ALAN B. WEDER, MD
Professor of Medicine
Department of Internal Medicine
The University of Michigan Medical Center
Ann Arbor, Michigan

MATTHEW R. WEIR, MD
Professor of Medicine
Department of Medicine
University of Maryland School of Medicine
Baltimore, Maryland

GORDON H. WILLIAMS, MD
Professor of Medicine;
Director, Specialized Center of Research in
  Hypertension;
Chief, Hormonal Mechanisms of Cardiovascular
  Risk Laboratory
Harvard Medical School
Boston, Massachusetts

CONTENTS

PATHOGENESIS OF HYPERTENSION: GENETIC AND ENVIRONMENTAL FACTORS

Alan B. Weder

Like obesity and diabetes, essential hypertension is one of the "diseases of civilization" that results from the collision of a modern lifestyle with Paleolithic genes.

Genetic analyses of communities, families, twins, and individuals all support the tenet of a genetic contribution to blood pressure regulation, but the identification of specific genes that cause hypertension has only just begun. The use of segregating populations derived from inbred hypertensive and normotensive animals, which permits tracing the linkage of genetic markers with blood pressure, has led to the detection of several genes that may contribute to hypertension. It was hoped that such studies would identify candidate genes that cause essential hypertension, but none of the specific genes identified in rat models has been proven to cause disease in humans. The applicability of congenic and transgenic methods to rats has permitted studies of candidate loci and individual genes in relatively well-defined settings, and it is hoped that such models will define the effects of mutant genes on the control of blood pressure.

It should not be assumed that the effects of single-gene insertions or knockouts of candidate alleles will always have straightforward phenotypic effects. An example is the hypertensive rat created by insertion of the mouse renin gene. These rats are characterized by low levels of plasma renin and renal renin gene expression but also by high adrenal renin gene expression and fulminant hypertension. Such unpredictable phenotypic effects arising from seemingly "simple" genetic manipulations serve to emphasize the complexity of genomic dynamics.

The task of identifying genes that contribute to essential hypertension in humans is a great challenge, and the genetic architecture of human hypertension is only dimly perceived. Several notable successes have been achieved recently, however. The rare mendelian-dominant hypertensive syndrome of glucocorticoid-remediable hyperaldosteronism has been proven to result from a genetic chimerism of the genes for 11β-hydroxylase and aldosterone synthase, and several other mendelian genes associated with hypertension have been identified using similar methods. The more difficult problem of essential hypertension has also witnessed progress lately with the recently described link between the angiotensinogen gene and both essential hypertension and hypertension of pregnancy. A major problem in defining the genetics of essential hypertension is heterogeneity of the phenotype, and further advances may depend on refinements in subtyping hypertension. In addition to classic characterizations based on measurements of biochemical regulators of cardiovascular function, promising approaches include subtyping by membrane transport characteristics and definitions based on multivariate hypertension-related syndromes.

Regardless of its genetic substrate, hypertension is clearly an ecogenic disease, that is, environmental factors interact with genes to cause high blood pressure. Because the prevalence of hypertension is directly related to the mean blood pressure of the population, studies of environmental factors can rightly focus on factors that are universally active in societies (*eg*, high salt intake, calorie excess, and social stress) as well as specific factors (*eg*, alcohol excess) whose impacts are limited to at-risk individuals. There may be genetic subtypes of hypertensive individuals who are particularly sensitive to specific environmental factors, *eg*, dietary sodium and calcium, although interventional studies have not yielded conclusive evidence on which to base preventive approaches to hypertension.

GENETIC FACTORS IN HYPERTENSION

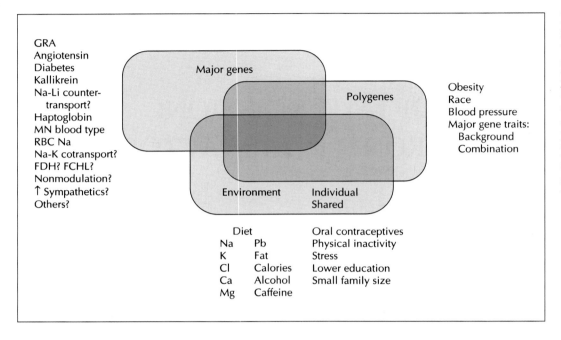

FIGURE 1-1. A model indicating the mechanisms by which essential hypertension could result from the combined effects of individual major genes that have a large impact on blood pressure, blended polygenes with small individual contributions, and environmental effects operating on individuals or within families. FCHL—familial combined hyperlipidemia; FDH—familial dyslipidemic hypertension; GRA— glucocorticoid-remediable aldosteronism. (*Courtesy of* Roger R. Williams, MD.)

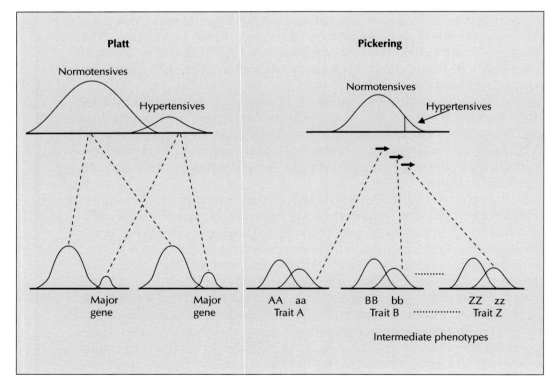

FIGURE 1-2. From the late 1940s through the 1960s, Sir George Pickering and Lord Platt of Grindleford debated the nature of the genetic basis of human essential hypertension. Platt, a prominent English internist, pointed to what he believed to be discontinuities in the distribution of blood pressure values in families of hypertensive individuals and postulated the existence of a major gene for hypertension, transmitted as a mendelian-dominant trait [1]. Pickering, who maintained that hypertensives have blood pressures in the upper end of a continuous, smooth distribution, argued that hypertension is a multigenic disease [2]. In such a construct, each gene has a small effect on a trait (intermediate phenotype) that contributes to increased blood pressure; the sum of all the trait effects, when sufficient to elevate blood pressure to some arbitrarily high value, is the genetic basis of essential hypertension. The consensus now supports Pickering's view, but the debate was of most importance because it sparked interest in the genetic basis of human essential hypertension.

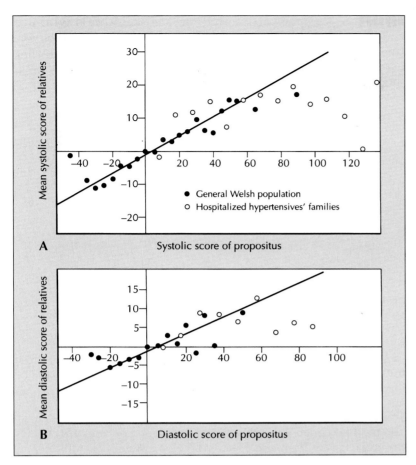

FIGURE 1-3. Relationship of systolic (**A**) and diastolic (**B**) age- and sex-adjusted blood pressure (referred to as "score") in hypertensive individuals and first-degree relatives selected from the general Welsh population and from the families of hospitalized hypertensives. The regression line applies to the population data. The continuous linear relationship supports a multifactorial mode of inheritance. (*Adapted from* Ledingham [3].)

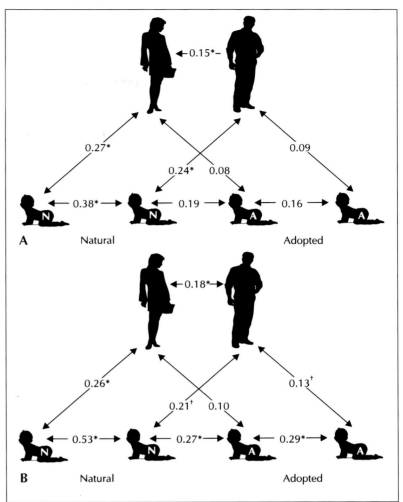

FIGURE 1-4. Correlation coefficients for relationships in systolic (**A**) and diastolic (**B**) blood pressure among parents, natural (biological) children, and adopted children. The weak correlations between parents, parents and adopted children, and adopted and natural children primarily reflect the effects of environment on blood pressure. The stronger correlations between parents and their biological children as well as between biological siblings reflect the additive effects of shared genes and environment [4]. In general, blood pressure correlation between siblings is weaker than that between nonidentical (dizygotic) twins (*see* Fig. 1-5), although both groups would be expected to share the same proportion of parental genes (50%). A recent study from Norway that examined the correlation between blood pressure in 43,751 parent-offspring pairs, 19,140 sibling pairs, and 169 pairs of twins suggests that this difference is partially due to age-dependent genetic effects on blood pressure. Age-dependent effects are absent in twins but can somewhat degrade the apparent strength of correlations between nontwin siblings and between parents and offspring [5]. *Asterisks* indicate $P < 0.001$; *daggers*, $P < 0.01$. (*Adapted from* Mongeau *et al.* [4].)

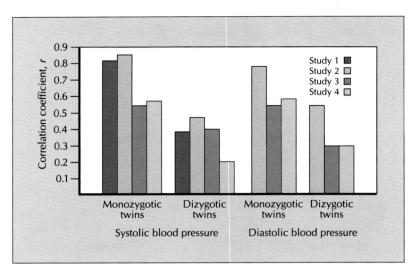

FIGURE 1-5. Comparison of correlation coefficients for systolic and diastolic blood pressure between monozygotic and dizygotic twins in four studies. All studies show a stronger relationship between blood pressure in monozygotic than in dizygotic twins, thereby suggesting that genes and environmental effects are important contributors to the level of blood pressure [6]. Diastolic blood pressure was not reported for study 1.

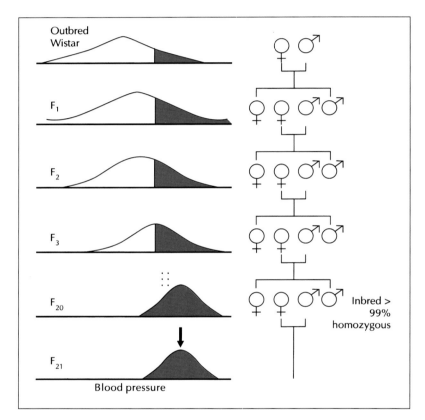

FIGURE 1-6. Schema for the development of inbred hypertensive rat strains. Beginning with animals from the upper end (*shaded*) of the blood pressure distribution of a colony of Wistar rats, offspring are selected based on blood pressure level in successive brother-sister inbreedings. As genes for high blood pressure are selected (and those for low blood pressure progressively eliminated), the population mean moves to higher values and the variability decreases. After approximately 20 generations, animals become more than 99% homozygous for all loci, including those controlling blood pressure. The residual variability in this inbred population presumably reflects the impact of environmental factors on blood pressure. *F* indicates the number of generations; the vertical line in each population indicates the level of blood pressure defining hypertension.

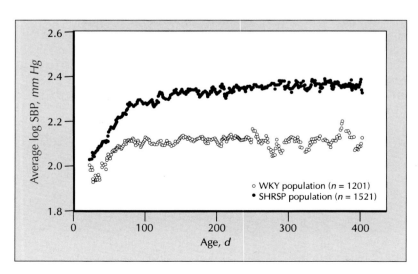

FIGURE 1-7. An example of stabilization of a hypertensive phenotype by inbreeding. Shown is a comparison of average systolic blood pressure (SBP) obtained by the tail cuff method in normotensive Wistar-Kyoto (WKY) rats and spontaneously hypertensive stroke-prone (SHRSP) rats. Curves are constructed using moving averages and are expressed on a log scale. Blood pressure diverges during the first 100 days of life but maintains a relatively constant difference thereafter. Investigations of the development of hypertension in these inbred models suggest that critical events occurring during the development of hypertension (before 100 days of age) influence the level of blood pressure that is ultimately achieved (*see* Fig. 1-11) [7].

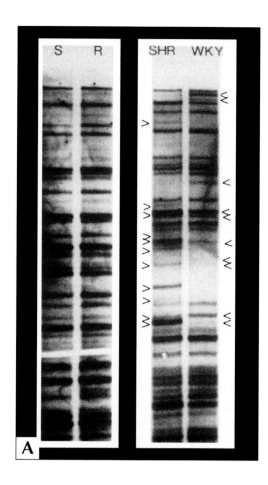

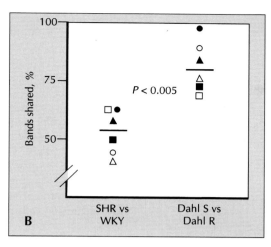

FIGURE 1-8. DNA fingerprinting is a method of estimating the genetic relatedness of inbred strains. **A,** Southern blot showing DNA finger-prints of inbred Dahl salt-sensitive (S) and salt-resistant (R) rats (*left*) and an inbred spontaneously hypertensive rat (SHR) and Wistar-Kyoto (WKY) rat (*right*). The fingerprinting was generated by probing HinfI-digested DNA with an oligonucleotide corresponding to the consensus repeat sequence of the human myoglobin 33.15 minisatellite. *Arrowheads* designate bands not shared between the hypertensive strains and the normotensive controls [8]. **B,** The percentage of bands shared between normotensive and hypertensive rats. Each symbol represents the percentage of bands shared between two inbred strains for a single restriction enzyme-probe combination. As shown by the horizontal bars for the means, SHR and WKY rats share an average of about 50% of the bands, while Dahl SS/Jr and Dahl SR/Jr share an average of about 80% [8]. Most of the genetic differences are unrelated to factors that influence blood pressure. Studies that simply compare the two strains become less informative as the percentage of shared bands diminishes.

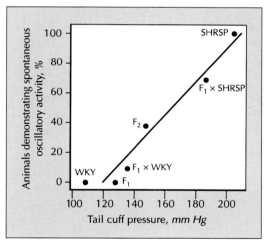

FIGURE 1-9. Relating the prevalence or strength of one phenotypic trait to another in segregating populations yields evidence that supports the degree of genetic relatedness of the traits. In this study, normotensive Wistar-Kyoto (WKY) rats were crossed with spontaneously hypertensive stroke-prone rats (SHRSP) to produce first-generation (F_1) offspring. These offspring were then inbred to produce F_2 offspring as well as back-crossed to parental WKY and SHRSP rats. Spontaneous oscillatory activity of tail artery strips in a muscle bath preparation was closely related to blood pressure obtained by the tail artery method [9]. This relationship supports the idea that spontaneous oscillatory activity and hypertension have a close genetic relationship. (*Adapted from* Bruner *et al.* [9].)

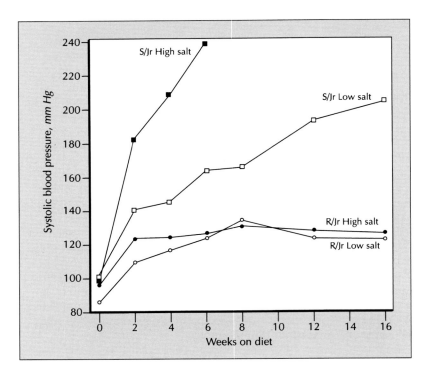

FIGURE 1-10. Genes for hypertension may require exposure to an environmental condition for full expression. In this study, the blood pressure response of inbred Dahl salt-sensitive (S/Jr) and salt-resistant (R/Jr) rats to high- (8%) and low- (0.3%) salt diets was monitored after weaning (30 days of age). Feeding a high-salt diet to S/Jr rats resulted in a rapid rise in blood pressure and was fatal to all 10 rats in the group. S/Jr rats fed a low-salt diet showed a slower rise in blood pressure, and all 10 rats survived for the 16 weeks of observation. Dietary salt had virtually no effect on blood pressure in R/Jr rats, and both high- and low-salt treated R/Jr rats had blood pressure lower than either S/Jr group [10]. S/Jr rats therefore have genes capable of raising blood pressure even in the absence of dietary salt excess, but the mechanisms promoting hypertension are markedly intensified by salt loading. (*Adapted from* Rapp [10].)

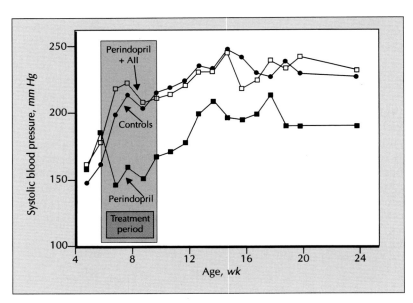

FIGURE 1-11. Some genes that promote hypertension may be only transiently activated during development. In this experiment, comparison was made of untreated controls versus spontaneously hypertensive rats treated for 4 weeks (from 6 through 10 weeks of age) with an angiotensin-converting enzyme inhibitor (perindopril, 3 mg/kg/d) or perindopril plus angiotensin II (AII, 200 ng/kg/min) administered subcutaneously. Systolic blood pressure was monitored by the tail cuff method. Treatment with perindopril alone lowered blood pressure during treatment; after perindopril was discontinued, blood pressure rose but never reached control levels. Combined treatment with perindopril and AII resulted in blood pressure similar to controls both during and after treatment [11]. The results suggest that there is a critical period in the 6- to 10-week age range during which AII promotes processes necessary for the full expression of hypertension during adulthood. (*Adapted from* Harrap *et al.* [11].)

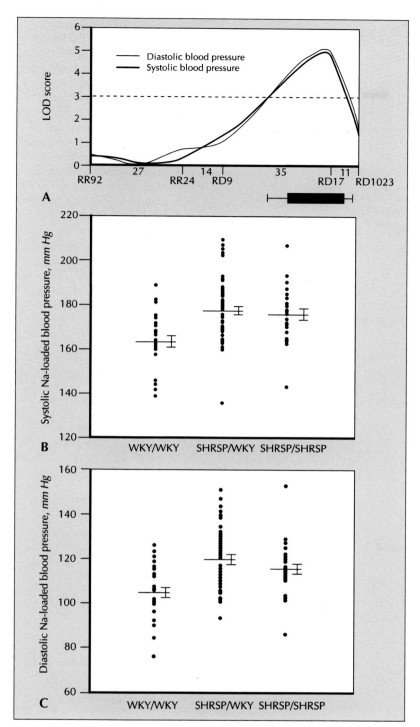

Figure 1-12. Genetic linkage can be used to identify genomic sites contributing to such quantitative traits as blood pressure. In this study, F_2 progenies were derived by cross-breeding normotensive Wistar-Kyoto (WKY) and spontaneously hypertensive stroke-prone (SHRSP) rats. Blood pressure was determined during dietary salt loading (1% NaCl in drinking water for 12 days) by direct intra-arterial recording. Genetic linkage to a series of genomic markers of known location was undertaken. Results of the linkage analysis are expressed as logarithm of the odds (LOD) scores, which represent the log of the odds ratio; by convention, an LOD score of 3.0 (*horizontal dashed line*) or greater is considered significant. **A,** The highest LOD scores are found in association with a chromosome 10 marker designated RD17, which was derived from a microsatellite of the growth hormone (GH) gene and is adjacent to the gene for angiotensin-converting enzyme (ACE). Systolic (**B**) and diastolic (**C**) Na-loaded blood pressure of individual animals genotyped for the SHRSP and WKY alleles of the RD17 locus. Group means are indicated by the *horizontal lines*, and standard errors are shown by the *t bars* bracketing the means. Rats that are homozygous for the SHRSP allele and those that are heterozygotes have higher blood pressures than those that are homozygous for the WKY allele [12]. It should be emphasized that linkage with a site adjacent to the ACE and GH genes does not prove that either gene necessarily causes hypertension. Hilbert *et al.* [13] found a similar linkage for this cross. (*Adapted from* Jacob *et al.* [12].)

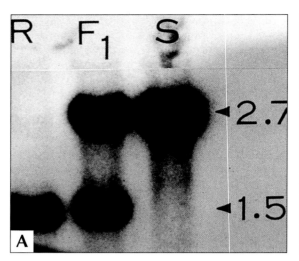 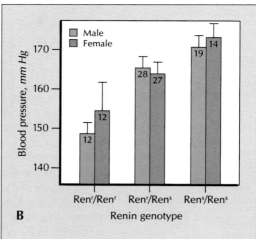

rats and their offspring. After digestion with the restriction enzyme Bgl II the fragments were separated by gel electrophoresis, and probed with a radioactive cDNA probe for the renin gene. Two bands of different size were detected: a 2.7-kb fragment in S rats and a 1.5-kb fragment in R rats (**A**). Heterozygotes (F_1) have both bands. Blood pressure obtained by the tail cuff method after dietary salt loading is shown for F_2 male and female rats classified by genotype at the renin locus (**B**). Each dose of the S allele raises blood pressure by approximately 10 mm Hg; heterozygotes are about 10 mm Hg higher than are homozygous RR F_2 rats, while SS homozygotes are about 20 mm Hg higher than RR [14]. There are no important sex differences. *Numbers inside bars* indicate the number of rats studied.

FIGURE 1-13. Genes suspected to play a role in hypertension are referred to as *candidate genes*. Because the renin-angiotensin-aldosterone (RAA) system is thought to be of pathogenetic importance in hypertension, genes for RAA elements are among the best studied candidates. In this experiment, genomic DNA was derived from Dahl salt-sensitive (S) and salt-resistant (R)

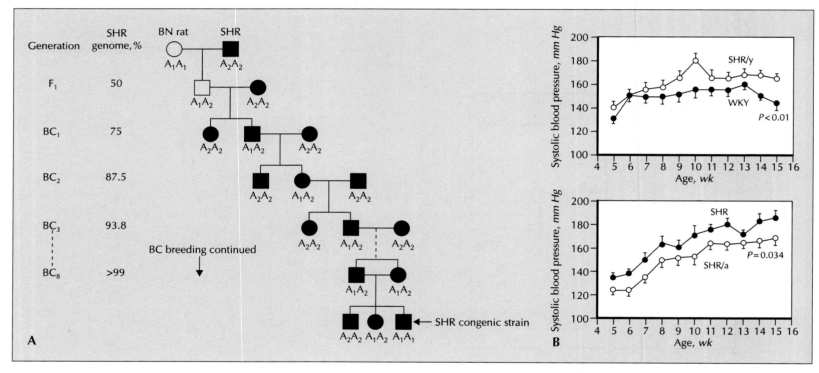

FIGURE 1-14. Derivation of a congenic strain in which a chromosomal locus on the Brown-Norway (BN) rat is transferred into the spontaneously hypertensive rat (SHR) genome. **A,** In this example, the BN strain is homozygous for the A_1 allele, while the SHR strain is homozygous for the A_2 allele. An F_1 offspring from a BN × SHR cross will carry one A_1 and one A_2 allele. Back-crossing this F_1 rat to an SHR yields progeny (BC_1) that have either a homozygous A_2 genotype or are heterozygotes at the A locus. Random transmission of other genes enriches the proportion of SHR genes at other loci; and by repeated back-crossing of offspring carrying the A_1 locus, after eight generations have been back-crossed, more than 99% of the genes not linked to the A locus are derived from the SHR. Heterozygotes at the A locus in the BC_8 generation are mated, and homozygotes for the A_1A_1 genotype are selected for further inbreeding to establish a congenic strain [15]. The phenotypic action

of the A_1 allele operating in the SHR genetic background can then be assessed. By means of direct genotyping of offspring at the locus of interest, the efficiency of the development of congenics can be increased. The congenic paradigm has been used to study the effects of the Y chromosome of the SHR. **B,** Tail cuff systolic blood pressure for F_{11} male rats with a Y chromosome derived from SHR and a genome derived from normotensive Wistar-Kyoto (WKY) rats (SHR/y; $n = 8$) compared with WKY males ($n = 8$; *top panel*). The blood pressure difference averages 12 mm Hg, which can be thought of as the hypertensive effect of the SHR/y chromosome. F_{11} males with a normotensive Y chromosome in an SHR genome (SHR/a; $n = 8$) were compared with male SHR rats ($n = 8$; *bottom panel*). The SHR/a males have blood pressures that are, on average, 14 mm Hg lower than those of the SHR rats, thereby suggesting that this effect results from the absence of the hypertensive Y chromosome [16].

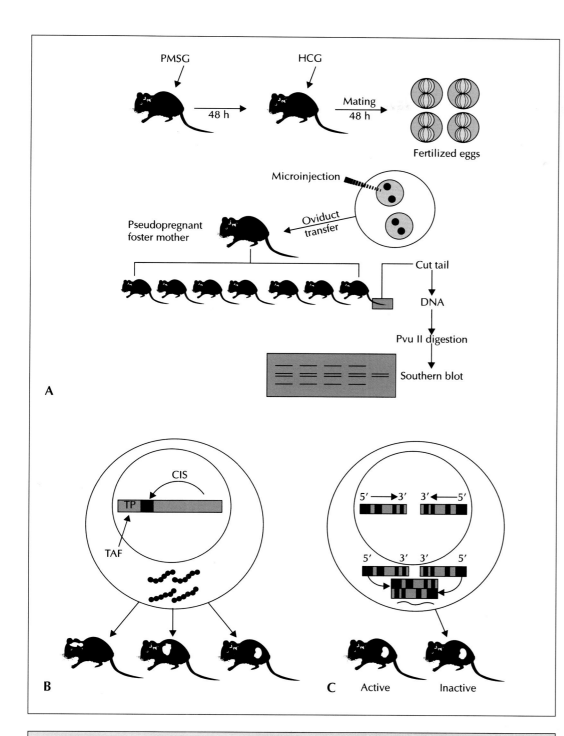

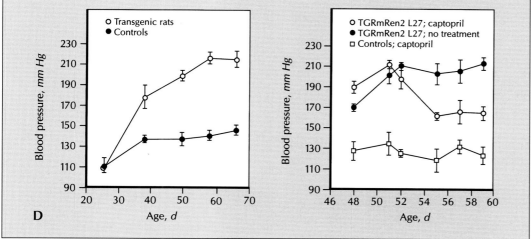

FIGURE 1-15. Methods involved in the production of transgenic animals by microinjection. **A,** Female hosts are prepared by injection of pregnant mare's serum gonadotropin (PMSG) and 48 hours later with human chorionic gonadotropin (HCG). Mating occurs 12 hours after injection of HCG, and fertilized eggs are removed and placed into tissue culture. Under the microscope, transgene DNA is microinjected into the male pronucleus, and the fertilized eggs are transferred into the oviduct of a pseudopregnant foster mother. Offspring are analyzed for the presence or absence of the transgene in DNA samples extracted from tail biopsies [17]. **B,** Transgenic techniques can be used to make insertional constructs with tissue-specific expression. Specificity is conferred by linking the transgene to tissue-specific or cell-specific promoters. Such hybrid genes are then active only in cells in which the particular promoter is active [17]. **C,** Gene activity can be suppressed by microinjection of a gene construct oriented in the reverse (antisense) orientation. The endogenous gene is transcribed in the 5′-3′ orientation while the antisense gene is transcribed 3′-5′. The two cRNA transcription products hybridize and block translation, resulting in suppression of gene expression in the phenotype [17]. **D,** Effects on blood pressure of introduction of a mouse renin gene (Ren2) into rats. The transgenic founder line is designated TGRmRen2 L27. Blood pressure in the transgenic animals and controls (mean ± SE) are compared (*left*), and the effect of treatment with captopril on blood pressure of the transgenic animals is shown (*right*) [18]. In TGRmRen2 L27 rats receiving captopril, the dose was 10 mg/kg/d in drinking water. CIS—cis acting factor; TP—tissue-specific promoter; TAF—*trans*-acting factor.

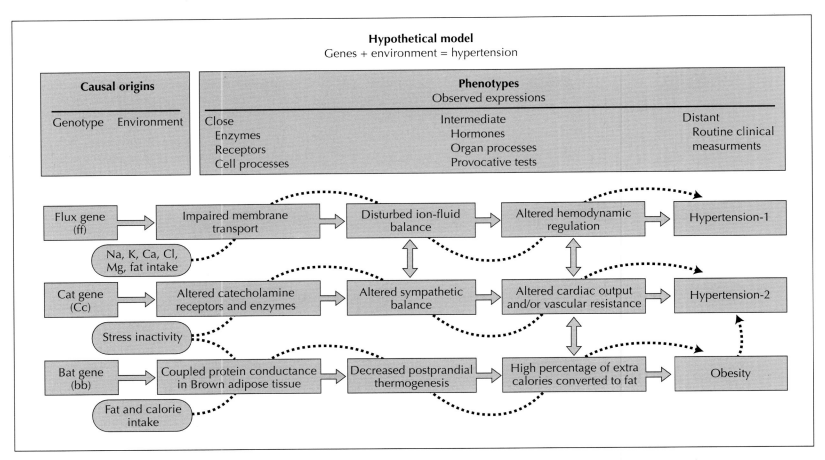

FIGURE 1-16. The flow of events from genes to their ultimate phenotypic expression. In this depiction, it is assumed that there are discrete hypertension-promoting genes (*eg*, Flux [ion transport], catecholamine [Cat], and brown adipose tissue [Bat] genes) that interact with environmental factors. Describing effects related directly to such genes, that is, close phenotypes, may help to identify the genes. As further higher-order interactions occur among genes, environment, and phenotypes, the remote phenotypic expression of individual genes that promote hypertension becomes more complex (intermediate phenotypes). Final or distant phenotypes, such as blood pressure itself (hypertension-1 and hypertension-2), appear similar and multifactorial because of the large number of interactions that intervene between genotype and phenotype. Backtracking to specific genes from this level is usually impossible [19]. (*Adapted from* Williams *et al.* [19].)

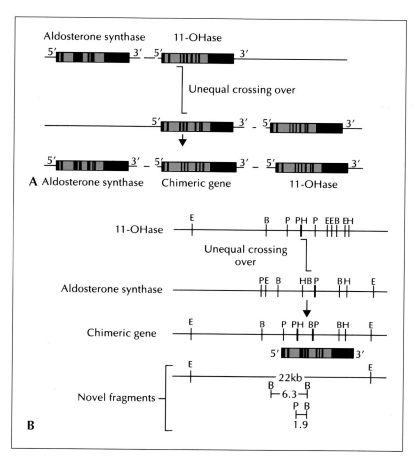

FIGURE 1-17. Glucocorticoid-remediable hyperaldosteronism is a rare, mendelian-dominant cause of hypertension. Molecular genetic analysis reveals that the defect results from the action of a hybrid or chimeric gene containing a glucocorticoid-responsive element derived from the 11-OHase gene and a synthetic element derived from the aldosterone synthase gene. The chimera is apparently the product of an unequal crossover; such a crossover leads to a chimeric gene positioned between the normal aldosterone synthase gene and the normal 11-OHase gene in one of the two elements. **A,** The unequal crossing over occurs in the intron between exons 3 and 4. **B,** Restriction enzyme sites for EcoRI (E), HindIII (H), and PvuII (P) and the location of the exons of the chimeric gene on the restriction enzyme map. The map predicts that digested DNA from affected subjects with the enzymes indicated (either alone or in combination with BamHI [B]) should together give three novel fragments hybridizing to probes directed to exon 3-4. Other fragments should be identical to those derived from the normal 11-OHase and aldosterone synthase genes. The origin of each of the novel fragments is indicted on the map of the chimeric gene [20]. (*Adapted from* Lifton *et al.* [20].)

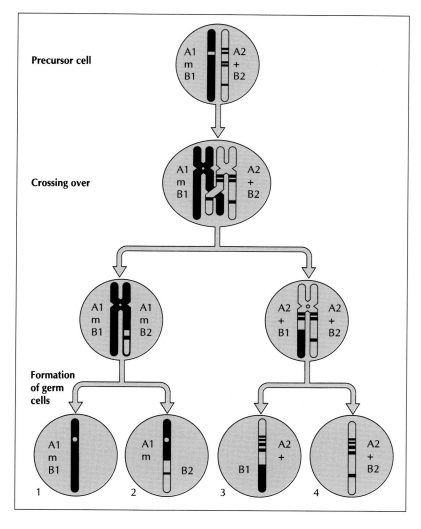

FIGURE 1-18. Genetic linkage follows the transmission of genetic markers and disease through several generations to find markers that travel closely with disease genes. Recombination during meiosis makes it possible to detect genetic linkage. An idealized pair of homologous chromosomes (*top*) carries two markers (A and B) and a mutant, disease-producing gene (m) or its normal allele (+). In the precursor cell, m is associated with allele 1 at both the A and B marker loci. In the first phase of meiosis, chromosomes are replicated. The homologous chromosomes may then cross over and exchange segments of chromosomal material by recombination. In this example, crossing over occurs at a site between A and B. The ultimate result of this event is the creation of four germ cells (sperm or eggs), two of which carry the original parental combinations of alleles (*1,3*) and two of which contain recombinant chromosomes (*2,4*). In cell 2, the mutant gene is associated with allele 1 at locus A but now joins allele 2 at locus B. The probability of a crossover event is a measure of the genetic distance between the marker locus and the mutant gene; a low frequency of crossovers indicates that the disease gene and marker locus are closely linked. The demonstration of close linkage can be used to localize the chromosomal location of the disease gene and direct further studies aimed at its identification [21]. (*Adapted from* White and Lalouel [21].)

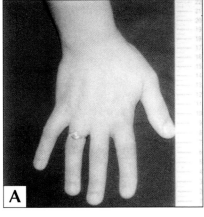

A

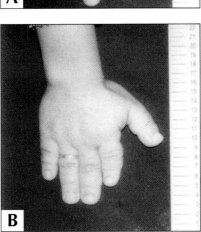

B

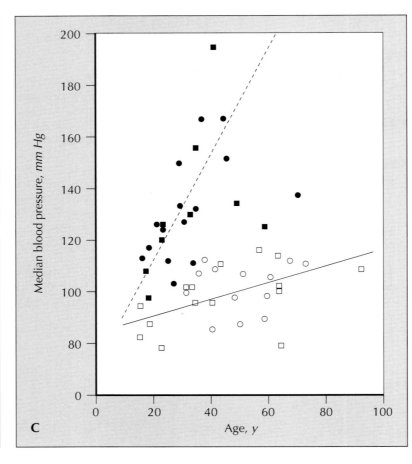

C

FIGURE 1-19. In 1973, a family with autosomal dominantly inherited brachydactyly and severe hypertension with complete cosegregation of both traits was described, and the genetic basis of this essential form of hypertension has now been studied [22]. **A,** An unaffected individual compared with **B,** an affected individual with characteristic shortening of the index finger. **C,** The relationship between median arterial blood pressure and age in affected (*filled circles*) and unaffected (*open circles*) family members. Using the ratio of index-finger-to-middle-finger length, a linkage analysis revealed a tightly linked marker on chromosome 12. Although the syndrome is thought to result from a single pleiotropic gene or two closely situated genes, no candidate genes have been identified as yet. (*Adapted from* Schuster *et al.* [22].)

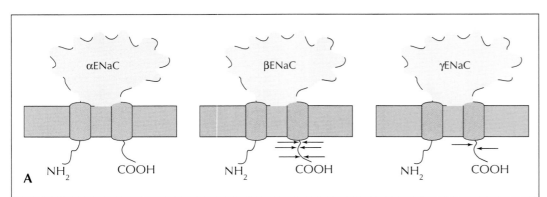

A

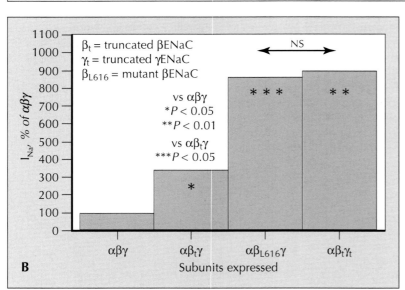

B

FIGURE 1-20. Liddle's syndrome is a mendelian autosomal recessive form of moderate to severe hypertension [23]. Hypertension results from increased renal tubular sodium and water reabsorption, and because renal transplantation cures the syndrome, the pathogenic abnormality is intrinsic to the kidney [24]. A specific genetic basis of the disorder was suggested by linkage analysis that identified a site on chromosome 16 [25] known to contain genes for the β and γ subunits of the amiloride-sensitive epithelial sodium channel (ENaC). The ENaC is a hetero-trimer (the gene for the α subunit is located on chromosome 12). **A,** Each subunit spans the plasma membrane twice and has intra-cellular NH_2- and COOH-termini. Examination of the primary sequence of genes encoding the β and γ subunits revealed several mutations (*arrows*) that result in truncations of the COOH-terminus or substitutions of amino acids in a proline-rich segment of the COOH-terminus [26,27]. **B,** Effect of mutation of the β subunit of the epithelial Na^+ channel on amiloride-sensitive Na^+ current in *Xenopus* oocytes [27]. Subsequent experiments in which ENaC containing normal or mutant subunits were expressed in *Xenopus* oocytes demonstrated that the COOH-terminus mutations markedly increase whole-cell sodium current [28]. The β and γ subunit mutations responsible for Liddle's syndrome are thought to impair removal of active channels from apical cell membranes [29], resulting in excessive renal sodium and water reabsorption, and ultimately in hypertension. These mutations keep the gate open, and thus increase sodium current. (**A** *adapted from* Lifton [29]; **B** *adapted from* Hansson *et al.* [27].)

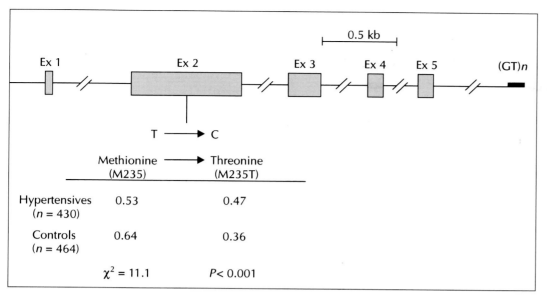

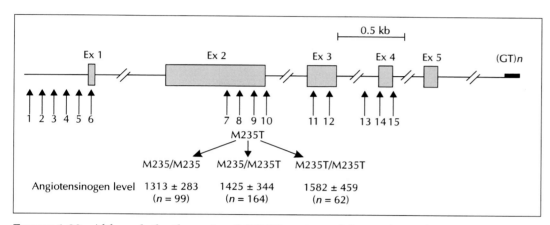

FIGURE 1-21. The angiotensinogen (renin substrate) gene has been linked to essential hypertension in genetic studies of two large panels of hypertensive sibships from Utah and Paris. Further molecular analysis identified a point mutation at position 704 in exon 2 in which cytosine replaces thymidine. This allele codes for threonine (M235T) instead of the normal methionine (M235) at amino acid position 235 in the angiotensinogen molecule. The allele frequencies in hypertensive individuals and normotensive controls are shown. There is a highly significant excess of the M235T variant associated with hypertension [30]. A recent study has also associated the M235T variant with an increased risk of preeclampsia in white women [31].

FIGURE 1-22. Although the threonine (M235T) variant of the angiotensinogen gene (the ninth of 15 mutations in the original report) results from a change in an exon, it is not known whether molecular variants at this locus directly affect angiotensinogen function. It does appear that the different genotypes encoding the amino acid at position 235 are associated with different plasma levels of angiotensinogen. Plasma angiotensinogen concentrations (ng/mL, mean ± SD) for homozygotes for the methionine-coding allele (M235/M235), homozygotes for the threonine substitution (M235T/M235T), and eterozygotes (M235/M235T) are shown. Because circulating levels of angiotensinogen are close to the Michaelis constant for the enzymatic reaction between renin and angiotensinogen, it is probable that the M235T allele is associated with higher circulating levels of angiotensin II, which could play a role in promoting hypertension [30,31].

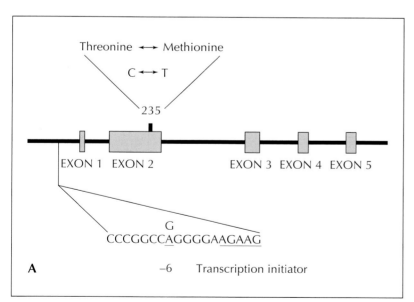

A

FIGURE 1-23. A nucleotide substitution in the promoter of human angiotensinogen is associated with essential hypertension and affects basal transcription in vitro. A, Schematic representation. Further investigation of molecular variation in the proximal promoter region of the angiotensinogen gene has identified a variant (an adenosine instead of a guanine) six nucleotides upstream from the site of transcription initiation.

Continued on next page

B. FREQUENCY OF HAPLOTYPE AMONG VARIOUS RACES

HAPLOTYPE	WHITES	JAPANESE	AFRICAN-CARIBBEANS
G(-6) - M235	0.610	0.242	0.173
G(-6) - T235	0.004	0.015	0.006
A(-6) - M235	0.010	0.000	0.000
A(-6) - T235	0.376	0.743	0.821

FIGURE 1-23. *(Continued)* **B**, The A(-6) allele is in very tight linkage disequilibrium with the T235 allele and represents the original form of the gene, as evidenced by the higher frequency of both alleles in African-Caribbeans than in whites. Tests of promoter function strongly suggest that the A(-6) allele increases the basal transcription rate of the gene, consistent with the observation that individuals with the T235 allele have increased plasma levels of angiotensinogen [32].

A. ASSOCIATION OF THE α-ADDUCIN LOCUS WITH ESSENTIAL HYPERTENSION*

460 GENOTYPE	CONTROL, n=332	HYPERTENSIVE PATIENTS, n=477
Gly/Gly	243 (73.2%)	289 (60.6%)
Gly/Trp	78 (23.5)	166 (34.8%)
Trp/Trp	11 (3.3)	22 (4.6%)

*$P=0.001$ between control group and hypertensive group.

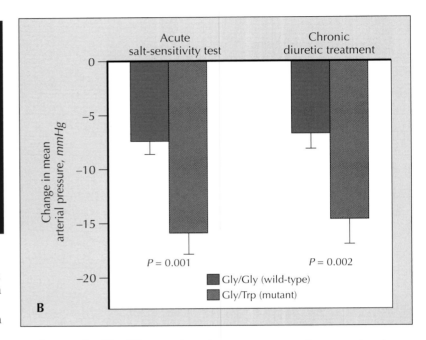

B

FIGURE 1-24. Association of the α-adducin locus with essential hypertension. Adducin is a heterodimeric (α/β) protein expressed in renal tubules, which is thought to regulate sodium transport through changes in the actin cytoskeleton. Point mutations (one each in the α- and β-adducin subunits) account for up to 50% in the difference in blood pressure between the hypertensive and normotensive strains of the Milan inbred rat strain. There is close (~94%) homology between rat and human α-adducin genes, and genomic markers near the α-adducin gene are associated with hypertension in humans [33]. **A**, Studies of the association of an α-adducin polymorphism (C → A transversion at residue 460, resulting in a Gly → Trp substitution) were carried out in two populations: 195 patients with essential hypertension and 181 normotensive control subjects from France; and 282 patients with essential hypertension and 151 normotensive control subjects from Italy. In both populations, the Trp allele was more common in those patients with hypertension than in control subjects ($P = 0.01$ in France; $P = 0.009$ in Italy). Because country of origin was not a confounding stratifer, the data were pooled and, as shown, the Gly/Gly genotype is more common in normotensive control subjects than in patients with hypertension. **B**, The functional significance of this allelic difference for sodium handling was investigated by comparing two measures of blood pressure responsiveness to manipulation of sodium balance. *Left*, The Weinberger acute salt-sensitivity protocol; *right*, the effect of chronic diuretic treatment in subjects with Gly/Gly versus Gly/Trp genotypes (subjects with the Trp/Trp genotype were too uncommon to study as a separate group). For both interventions, individuals with one copy of the Gly allele demonstrated significantly greater depressor responses to the intervention than those homozygous for the wild-type allele [34].

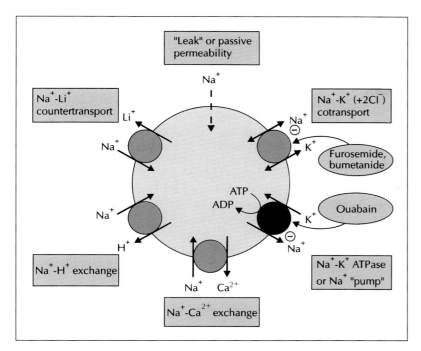

FIGURE 1-25. There has been considerable interest in the association of cellular Na⁺ transport differences with hypertension [35]. This figure demonstrates most of the pathways for Na⁺ transport for which hypertension-related abnormalities have been described; studies have been carried out primarily in such circulating cells as red and white blood cells and platelets. The Na⁺-K⁺ pump (*black circle*) is referred to as *active transport* because it requires the consumption of ATP. The energy expended by the pump is converted to a transmembrane gradient for Na⁺ (low intracellular Na⁺), which can be used to effect transmembrane Na⁺ movements via other passive (non–ATP requiring) transport systems (*red circles*). Inhibition of the pump results in an accumulation of intracellular Na⁺ and a decreased transmembrane Na⁺ gradient, which has been hypothesized to inhibit Na⁺-Ca²⁺ exchange, raise intracellular Ca²⁺, and cause vasoconstriction and hypertension [36]. A similar increase in cell Na⁺ could promote hypertension if increased passive Na⁺ influx occurred through the so-called leak pathway. Alternatively, pump inhibition may partially depolarize the membranes of smooth muscle cells and promote vasoconstriction via activation of voltage-sensitive Ca²⁺ channels [37]. Increased activity of the Na⁺-Li⁺ countertransporter has been consistently associated with hypertension [38], but its physiologic function is unknown. Na⁺-Li⁺ countertransport may be a mode of Na⁺-H⁺ exchange, which could promote hypertension via alteration of intracellular pH. Cotransport of loop-diuretic–sensitive Na⁺-K⁺-2Cl⁻ by a loop-diuretic–sensitive system has been variably associated with hypertension, and studies in the Milan hypertensive rat strain indicate that alterations in the activity of this system may affect renal sodium reabsorption [39].

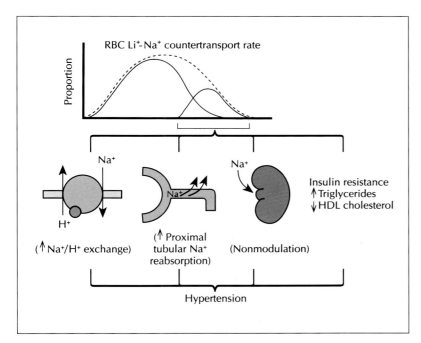

FIGURE 1-26. Increased red blood cell (RBC) Na⁺-Li⁺ countertransport consistently has been associated with essential hypertension [38]. Although the cellular role of Na⁺-Li⁺ countertransport is unknown, it has been linked to a number of physiologic abnormalities that could contribute to hypertension. The distribution of RBC Na⁺-Li⁺ countertransport in the population is a mixture of two subdistributions. Individuals with the high RBC Na⁺-Li⁺ countertransport phenotype may have abnormal activity of membrane Na⁺-H⁺ exchange [40]; as a result, cellular functions, such as pH regulation, could be altered. Increased RBC Na⁺-Li⁺ countertransport has also been associated in some studies with enhanced proximal tubular sodium reabsorption [41] and with impaired renal blood flow modulation in response to dietary salt loading, which results in salt-sensitive hypertension [42] (*see* Fig. 1-30). Finally, there is a clear association between increased RBC Na⁺-Li⁺ countertransport and a metabolic syndrome of insulin resistance, hypertriglyceridemia [43], and low plasma high-density lipoprotein cholesterol. One or more of these physiologic and biochemical mechanisms may contribute to the increased incidence of hypertension found in high RBC Na⁺-Li⁺ countertransport groups.

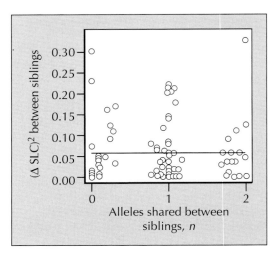

FIGURE 1-27. The association of cellular Na$^+$ transport abnormalities with hypertension does not indicate that transport disorders cause hypertension, but causality can be tested by determining whether abnormalities in membrane transport are genetically linked to hypertension or its intermediate phenotypes. In this study, blood pressure and red blood cell (RBC) Na$^+$-Li$^+$ countertransport (SLC) were measured in pairs of siblings. These siblings underwent further genetic characterization by determining which of two alleles for a gene encoding a Na$^+$-H$^+$ antiporter was carried by each. The relationship between genotypic and phenotypic similarities was then examined. Pairs of individuals sharing similar inherited genes should be phenotypically closer (phenotypic differences between genotypically similar siblings should be less) than pairs in whom fewer inherited genes are shared. If there are two alleles, pairs of siblings can share zero, one, or two alleles inherited from their parents. A significant genetic relationship between the number of shared alleles and the square of the difference in blood pressure or SLC should yield a significant inverse linear regression. There was no evidence for a linkage between allelic differences at the antiporter locus with hypertension, and (as shown) there is no significant relationship between genotype and the RBC SLC phenotype. These findings effectively exclude this Na$^+$-H$^+$ antiporter locus as a candidate gene for hypertension or elevated RBC SLC activity [44]. (*Adapted from* Lifton *et al.* [44].)

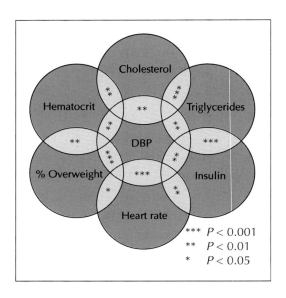

FIGURE 1-28. Hypertension may be only one element of a complex syndrome. This figure illustrates the clustering of risk factors associated with diastolic blood pressure (DBP) in the Tecumseh Blood Pressure Study [45]. The observed correlations may result from the dependence of all factors on some common element, such as one gene with pleiotropic effects on multiple phenotypic characteristics, or may represent interactions of many genetic and environmental factors. Clustering may provide clues to the underlying pathophysiology of disease, and such clusters may be used as complex phenotypes in genetic studies. (*Adapted from* Julius *et al.* [45].)

FAMILIAL DYSLIPIDEMIC HYPERTENSION

Definition: Two or more siblings having *both* the onset of hypertension/high blood pressure (HBP) before age 60 y *and* abnormal blood lipids (total cholesterol, LDL cholesterol, or triglycerides > 90th percentile or HDL cholesterol < 10th percentile)

ALL ADULTS, %	ADULTS WITH HBP, %	SUBGROUPS
11	100	HBP at any age
6	51	HBP before age 60 y
3	25	HBP before age 60 y in ≥ 2 subgroups
1	12	Familial dyslipidemic hypertension

FIGURE 1-29. The complex phenotype of familial dyslipidemic hypertension (FDH) is an example of how analysis of clustering can contribute to understanding the pathophysiology of disease. FDH, a syndrome consisting of early-onset hypertension combined with one or more lipid disturbances in at least two siblings, is present in approximately 12% of all hypertensive individuals. Although its genetic basis is unknown, FDH may be useful as a complex phenotype for genetic studies of hypertension. In addition, individuals in families with FDH can be screened intensively for cardiovascular risk factors in an attempt to prevent progression of atherosclerosis [46]. HDL—high-density lipoprotein; LDL—low-density lipoprotein.

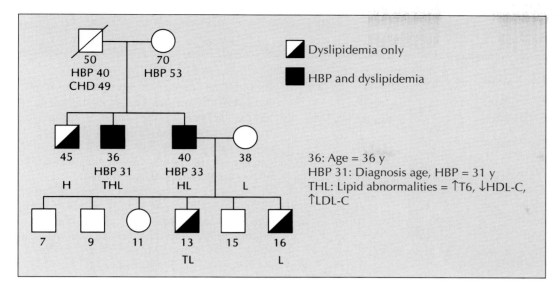

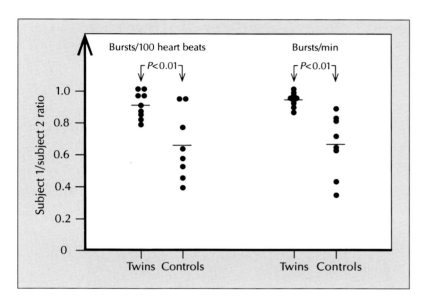

FIGURE 1-30. A three-generation pedigree with familial dyslipidemic hypertension (FDH). Not all individuals of the family are affected, and not all affected individuals have every element of the syndrome. Hypertension and lipid abnormalities were seen in two second-generation brothers (aged 36 and 40 years at diagnosis), and another brother had only lipid abnormalities (aged 45 years at diagnosis). The father developed hypertension at the age of 40 and coronary heart disease (CHD) at the age of 49; he died at age 50 (*diagonal line*). In the third generation, early screening detected lipid abnormalities in two teenage offspring [47]. H—low HDL cholesterol; HBP—high blood pressure; HDL—high-density lipoprotein; L—high LDL cholesterol; LDL—low-density lipoprotein; T—high triglycerides.

FIGURE 1-31. Technologic advances will increase the precision of physiologic measurements and the delineation of intermediate phenotypes. Recording muscle sympathetic nerve activity (MSNA) by microneurography provides more direct assessment of the sympathetic nervous system than was previously possible with physiologic (*eg*, heart rate), biochemical (*eg*, plasma catecholamines), or pharmacologic (responses to α- and β-blockers) approaches. Comparison of nine pairs of male monozygotic twins (aged 25 to 45 years) with eight pairs of healthy, age-matched unrelated males (aged 26 to 42 years) revealed that the intrapair MSNA difference was far less in twins than in controls. This finding suggests that MSNA may be genetically controlled [48].

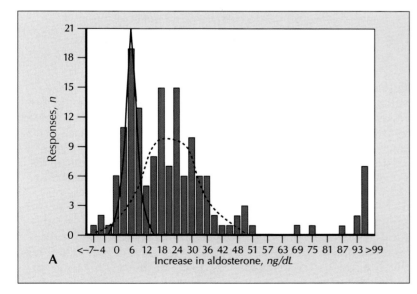

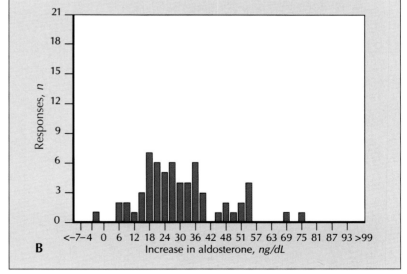

FIGURE 1-32. Other complex intermediate phenotypes may have monogenic determinants. Nonmodulation is a trait characterized by abnormal angiotensin-mediated control of aldosterone release and renal blood flow, abnormal renal sodium handling, and salt sensitivity of blood pressure in hypertensive individuals with normal and high levels of renin. **A,** In a study of 150 hypertensive subjects who were infused with angiotensin II (3 ng/kg/min) while consuming 10 mEq of sodium, increases in plasma aldosterone were bimodally distributed (*P* < 0.00009 for bimodal versus unimodal distribution). **B,** Responses of 61 normotensive subjects without a family history of hypertension [49]. Bimodality is consistent with, but not proof of, the action of a single gene underlying the phenomenon of nonmodulation. (*Adapted from* Williams *et al.* [49].)

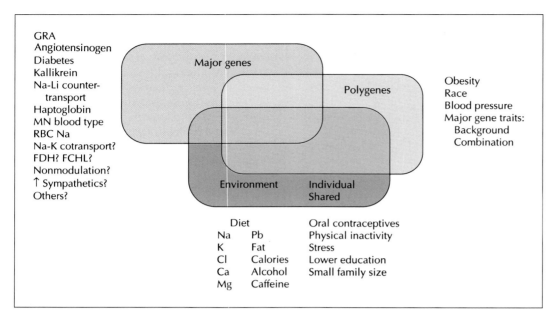

GRA
Angiotensinogen
Diabetes
Kallikrein
Na-Li counter-
    transport
Haptoglobin
MN blood type
RBC Na
Na-K cotransport?
FDH? FCHL?
Nonmodulation?
↑ Sympathetics?
Others?

Major genes

Polygenes

Obesity
Race
Blood pressure
Major gene traits:
    Background
    Combination

Environment   Individual
               Shared

Diet
Na   Pb
K   Fat
Cl   Calories
Ca   Alcohol
Mg   Caffeine

Oral contraceptives
Physical inactivity
Stress
Lower education
Small family size

Figure 1-33. Hypertension results from the impact of environmental factors complemented by a genetic predisposition. In some individuals, single environmental factors, such as alcohol, may be sufficient to cause hypertension; in others, the cumulative effect of many factors is required. FCHL—familial combined hyperlipidemia; FDH—familial dyslipidemic hypertension; GRA—glucocorticoid-remediable aldosteronism; RBC—red blood cells. (*Courtesy of* Roger R. Williams, MD.)

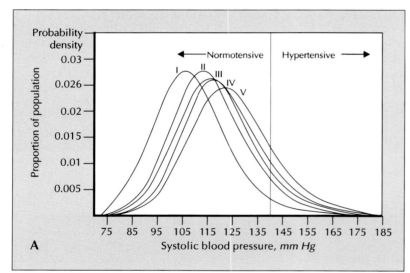

A

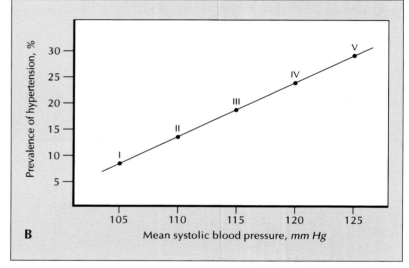

B

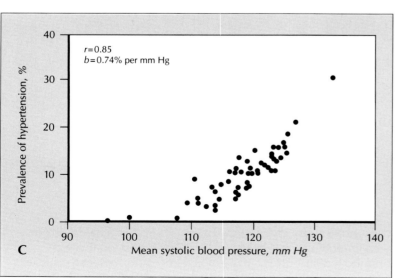

C

Figure 1-34. Environmental factors can cause hypertension by shifting the distribution of blood pressure in an entire population toward higher values [50]. **A,** Systolic blood pressure data collected in the INTERSALT Study (*see* Fig. 1-33) in 10,079 individuals (men and women aged 20 to 59 years) from 52 populations [51]. To illustrate the effect of populational blood pressure shifts on the prevalence of hypertension, these populations were divided into quintiles based on populational mean values. Five frequency distributions are shown for the aggregated individual values for the population quintiles. **B,** The populations shift as a whole, and the mean value determines the prevalence of hypertension (systolic blood pressure >140 mm Hg). **C,** The prevalence of hypertension in the 52 individual centers of the INTERSALT Study. Prevalence of hypertension is closely related to the populational mean systolic blood pressure [52]. **A** also demonstrates the considerable overlap between blood pressure values in populations characterized by different prevalences of hypertension [50].

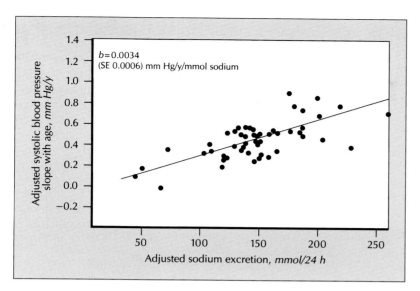

FIGURE 1-35. The INTERSALT Study [51] was undertaken to determine the relationship between urinary sodium excretion (which reflects dietary sodium intake) and blood pressure. Two hundred individuals were studied at each of 52 centers throughout the world. Averages for urinary sodium excretion (adjusted for age, sex, body mass index, and alcohol consumption) and blood pressure rise with age are shown. Each point represents one center. From the slope of the regression line (0.0034 ± 0.00006 mm Hg/y/mmoL Na$^+$) the magnitude of the effect of urinary sodium excretion can be estimated; reduction of sodium intake by 100 mmoL/d could reduce the rise in systolic blood pressure by 3.4 mm Hg for a period of 10 years [51].

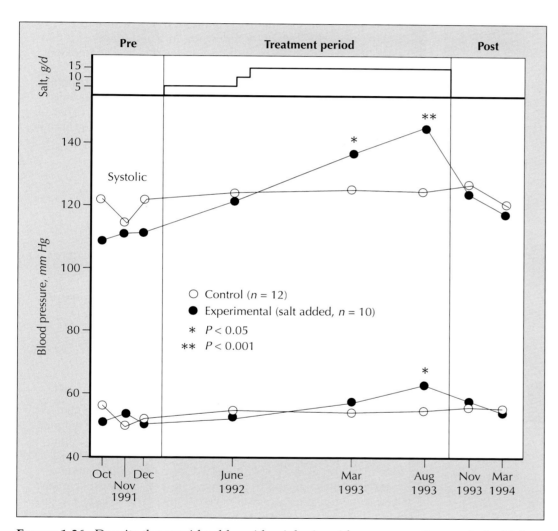

closest to humans, chimpanzees, that strongly support a causal role for sodium chloride in essential hypertension.

The study reported results in a group of 22 chimpanzees maintained in small long-term stable social groups and fed a vegetable and fruit diet to which infant formula was added as a calorie, protein, calcium, and vitamin supplement. Ten experimental animals were further supplemented with NaCl (5 g/d for 19 weeks, 10 g/d for 3 weeks, and 15 g/d for 67 weeks). After the experimental period, salt supplements were discontinued, and blood pressure was monitored after 20 weeks. Blood pressure was measured with an automated recorder (Dynamap) while the animals were anesthetized with ketamine and diazepam.

During the 2.5 years of experiment, the control group showed no significant change in average systolic, diastolic, or mean blood pressure. By the end of the 84 weeks of sodium supplementation, chimpanzees in the experimental group demonstrated average increases of 33 mm Hg systolic ($P < 0.001$ versus baseline and control), 10 mm Hg diastolic ($P < 0.01$ versus baseline, $P < 0.05$ versus control), and 15 mm Hg mean ($P < 0.01$ versus baseline, $P < 0.05$ versus control). Following sodium chloride withdrawal, blood pressures returned to baseline in the treated animals [51]. These data strongly support the hypothesis that increased salt consumption associated with the transition from hunter–gatherer to agricultural lifestyles causes blood pressure to increase. (*Adapted from* the INTERSALT Cooperative Research Group. [51].)

FIGURE 1-36. Despite the considerable epidemiologic evidence supporting a role for high sodium chloride intake in the etiology of hypertension, experimental manipulation of dietary sodium over prolonged periods is not possible in humans, and the salt hypothesis remains unproved. Recently, experiments were carried out in the species phylogenetically

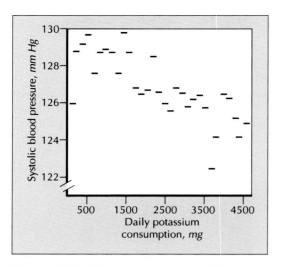

FIGURE 1-37. Dietary potassium intake is inversely related to systolic blood pressure. Displayed are values for systolic blood pressure and daily intake of potassium, as determined from dietary recall by participants in the National Health and Nutrition Examination Survey-I cohort (a national population-based sample) [54].

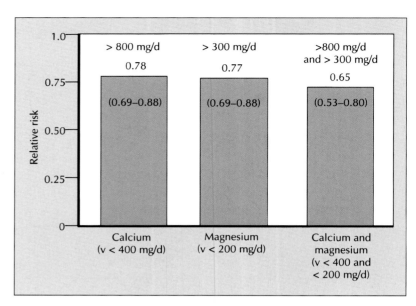

FIGURE 1-38. Effect of dietary calcium and magnesium intake on the 4-year relative risk of hypertension in women in the United States. Relative risks for the highest versus the lowest intake of calcium and magnesium as well as the combined intake of calcium and magnesium are depicted. Higher intake of calcium and magnesium is associated with a lower risk of developing hypertension. Lowest relative risk is associated with a high intake of both calcium and magnesium [55]. Values are adjusted for age, Quetelet's index, and alcohol consumption. (*Adapted from* Witteman *et al.* [55].)

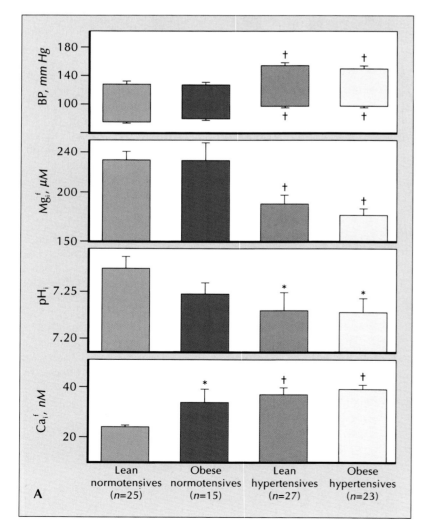

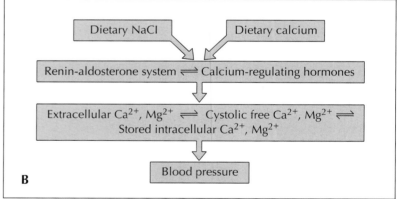

FIGURE 1-39. The effects of dietary electrolytes may be mediated by their impact on cellular electrolyte handling. **A,** Nuclear magnetic resonance spectroscopy was used to measure free intracellular calcium (Ca_i^f), magnesium (Mg_i^f), and pH (pH_i); spectroscopy was done in erythrocytes freshly obtained from untreated lean and obese normotensive and hypertensive individuals. Both lean and obese hypertensive individuals were found to have higher levels of intracellular calcium and lower levels of pH and Mg_i^f compared with lean normotensive individuals. Obese normotensive individuals were also found to have significantly higher Ca_i^f in the erythrocytes than do lean normotensive individuals [56]. *Asterisks* indicate $P = 0.05$ versus lean normotensives; *daggers* indicate $P = 0.001$ versus lean normotensives. **B,** A theoretic schema of the possible impact of dietary electrolytes on hormones, cellular electrolytes, and ultimately, blood pressure [57].

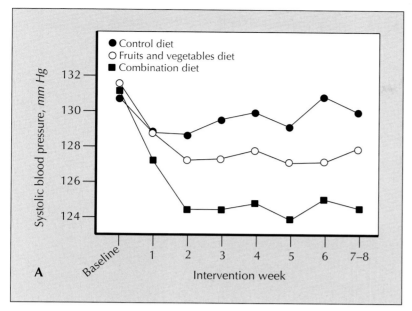

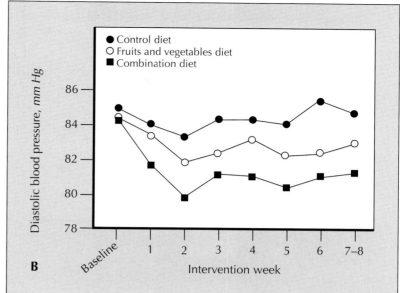

FIGURE 1-40. Mean systolic blood pressure (SBP) and diastolic blood pressure (DBP) at baseline and during each intervention week, according to diet, for 379 subjects with complete sets of weekly blood pressure measurements. **A,** Mean SBP. **B,** Mean DBP. Dietary sodium restriction may not be the key dietary intervention for controlling hypertension. The Dietary Approaches to Stop Hypertension (DASH) trial, a multicenter, randomized feeding study, tested the effects of dietary patterns on blood pressure [58]. Study subjects were healthy, middle-aged adults, average age 44 to 45 years, with borderline or stage 1 hypertension (entry criteria: SBP < 160 mm Hg, DBP 80 to 90 mm Hg) in the absence of treatment with antihypertensive drugs. Following screening, all participants were given a control diet with a macronutrient profile and fiber content near averages in the United States, and potassium, magnesium, and calcium levels close to the 25th percentile for Americans. After 3 weeks on this control diet, subjects were randomly allocated to 8-week periods of either the control diet, a fruits-and-vegetables diet that provided potassium and magnesium levels near the 75th percentile for the United States (along with an

increased fiber content), or a combined diet rich in fruits and vegetables, but also reduced in saturated fat, total fat, and cholesterol. Of note, the sodium content of all three diets was similar (approximately 3 g/d). Both dietary interventions resulted in a lowering of blood pressure compared with the results from the control subjects. The combination diet generally outperformed the fruits-and-vegetables diet, and both diets were more effective in treating patients with hypertension than those without. Compared with the run-in phase, urinary potassium excretion approximately doubled in both dietary intervention groups with little change in urinary sodium. Magnesium excretion increased in the combined dietary intervention while calcium excretion fell rather dramatically with the fruits-and-vegetables diet. All diets were well tolerated, and self-reported adherence was excellent, with over 93% of the patients following the diets as directed. Because no other factors such as alcohol, body weight, and sodium excretion (all known to affect blood pressure) changed systematically, the authors ascribed the observed changes in blood pressure to the dietary interventions.

Continued on next page

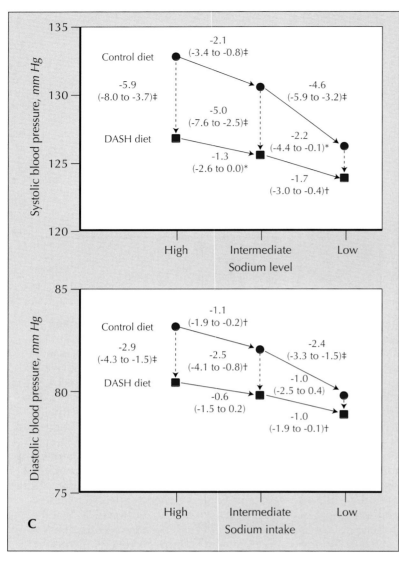

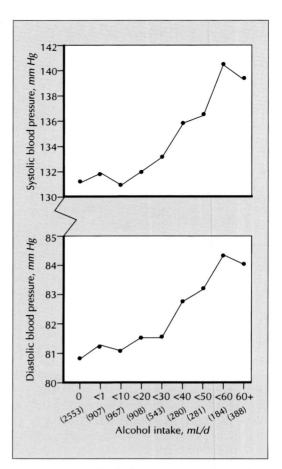

FIGURE 1-41. Alcohol is an environmental cause of hypertension that demonstrates a threshold effect. In this survey, alcohol intake showed no effect on systolic or diastolic blood pressure until consumption exceeded 10 mL/d. An intake of 20 mL/d or more resulted in a linear relationship between both systolic and diastolic blood pressure and consumption. If intake is very high (> 60 mL/d), the effect on blood pressure may reach a plateau [47]. Numbers in parentheses indicate the numbers of subjects reporting various average daily intakes in this survey. (*Adapted from* Criqui *et al.* [60].)

FIGURE 1-40. (*Continued*) **C,** The effect of varying sodium intake with control and DASH diets. In this study, patients were at least 22 years of age and had average screening blood pressures (three visits) of 120 to 159 mm Hg systolic and 80 to 95 mm Hg diastolic. Three levels of sodium intake were examined: 1) high (target of 150 mmol/d, reflecting typical consumption in the United States), 2) intermediate (target of 100 mmol/d, reflecting the upper limit of current national recommendations), and 3) low (50 mmol/d). In this study, the DASH diet was the same as the "combination diet" in **A** and **B**. Patients were randomly assigned to one of the two diets in a parallel-group design and then randomly assigned to one of the three sodium levels, each of which was consumed for 30 consecutive days. The primary outcome was SBP (*upper panel*) at the end of each 30-day period; DBP (*lower panel*) was a secondary outcome. Mean differences and 95% CIs in blood pressure at each sodium level (*solid lines*) and mean differences between diets (*dashed lines*). *Asterisks* indicate $P < 0.05$, *daggers* indicate $P < 0.01$, and *double daggers* indicate $P < 0.001$; these indicate significant differences in blood pressure between control and DASH diet groups or between dietary sodium intakes. Effects were greater in hypertensive subjects (SBP 140 to 159 mm Hg or DBP 90 to 95 mm Hg) than normotensive subjects and in women than in men. Reduction of dietary sodium augments the reduction in blood pressure produced by the DASH diet. Realizing long-term health benefits will depend on the ability of people to make long-lasting changes in dietary composition. (**C** *adapted from* Sacks *et al.* [59].)

EFFECTS OF SKIN COLOR, SOCIOECONOMIC STATUS, AND EDUCATION ON BLOOD PRESSURE

| | SOCIOECONOMIC STATUS* | | | HIGH SCHOOL EDUCATION | |
| | Blood pressure, *mm Hg* | | | Blood pressure, *mm Hg* | |
QUARTILE OF SKIN REFLECTANCE	LOW (*n* = 142)	MEDIUM (*n* = 168)	HIGH (*n* = 147)	NO (*n* = 288)	YES (*n* = 169)
I (darkest) (*n* = 125)	148/99	142/92	128/81	143/94	128/81
II (*n* = 115)	136/86	139/88	134/87	141/88	131/85
III (*n* = 115)	136/91	136/87	142/91	140/91	136/87
IV (lightest) (*n* = 102)	133/84	139/86	128/84	131/84	136/86

*Green index.

FIGURE 1-42. It is widely perceived that stress contributes to hypertension, but measurements of stress are imprecise and the impact of stress is often difficult to quantify. Stress is thought to contribute to differences in blood pressure between blacks and whites in the United States. In this study, skin color was measured by reflectometry in blacks in three US cities. Blood pressure was higher in darker-skinned individuals; however, there was also a strong correlation between socioeconomic status, as measured by the Green index (which classifies education, income, and occupation [61]) and high blood pressure, as well as between educational level and high blood pressure. Higher systolic and diastolic blood pressures were significantly associated with darker skin color independent of age, body mass index, blood glucose concentration, urea nitrogen, uric acid, and urinary sodium and potassium in a multiple linear-regression analysis. These findings may indicate the inability of blacks in a low socioeconomic strata to cope with the increased social stress associated with darker skin color [62].

GENE-ENVIRONMENT INTERACTIONS IN HYPERTENSION

ESTIMATED DIET OF LATE PALEOLITHIC MAN VERSUS THAT OF CONTEMPORARY AMERICANS*

	LATE PALEOLITHIC DIET (ASSUMING 35% MEAT)	CURRENT AMERICAN DIET
Total dietary energy, %		
Protein	33	12
Carbohydrate	46	46
Fat	21	42
Polyunsaturated:saturated fat ratio	1.41	0.44
Sodium, *mg*	690	3400
Potassium, *mg*	11,000	2400
K:Na ratio	16:1	0.7:1
Calcium, *mg*	1500–2000	740.0

FIGURE 1-43. Mankind evolved as hunters and gatherers. At that stage, food was often scarce and consisted largely of fruits, vegetables, and lean meats; and energy expenditure through physical activity was high. This way of life persisted until late Paleolithic times, approximately 10,000 years ago. The emergence of agriculture and later of urbanization resulted in marked changes in dietary composition, and patterns of activity occurred at a pace that precluded genetic adaptation via natural selection. The modern diet is characterized by relative excesses of calories, fat, and sodium and relative deficiencies of protein, potassium, and calcium, while the modern lifestyle is becoming increasingly sedentary. All such factors may contribute to the rise of "diseases of civilization," including hypertension, diabetes, and atherosclerosis [63,64]. (*Adapted from* Eaton *et al.* [64].)

COMPARISON OF FOUR LOW-SODIUM CENTERS AND REMAINING 48 INTERSALT CENTERS

VARIABLES	YANOMANO	XINGU	PAPUA NEW GUINEA	KENYA	REMAINING 48 CENTERS
Lifestyle factors					
24-H sodium (median), *mmol*	< 1	6	27	51	160
Sodium/potassium ratio (median)	< 0.01	0.08	0.48	1.8	3.4
BMI	21.2	23.4	21.7	20.8	25.2
Alcohol drinkers, %	0	0	8.7	30.7	53.0
Blood pressure					
Systolic (median), *mm Hg*	95.4	98.9	107.7	109.9	118.7
Diastolic (median), *mm Hg*	61.4	61.7	62.9	67.9	74.0
Hypertensive, %	0	1.0	0.8	5.0	17.4
Systolic slope with age, *mm Hg/10 y*	-1.1	+0.6	-1.4	+2.4	+5.0

FIGURE 1-44. Cross-cultural differences between acculturated and less acculturated societies demonstrate the impact of the modern lifestyle on blood pressure. Four relatively primitive populations with a lifestyle and diet probably similar to that of Paleolithic man were included in the INTERSALT Study [51]. The studied populations were characterized by relative leanness, low sodium and high potassium intakes, and little if any alcohol consumption. As shown, such societies are virtually free of hypertension and do not demonstrate the progressive rise in systolic blood pressure that is evident in western societies [64]. Hypertension was defined as a systolic blood pressure of 140 mm Hg or more, a diastolic blood pressure of 90 mm Hg or more, or receiving antihypertensive therapy. BMI—body mass index. (*Adapted from* Stamler *et al.* [65].)

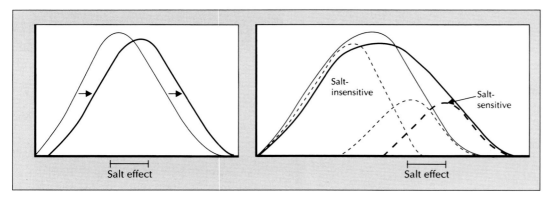

FIGURE 1-45. Although many investigators divide subjects into *salt-sensitive* and *salt-resistant* (salt-insensitive) subtypes, others believe that there is a continuous range of blood pressure responsiveness to dietary salt excess. These two views have implications for recommendations regarding dietary salt intake. If there are two distinct subtypes, dietary salt restriction should ideally be directed only toward individuals who would benefit from an antihypertensive blood pressure response; dietary salt restriction would be wasted in salt-resistant hypertensive individuals. If the entire population is sensitive to dietary salt restriction, however, universal salt restriction would decrease the prevalence of hypertension by lowering the population mean. Current markers of salt sensitivity (*eg*, age, race, and renin status) are not precise enough to have clinical usefulness in individual patients [66]; genetic markers hold greater promise for identifying salt-sensitive hypertensive individuals.

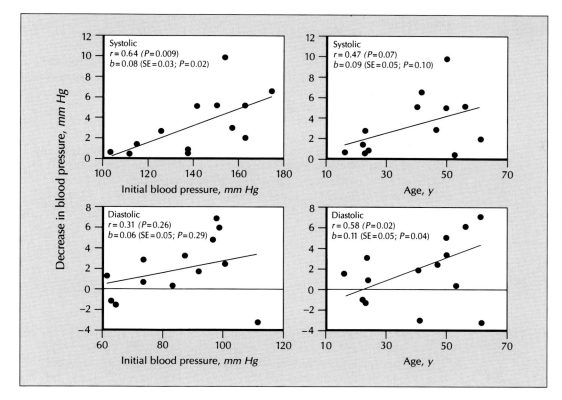

FIGURE 1-46. Data from 13 randomized trials suggest that sodium restriction has a greater impact on systolic blood pressure than on diastolic pressure. The relationships of blood pressure change induced by salt restriction to both initial blood pressure level and age imply that dietary salt restriction may be most useful in older hypertensive individuals with systolic accentuation of blood pressure [67]. These interventional data support the cross-sectional findings of the INTERSALT study in which salt intake seemed most closely related to the rise in systolic blood pressure associated with age [51,65].

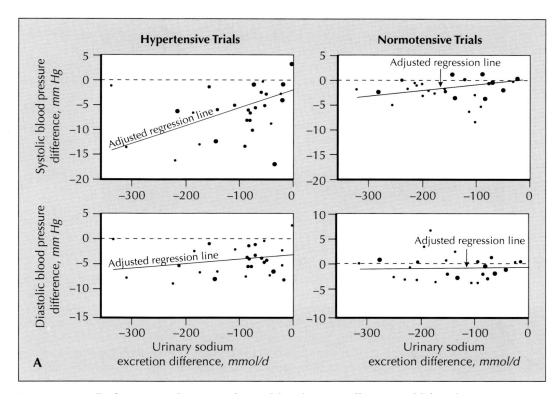

FIGURE 1-47. Reduction in dietary sodium chloride is a well-accepted lifestyle recommendation for the treatment of hypertension and also has been recommended for prevention of hypertension [68]. However, despite the results reported in Figure 1-45, there remains considerable debate about the feasibility and antihypertensive efficacy of dietary

salt reduction in Westernized societies. A recent meta-analysis of 56 trials of dietary salt modification (28 in hypertensive and 28 in normotensive individuals) suggests that the effects on blood pressure are modest and largely confined to elderly hypertensive persons [69].

A, Regression lines for systolic (*top panels*) and diastolic (*bottom panels*) blood pressure change as a function of change in urinary sodium excretion. Regressions are adjusted for the number of urinary sodium measurements, and the size of the data points reflects the effective sample size of the trial, where the *largest dot* represents trials with over 150 participants and the *smallest dot*, trials of 15 or less subjects. In the hypertensive trials, slopes of the regression were 3.7 mm Hg/100 mmol Na$^+$/day for systolic pressure ($P < 0.001$), and 0.9 mm Hg/100 mmol Na$^+$/day for diastolic pressure ($P = 0.09$). In normotensive trials, regression slopes were 1.0 mm Hg/100 mmol Na$^+$/day for systolic pressure ($P < 0.001$), and 0.1 mm Hg/100 mmol Na$^+$/day for diastolic pressure ($P = 0.64$). Note that regression lines do not pass through the origins, suggesting that there was a decrease in blood pressure even in the absence of a change in urinary sodium excretion.

Continued on next page

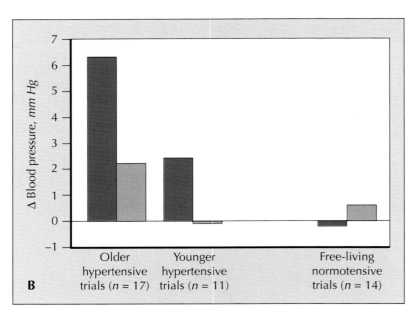

FIGURE 1-47. *(Continued)* **B,** Results of two subgroup analyses. In the first, the effect of changing sodium intake was shown to be greater in trials of older (aged 45 years or over), 6.3/2.2 mm Hg (95% CI, 4.11 to 8.44/1.58 to 3.87), than younger (under age 45 years) persons, 2.4/-0.1 mm Hg (95% CI, 0.35 to 4.38/-1.61 to 1.37). In the second, examination of 14 trials in normotensive persons who prepared and ate food outside of an institutional setting demonstrated no evidence of a systematic change in blood pressure, -0.2/0.6 mm Hg (95% CI, -1.48 to 1.01/-0.88 to 2.07).

The meta-analysis suggests that in the range of dietary sodium change achievable in controlled trials, the antihypertensive effect is modest and greatest in elderly hypertensive persons. (*Adapted from* Midgley *et al.* [69].)

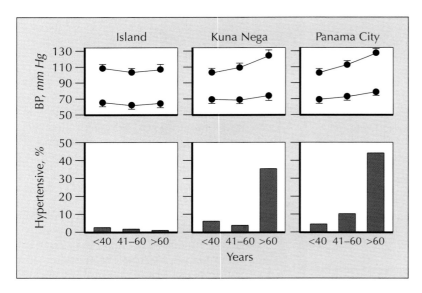

FIGURE 1-48. Dietary sodium intake may interact with other social and cultural factors to affect blood pressure (BP). An interesting situation has been described in Kuna Indians, who traditionally have lived in the isolated San Blas Island chain off Panama, but who have also migrated to mainland areas where they live both in predominantly Kuna communities (Kuna Negra, a suburb of Panama City) where they maintain many of their traditional cultural practices, and in urban areas of Panama City where they are more affected by acculturation. Dietary sodium intake is relatively high in Kuna living on San Blas Island, averaging 135±15 mEq/g creatinine, but the prevalence of hypertension is very low, and blood pressure does not rise with age. Kuna who live in Panama City show the highest prevalence of hypertension and the greatest rise of blood pressure with age. Thus, cultural factors may protect Kuna who live on the island from hypertension, despite their relatively high sodium intake [70].

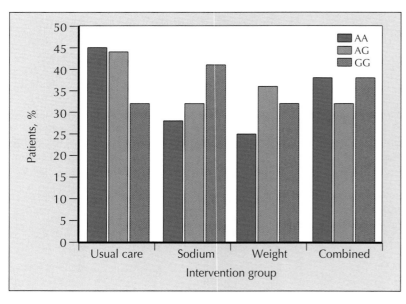

FIGURE 1-49. The effect of angiotensinogen genotypes on incident hypertension in response to reduction of dietary sodium intake, weight loss, or both in a substudy of the Trials of Hypertension Prevention. Subjects were men and women between the ages of 30 and 54 years who were moderately overweight (110% to 160% of

desirable body weight) and had a mean diastolic blood pressure between 83 and 89 mm Hg (three visits). Subjects were randomly assigned to a usual-care group, a sodium-reduction group (goal ≤ 80 mmol/d), a weight-reduction group (goal of 4.5-kg weight reduction), or a combined intervention group (both goals). Genotypes (AA, AG, and GG) were determined at the –6 position of the angiotensinogen gene, a site associated with higher blood pressure and angiotensinogen levels. Shown are 3-year incidences of hypertension by genotype for each of the four interventions. Subjects with the AA genotype had the highest incidence of hypertension after 3 years in the usual care group but the lowest incidence in the sodium-reduction and weight-loss groups. Differences in the AA and AG genotypes of the sodium-reduction group were significant, while those for the GG group were not. Individuals with the AA and AG genotypes showed similarly significant decreases in hypertension incidence in the weight-loss group, whereas the GG subjects did not. The combined intervention did not show a significant reduction in the AA group but did in the heterozygote group. These findings suggest that although people with the AA genotype develop hypertension to a greater degree without intervention, they respond more favorably to salt reduction or weight loss. It appears that the GG genotype may distinguish individuals who are primarily salt-insensitive. Understanding genotype-environment interactions such as these may improve targeting of specific interventions to susceptible individuals. (*Adapted from* Hunt *et al.* [71].)

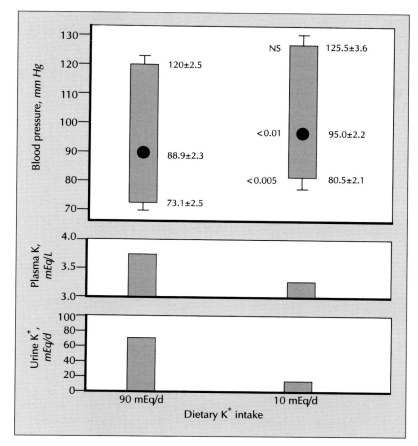

Figure 1-50. Blood pressure increases during dietary potassium restriction. In this study of normotensive men, lowering the potassium intake from a usual level (90 mEq/d) to a very low level (10 mEq/d) induced an increase in blood pressure and a decrease in plasma potassium concentration [72]. The mechanisms that mediate the effect of potassium restriction on blood pressure are not known but may include sodium retention, hormonal changes, and inhibition of membrane Na^+-K^+ ATPase. (*Adapted from* Krishna *et al.* [72].)

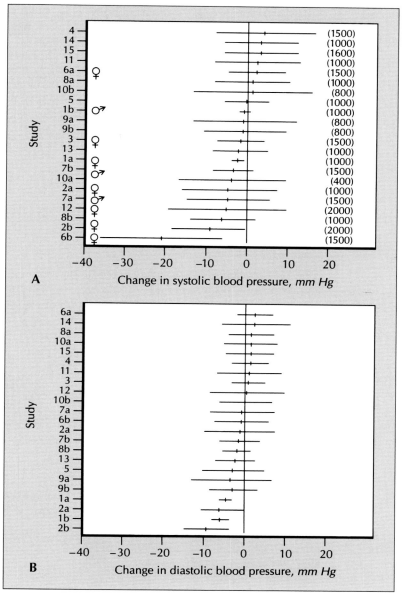

Figure 1-51. Because epidemiologic evidence suggests that dietary calcium deficiency is related to hypertension, many trials of the effects of dietary calcium supplementation on blood pressure have been undertaken. This figure depicts the difference from baseline to the final measurement of systolic (**A**) and diastolic (**B**) blood pressure in 15 double-blind, placebo-controlled intervention trials. Studies are displayed according to effect on systolic pressure. For studies of men or women only, gender is indicated; no designation means that both men and women were included. Doses of supplements (in mg/d) are given in parentheses on the right. The overall average effect of calcium supplements on blood pressure appears small, but it may be possible to identify subgroups in which such supplementation would be beneficial [73]. For additional details about each study, refer to Grobbee and Waal-Manning [73].

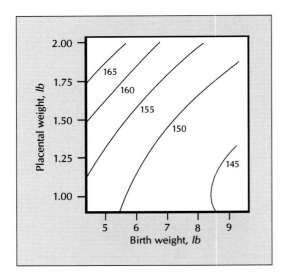

FIGURE 1-52. Relationship of birth weight and placental weight to blood pressure in adulthood. The subjects were men and women aged 46 to 54 years who were born in Preston, Lancashire, between 1935 and 1943 (*n* = 449). Isobars of systolic pressure depict the relationships among systolic blood pressure, placental weight, and birth weight. High placental weight and low birth weight are associated with high blood pressure, implying that factors in utero affect blood pressure throughout life [74]. The mechanisms by which placental and fetal weight influence blood pressure in later life are unknown. (*Adapted from* Barker *et al.* [74].)

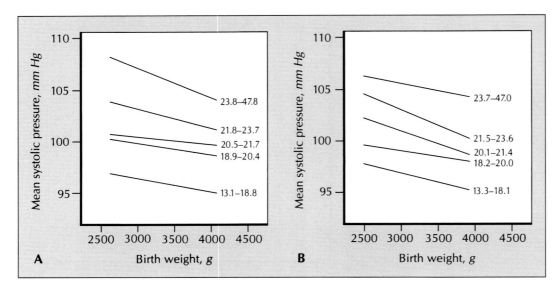

FIGURE 1-53. In utero effects on growth appear to influence the subsequent expression of blood pressure in children and adults. Shown are regression lines relating blood pressure to birth weight in 3591 British children aged 5 to 7.5 years. The data are stratified by quintiles of weight (in kg) at ages 5 to 7.5 for boys (**A**) and girls (**B**). Birth weight has a significant inverse relationship with systolic and diastolic blood pressure of childhood when standardized for contemporaneous weight (weight ranges for each quintile are to the right of the regression lines). This relationship may reflect the rate of weight gain during infancy and early childhood [75]. (*Adapted from* Whincup *et al.* [75].)

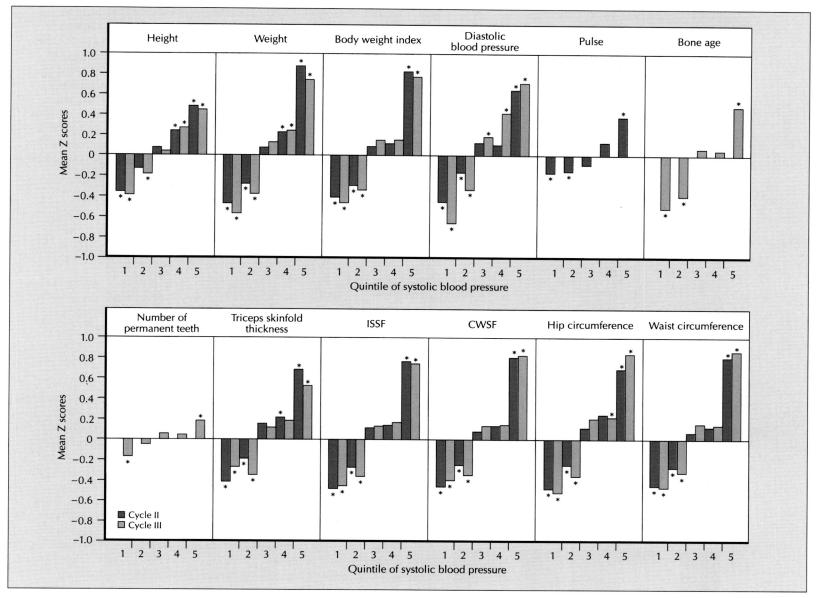

FIGURE 1-54. The level of blood pressure during childhood tends to maintain its rank order in a population, a phenomenon known as *tracking*. In a sample of 2165 children examined in the US National Center for Health Statistics Health Examination Surveys on two occasions separated by about 4 years (cycle II [1963–1965] at ages 6 to 12 and cycle III [1966–1970] at ages 12 to 17), children with blood pressure consistently in the highest quintile were taller, heavier, more obese, had greater bone age, greater numbers of permanent teeth, and were more sexually mature than their peers. Relationships between selected measures and systolic blood pressure quintiles at each cycle are depicted. Numbers of subjects in the first, second, third, fourth, and fifth quintiles were 166, 110, 104, 120, and 209, respectively [76]. *Asterisks* indicate $P < 0.05$. CWSF—chest wall skinfold thickness; ISSF—infrascapular skinfold thickness. (*Adapted from* Lauer *et al.* [76].)

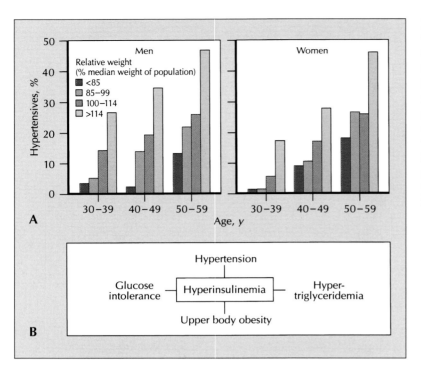

FIGURE 1-55. Epidemiologic observations worldwide agree that weight is directly and strongly related to blood pressure throughout adulthood. Data from the Framingham Heart Study show the relationship of relative weight to the prevalence of hypertension (systolic > 160 mm Hg or diastolic > 95 mm Hg) in men and women in three age groups (**A**). The relationship is consistent and all trends are significant at $P = 0.05$ [77]. The distribution of body fat also may play a role in hypertension, as upper body (central) fat seems to be more closely associated with hypertension than does peripheral fat. Because central obesity is also associated with insulin resistance, hyperinsulinemia has been proposed as a factor potentially linking obesity, glucose intolerance, and dyslipidemia to hypertension (**B**) [78].

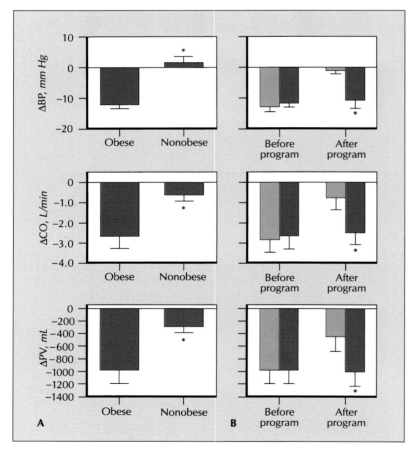

FIGURE 1-56. Obesity-related hypertension may be mediated partially through dietary salt excess. Sixty obese and 18 nonobese adolescents were tested for the effects of successive 2-week periods of high (> 250 mEq/d) and low (< 30 mEq/d) dietary salt intake on blood pressure (BP), cardiac output (CO), and plasma volume (PV). **A,** Compared with nonobese adolescents, obese individuals showed greater changes in BP (salt sensitivity), CO, and PV. **B,** Obese adolescents were then offered a 20-week weight-loss program. A total of 36 lost more than 1 kg of body weight (*light bars*), whereas 15 did not (*dark bars*). Compared with responses before the weight-loss program, individuals who lost weight became less salt-sensitive, that is, responses to dietary salt manipulation were less for BP, CO, and PV. Individuals who did not lose weight remained salt-sensitive [79]. (*Adapted from Rocchini et al.* [79].)

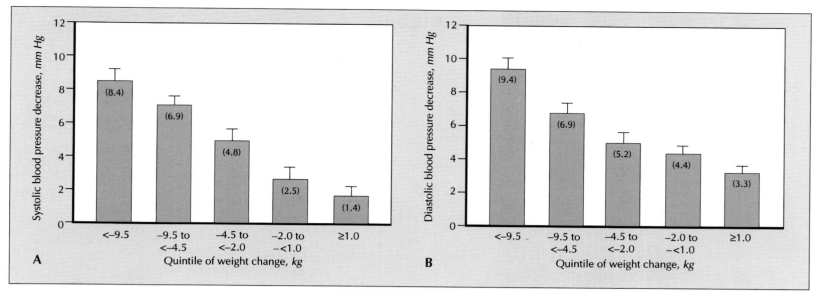

FIGURE 1-57. Weight and various measures related to obesity (Quetelet's index, skinfold thickness) have a strong correlation with the level of blood pressure. The effect of weight loss on blood pressure was studied in phase 1 of the Trials of Hypertension Prevention. Changes in both systolic (**A**) and diastolic (**B**) blood pressure were directly related to changes in weight, thereby supporting the concept that excess weight contributes to hypertension [80]. Average blood pressure decrease is listed in parentheses in each bar. (*Adapted from* Stevens *et al.* [80].)

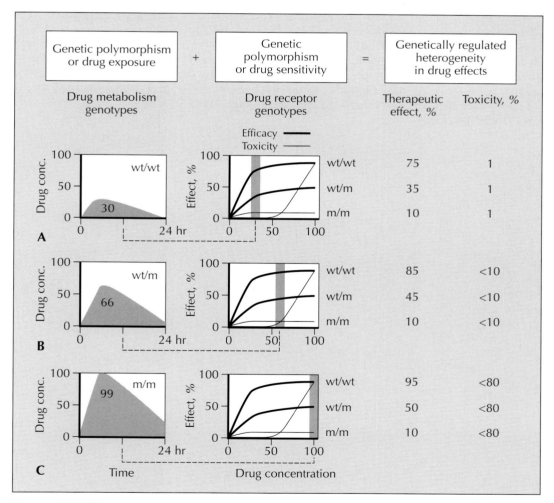

FIGURE 1-58. Pharmacogenomics is an emerging field seeking to relate genetic variation to drug effects. The complexity of the impact of genetic differences on therapeutic efficacy is illustrated, depicting the potential consequences of administering the same dose of medication to individuals with both different drug-metabolism genotypes and different drug-receptor genotypes. Active drug concentrations in the systemic circulation are determined by the individual's drug-metabolism genotype with (**A**) homozygous wild type (wt/wt) patients converting 70% of a dose to the inactive metabolite, leaving 30% to exert an effect on the target receptor. For the patient with heterozygous (wt/m) drug-metabolism genotype (**B**), 35% is inactivated, whereas the patient with homozygous mutant (m/m) drug metabolism (**C**) inactivates only 1% of the dose by the polymorphic pathway, yielding the three drug concentration-time curves. Pharmacologic effects are further influenced by different genotypes of the drug receptor, which have different sensitivity to the medication, as depicted by the curves of drug concentration versus effects, *middle*. Patients with a wt/wt receptor genotype exhibit a greater effect of any given drug concentration in comparison with those with a wt/m receptor genotype, whereas those with m/m genotypes are relatively refractory to drug effects at any plasma drug concentration. These two genetic polymorphisms (in drug metabolism and drug receptors) yield nine different theoretical patterns of drug effects, *right*. The therapeutic ratio (efficacy:toxicity) ranges from a favorable 75 in the patient with wt/wt genotypes for drug metabolism and drug receptors to < 0.13 in the patient with m/m genotypes for drug metabolism and drug receptors. (*Adapted from* Evans and Relling [82].)

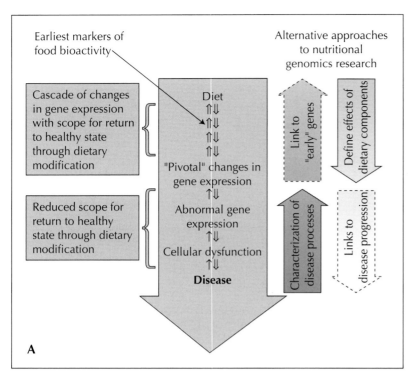

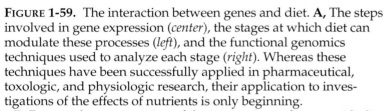

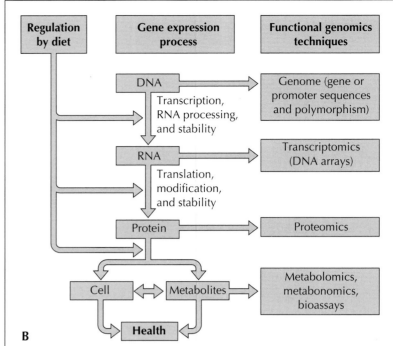

FIGURE 1-59. The interaction between genes and diet. **A,** The steps involved in gene expression (*center*), the stages at which diet can modulate these processes (*left*), and the functional genomics techniques used to analyze each stage (*right*). Whereas these techniques have been successfully applied in pharmaceutical, toxologic, and physiologic research, their application to investigations of the effects of nutrients is only beginning.

B, Proposed representation of the interactions of genes with diet that result in chronic diseases such as hypertension. Understanding the nutritional genomics of such diseases will require an understanding of how genes contribute to the genetic predisposition to the disease and how dietary factors interact with genetic predispositions. Studies of the effects of diet on patterns of gene expression could provide new insights into disease development processes. Lessons learned from the study of nutritional genetics may help to optimize the benefits of diet for populations and individuals. (*Adapted from* Hunt *et al.* [81].)

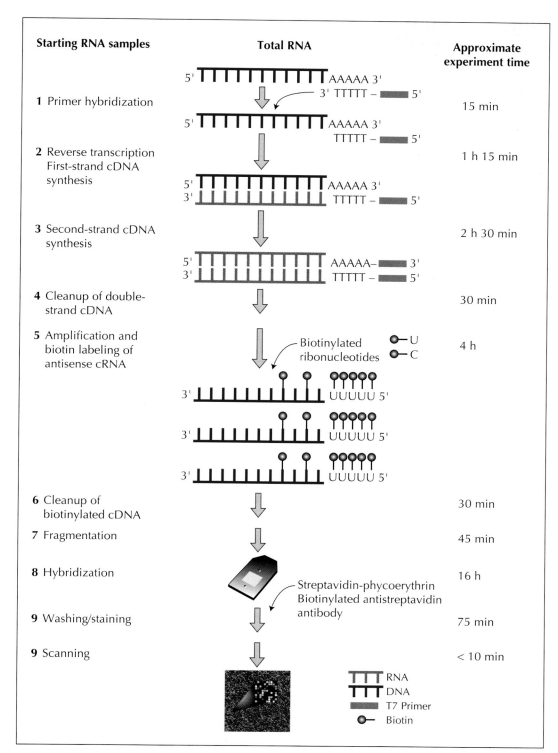

Starting RNA samples	Total RNA	Approximate experiment time
1 Primer hybridization	5' ▯▯▯▯▯▯▯▯ AAAAA 3' 3' TTTTT – ▮ 5' 5' ▯▯▯▯▯▯▯▯ AAAAA 3' TTTTT – ▮ 5'	15 min
2 Reverse transcription First-strand cDNA synthesis	5' ▯▯▯▯▯▯▯▯ AAAAA 3' 3' ▯▯▯▯▯▯▯▯ TTTTT – ▮ 5'	1 h 15 min
3 Second-strand cDNA synthesis	5' ▯▯▯▯▯▯▯ AAAAA– ▮ 3' 3' ▯▯▯▯▯▯▯ TTTTT – ▮ 5'	2 h 30 min
4 Cleanup of double-strand cDNA		30 min
5 Amplification and biotin labeling of antisense cRNA	Biotinylated ribonucleotides ●–U ●–C 3' ▯▯▯▯▯▯▯▯ UUUUU 5' 3' ▯▯▯▯▯▯▯▯ UUUUU 5' 3' ▯▯▯▯▯▯▯▯ UUUUU 5'	4 h
6 Cleanup of biotinylated cDNA		30 min
7 Fragmentation		45 min
8 Hybridization	Streptavidin-phycoerythrin Biotinylated antistreptavidin antibody	16 h
9 Washing/staining		75 min
9 Scanning		< 10 min

Legend:
▯▯▯ RNA
▯▯▯ DNA
▮ T7 Primer
●– Biotin

FIGURE 1-60. Expression array. The development of microarray technologies permits rapid and extensive analysis of gene expression under defined conditions. Shown is the method of producing arrays that can detect expression of thousands of genes. By monitoring expression of this many genes, global gene expression can be assessed and patterns of gene expression characterized for different conditions, *eg*, high- and low-salt diets. Whole-genome analyses also benefit studies in which the end goal is to focus on small numbers of genes, by providing an efficient tool to sort through the activities of thousands of genes, and to recognize the key players. The *inset* demonstrates color-coded sites, each representing a single gene. (*Adapted from* Affymetrix, Santa Clara, CA.)

1. Platt R: Heredity in hypertension. *Q J Med* 1947, 16:111–113.

2. Pickering GW: The genetic factor in essential hypertension. *Ann Intern Med* 1955, 43:457–464.

3. Ledingham JM: Genetics of human hypertension. In *Hypertensive Cardiovascular Disease: Pathophysiology and Treatment*. Edited by Amery A. The Hague/Boston/London: Martinus Nijhoff Publishers; 1982:206–216.

4. Mongeau J-G, Brion P, Sing CF: The influence of genetics and household environment upon the variability of normal blood pressure: the Montreal Adoption Survey. *Clin Exp Hypertens [A]* 1986, 8:653–660.

5. Tambs K, Eaves LJ, Moum T, *et al.*: Age-specific genetic effects for blood pressure. *Hypertension* 1993, 22:789–795.

6. Ward R: Familial aggregation and genetic epidemiology of blood pressure. In *Hypertension: Pathophysiology, Diagnosis, and Management*. Edited by Laragh JH, Brenner BM. New York: Raven Press Ltd; 1990:81–100.

7. Schork NJ, Jokelainen P, Grant EJ, *et al.*: Relationship of growth and blood pressure in inbred rats. *Am J Physiol* 1994, 266:R702–R708.

8. St. Lezin E, Simonet L, Pravenec M, *et al.*: Hypertensive strains and normotensive "control" strains: how closely are they related? *Hypertension* 1992, 19:419–424.

9. Bruner CA, Myers JH, Sing CF, *et al.*: Genetic association of hypertension and vascular changes in stroke-prone spontaneously hypertensive rats. *Hypertension* 1986, 8:904–910.

10. Rapp JP: Characteristics of Dahl salt-susceptible and salt-resistant rats. In *Handbook of Hypertension. Vol 4. Experimental and Genetic Models of Hypertension*. Edited by de Jong W. New York: Elsevier Science Publishers; 1984:286–295.

11. Harrap SB, Van Der Merwe WM, Griffin SA, *et al.*: Brief angiotensin-converting enzyme inhibitor treatment in young spontaneously hypertensive rats reduces blood pressure long-term. *Hypertension* 1990, 16:603–614.

12. Jacob HJ, Lindpaintner K, Lincoln SE, *et al.*: Genetic mapping of a gene causing hypertension in the stroke-prone spontaneously hypertensive rat. *Cell* 1991, 67:213–224.

13. Hilbert P, Lindpaintner K, Beckmann JS, *et al.*: Chromosomal mapping of two genetic loci associated with blood-pressure regulation in hereditary hypertensive rats. *Nature* 1991, 353:521–529.

14. Rapp JP, Wang S-M, Dene H: A genetic polymorphism in the renin gene of Dahl rats cosegregates with blood pressure. *Science* 1989, 243:542–544.

15. St. Lezin EM, Pravenec M, Kurtz TW: New genetic models for hypertension research. *Trends Cardiovasc Med* 1993, 3:119–123.

16. Ely DL, Daneshvar H, Turner ME, *et al.*: The hypertensive Y chromosome elevates blood pressure in F_{11} normotensive rats. *Hypertension* 1993, 21:1071–1075.

17. Ganten D, Lindpaintner K, Ganten U, *et al.*: Transgenic rats: new animal models in hypertension research. *Hypertension* 1991, 17:843–855.

18. Mullins JJ, Peters J, Ganten D: Fulminant hypertension in transgenic rats harbouring the mouse Ren-2 gene. *Nature* 1990, 344:541–544.

19. Williams RR, Hunt SC, Hasstedt SJ, *et al.*: Definition of genetic factors in hypertension: a search for major genes, polygenes, and homogeneous subtypes. *J Cardiovasc Pharmacol* 1988, 12(suppl 3):S7–S20.

20. Lifton RP, Dluhy RG, Powers M, *et al.*: A chimaeric 11β-hydroxylase/aldosterone synthase gene causes glucocorticoid-remediable aldosteronism and human hypertension. *Nature* 1992, 355:262–265.

21. White R, Lalouel J-M: Chromosomal mapping with DNA markers. *Sci Am* 1988, 258:40–48.

22. Schuster H, Wienker TF, Bähring S, *et al.*: Severe autosomal dominant hypertension and brachydactyly in a unique Turkish kindred maps to human chromosome 12. *Nat Genet* 1996, 13:98–100.

23. Liddle GW, Bledsoe T, Coppage WS: Aldosteronism but with negligible aldosterone secretion. *Trans Am Assoc Physiol* 1963, 76:199–213.

24. Botero-Velez M, Curtis JJ, Warnock DG: Brief report: Liddle's syndrome revisited: a disorder of sodium resorption in the distal tubule. *N Engl J Med* 1994, 330:178–181.

25. Shimkets RA, Warnock DG, Bositis CM, *et al.*: Liddle's syndrome: heritable human hypertension caused by mutations in the beta subunit of the epithelial sodium channel. *Cell* 1994, 79:407–414.

26. Hansson JH, Nelson-Williams C, Suzuki H, *et al.*: Hypertension caused by a truncated epithelial sodium channel gamma subunit: genetic heterogeneity of Liddle syndrome. *Nat Genet* 1995, 11:76–82.

27. Hansson JH, Schild L, Lu Y, *et al.*: A de novo missense mutation of the beta subunit of the epithelial sodium channel causes hypertension and Liddle syndrome, identifying a proline-rich segment critical for regulation of channel activity. *Proc Natl Acad Sci U S A* 1995, 92:11495–11499.

28. Schild L, Canessa CM, Shimkets RA, *et al.*: A mutation in the epithelial sodium channel causing Liddle disease increases channel activity in the Xenopus laevis oocyte expression system. *Proc Natl Acad Sci U S A* 1995, 92:5699–5703.

29. Lifton RP: Molecular genetics of human blood pressure variation. *Science* 1996, 272:676–680.

30. Jeunemaitre X, Soubrier F, Kotelevtsev YV, *et al.*: Molecular basis of human hypertension: role of angiotensinogen. *Cell* 1992, 71:1–20.

31. Ward K, Hata A, Jeunemaitre X, *et al.*: A molecular variant of angiotensinogen associated with preeclampsia. *Nature Genet* 1993, 4:59–61.

32. Inoue I, Nakajima T, Williams CS, *et al.*: A nucleotide substitution in the promoter of human angiotensinogen is associated with essential hypertension and affects basal transcription in vitro. *J Clin Invest* 1997, 99:1786–1797.

33. Casari G, Barlassina C, Cusi D, *et al.*: Association of the alpha-adducin locus with essential hypertension. *Hypertension* 1995, 25:320–326.

34. Cusi D, Barlassina T, Azzani T, *et al.*: Polymorphisms of alpha-adducin and salt sensitivity in patients with essential hypertension. *Lancet* 1997, 349:1353–1357.

35. Weder AB: Membrane sodium transport. In *Hypertension Primer. The Essentials of High Blood Pressure*. Edited by Izzo JL, Black HR. Dallas: American Heart Association; 1993: 36–37.

36. Blaustein M: Sodium ions, calcium ions, blood pressure regulation, and hypertension: a reassessment and a hypothesis. *Am J Physiol* 1977, 232:C165–C173.

37. Haddy FJ: Potassium, Na^+-K^+ pump inhibitor and low-renin hypertension. *Clin Invest Med* 1987, 10:547–554.

38. Canessa ML, Adragna NC, Solomon HS, *et al.*: Increased lithium-sodium countertransport in red cells of patients with essential hypertension. *N Engl J Med* 1980, 302:772–776.

39. Camussi A, Bianchi G: Genetics of essential hypertension: from the unimodal-bimodal controversy to molecular technology. *Hypertension* 1988, 12:620–628.

40. Canessa ML, Morgan K, Semplicini A: Genetic differences in lithium-sodium exchange and regulation of the sodium-hydrogen exchanger in essential hypertension. *J Cardiovasc Pharmacol* 1988, 12(suppl 3):92–98.

41. Weder AB: Red-cell lithium-sodium countertransport and renal lithium clearance in hypertension. *N Engl J Med* 1986, 314:198–201.

42. Redgrave J, Canessa M, Gleason R, *et al.*: Red blood cell lithium-sodium countertransport in non-modulating essential hypertension. *Hypertension* 1989, 13:721–726.

43. Doria A, Fioretto P, Avogaro A, *et al.*: Insulin resistance is associated with high sodium-lithium countertransport in essential hypertension. *Am J Physiol* 1991, 261:E684–E691.

44. Lifton RP, Hunt SC, Williams RR, *et al.*: Exclusion of the Na$^+$-H$^+$ antiporter as a candidate gene in human essential hypertension. *Hypertension* 1991, 17:8–14.

45. Julius S, Jamerson K, Meija A, *et al.*: The association of borderline hypertension with target organ changes and higher coronary risk: Tecumseh Blood Pressure Study. *JAMA* 1990, 264:354–358.

46. Williams RR, Hunt SC, Hopkins PN, *et al.*: Familial dyslipidemic hypertension: evidence from 58 Utah families for a syndrome present in approximately 12% of patients with essential hypertension. *JAMA* 1988, 259:3579–3586.

47. Williams RR, Hopkins PN, Hunt SC, *et al.*: Population-based frequency of dyslipidemic syndromes in coronary-prone families in Utah. *Arch Intern Med* 1990, 150:582–588.

48. Wallin G, Kunimoto MM, Sellgren J: Possible genetic influence on the strength of human muscle nerve sympathetic activity at rest. *Hypertension* 1993, 22:282–284.

49. Williams GH, Dluhy RG, Lifton RP, *et al.*: Non-modulation as an intermediate phenotype in essential hypertension. *Hypertension* 1992, 20:788–796.

50. Rose G: Population distributions of risk and disease. *Nutr Metab Cardiovasc Dis* 1991, 1:37–40.

51. INTERSALT Cooperative Research Group: INTERSALT: an international study of electrolyte excretion and blood pressure: results for 24 hour urinary sodium and potassium excretion. *BMJ* 1988, 297:319–328.

52. Rose G, Day S: The population mean predicts the number of deviant individuals. *BMJ* 1990, 301:1031–1034.

53. Denton D, Weisinger R, Mundy NI, *et al.*: The effect of increased salt intake on blood pressure of chimpanzees. *Nat Med* 1995, 1:1009–1016.

54. McCarron DA, Morris CD, Henry HJ, *et al.*: Blood pressure and nutrient intake in the United States. *Science* 1984, 224:1392–1398.

55. Witteman JCM, Willett WC, Stampfer MJ, *et al.*: A prospective study of nutritional factors and hypertension among US women. *Circulation* 1989, 80:1320–1327.

56. Resnick LM, Gupta RK, Bhargava KK: Cellular electrolytes in hypertension, diabetes, and obesity: a nuclear magnetic resonance spectroscopic study. *Hypertension* 1991, 17:951–957.

57. Resnick LM: Calciotropic hormones in human and experimental hypertension. *Am J Hypertens* 1990, 3(suppl):171–178.

58. Appel LJ, Moore TJ, Obarzanek E, *et al.*: A clinical trial of the effects of dietary patterns on blood pressure. DASH Collaborative Research Group. *N Engl J Med* 1997, 336:1117–1124.

59. Sacks FM, Svetkey LP, Vollmer WM, *et al.*: Effects on blood pressure of reduced dietary sodium and the Dietary Approaches to Stop Hypertension (DASH) diet. DASH-Sodium Collaborative Research Group. *N Engl J Med* 2001, 344:3–10.

60. Criqui MH, Langer RD, Reed DM: Dietary alcohol, calcium, and potassium: independent and combined effects on blood pressure. *Circulation* 1989, 80:609–614.

61. Green LW: Manual for scoring socioeconomic status for research on health behavior. *Public Health Rep* 1970, 85:815–827.

62. Klag MJ, Whelton PK, Coresh J, *et al.*: The association of skin color with blood pressure in US blacks with low socioeconomic status. *JAMA* 1991, 265:599–602.

63. Simopoulos AP: Dietary risk factors for hypertension. *Comp Ther* 1992, 18:26–30.

64. Eaton SB, Konner M, Shostak M: Stone agers in the fast lane: chronic degenerative diseases in evolutionary perspective. *Am J Med* 1988, 84:739–749.

65. Stamler J, Rose G, Elliott P, *et al.*: Findings of the international cooperative INTERSALT study. *Hypertension* 1991, 17(suppl I):9–15.

66. Grobbee DE: Methodology of sodium sensitivity assessment: the example of age and sex. *Hypertension* 1991, 17(suppl I):109–114.

67. Grobbee DE, Hofman A: Does sodium restriction lower blood pressure? *BMJ* 1986, 293:27–29.

68. Joint National Committee on Detection, Evaluation, and Treatment of High Blood Pressure: The Fifth report of the Joint National Committee on Detection, Evaluation, and Treatment of High Blood Pressure (JNC V). *Arch Intern Med* 1993, 153:154–183.

69. Midgley JP, Matthew AG, Greenwood CMT, Logan AG: Effect of reduced dietary sodium on blood pressure: a meta-analysis of randomized controlled trials. *JAMA* 1996, 275:1590–1597.

70. Hollenberg NK, Martinez G, McCullough M, *et al.*: Aging, acculturation, salt intake, and hypertension in the Kuna of Panama. *Hypertension* 1997, 171–176.

71. Hunt SC, Cook NR, Oberman A, *et al.*: Angiotensinogen genotype, sodium reduction, weight loss, and prevention of hypertension: trials of hypertension prevention, phase II. *Hypertension* 1998, 32:393–401.

72. Krishna GG, Miller E, Kapoor S: Increased blood pressure during potassium depletion in normotensive men. *N Engl J Med* 1989, 320:1177–1182.

73. Grobbee DE, Waal-Manning HJ: The role of calcium supplementation in the treatment of hypertension: current evidence. *Drugs* 1990, 39:7–18.

74. Barker DJP, Bull AR, Osmund C, *et al.*: Fetal and placental size and risk of hypertension in adult life. *BMJ* 1990, 301:259–262.

75. Whincup PH, Cook DG, Shaper AG: Early influences on blood pressure: a study of children aged 5–7 years. *BMJ* 1989, 299:587–591.

76. Lauer RM, Anderson AR, Beaglehole R, *et al.*: Factors related to tracking of blood pressure in children: U.S. National Center for Health Statistics Health Examination Surveys Cycles II and III. *Hypertension* 1984, 6:307–314.

77. Krieger DR, Landsberg L: Obesity and hypertension. In *Hypertension: Pathophysiology, Diagnosis, and Management*. Edited by Laragh JH, Brenner BM. New York: Raven Press, Ltd; 1990:1741–1757.

78. Kaplan NM: The deadly quartet: upper-body obesity, glucose intolerance, hypertriglyceridemia, and hypertension. *Arch Intern Med* 1989, 149:1514–1520.

79. Rocchini AP, Key J, Bondie D, *et al.*: The effect of weight loss on the sensitivity of blood pressure to sodium in obese adolescents. *N Engl J Med* 1989, 321:580–585.

80. Stevens VJ, Corrigan SA, Obarzanek E, *et al.*: Weight loss intervention in phase 1 of the Trials of Hypertension Prevention. *Arch Intern Med* 1993, 153:849–858.

81. Hunt SC, Cook NR, Oberman A, *et al.*: Angiotensinogen genotype, sodium reduction, weight loss, and prevention of hypertension: trials of hypertension prevention, phase II. *Hypertension* 1998, 32:393–401.

82. Evans WE, Relling MV:Pharmacogenomics: translating functional genomics into rational therapeutics. *Science* 1999, 286:487–491.

ROLE OF THE NERVOUS SYSTEM IN HUMAN HYPERTENSION

John Amerena and Stevo Julius

Despite early demonstrations that sympathetic activation elevates blood pressure and early clinical inklings that human hypertension may have a psychosomatic component, the pivotal role of the nervous system in human hypertension is only recently being clarified. There are two reasons for this delayed appreciation of the role the autonomic nervous system plays in the genesis and maintenance of blood pressure elevation in hypertension. The first deals with the complexities involved in the evaluation of autonomic function in humans, and the second is that hypertension is a dynamic process in which the manifestations of autonomic overactivity change with time.

This chapter gives a historical perspective of the role the nervous system plays in blood pressure regulation, followed by a sketch of the general organization of the autonomic control of blood pressure and a description of the methods used for assessment of autonomic nervous function in humans. None of the existing methods used alone can fully assess the overall autonomic function, which is the sum total of the central nervous tone, receptor properties, and organ responsiveness. The issue of measurement is further complicated by the fact that the central nervous tone to various organs is not regulated in a uniform fashion, so that activation in one organ can be associated with a decreased tone in another. Both the sympathetic and the para-sympathetic branches of autonomic control must be taken into consideration in measuring autonomic function as well as the negative feedback relationship that exists between the central nervous tone and the responsiveness of the peripheral organs.

Despite these difficulties, the mounting evidence of the crucial role of a combined increase in sympathetic tone and decrease in parasympathetic tone in human hypertension is beyond dispute. The evidence is particularly strong for younger patients with early, so-called *borderline* hypertension. The hallmark of the sympathetic overactivity in these patients is the so-called hyperkinetic state, which is best characterized by a fast heart rate and increased cardiac output. Close to 40% of all unselected patients with hypertension show such a hyperkinetic circulation. There is good biochemical, pharmacologic, and physiologic evidence of increased sympathetic and decreased parasympathetic tone in these patients, which is reviewed later in the chapter.

Both the hyperkinetic state and the sympathetic overactivity are less readily recognizable later in the course of hypertension. A large proportion of previously hyperkinetic patients later develop established hypertension, and questions arise as to the mechanisms involved in the hemodynamic transition from a fast heart rate/high cardiac output form of borderline hypertension to the later normal cardiac output/high vascular resistance profile that is characteristic of established hypertension. This transition is best explained by changes in cardiac and vascular responsiveness resulting from long-standing elevation of the blood pressure and sympathetic tone. The development of altered organ characteristics, in which cardiac responses are decreased and vascular reactivity is enhanced, also provides a basis for understanding why the sympathetic tone appears to become reset toward "normal" values during the development of established hypertension. These changes, their relationship to each other, and the mechanisms involved in their development, as well as their clinical significance, are outlined in the final section of this chapter.

FUNCTIONAL ORGANIZATION OF THE AUTONOMIC NERVOUS SYSTEM

CENTRAL CONTROL

REFLEX RISE IN BLOOD PRESSURE SHOWN IN THE 19TH CENTURY

STUDY	STIMULATION APPLICATION
von Bezold, 1863	Vagus and many other afferent nerves
Asp, 1867	Posterior roots and splanchnic nerves
Ganz, 1870	Gastric nerves
Grutzner and Heidenhain, 1877	Skin
Heger, 1887	Arteries (irritants applied)
Grossman, 1897	Radial, median, and ulnar nerves

FIGURE 2-1. A historical perspective of the research into the role of the central nervous system in controlling blood pressure. Clinical blood pressure measurement became available early in the 20th century, but scientists were able to measure intra-arterial blood pressure in animals in the middle of the 19th century. It was recognized very early that stimulation of the peripheral sensory nerves elicited a transient reversible reflex elevation in blood pressure.

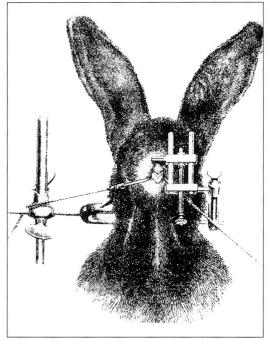

FIGURE 2-2. Surgical technique used by Owsjannikow [1] to cut through the midbrain of curarized rabbits. In the late 19th century, Owsjannikow studied the role of central nervous connections in the control of blood pressure in rabbits. He developed his own specialized microtome, which permitted well-defined cuts (by depth and in cranial vs dorsal directions) in the midbrain. (*Reproduced from* Owsjannikow [1].)

OWSJANNIKOW'S DATA

RESTING BLOOD PRESSURE, *mm Hg*	CUT C-QUAD LEFT TO RIGHT	CUT JUST BEHIND C-QUAD	CUT 2 mm POSTERIOR
77	105–97	↑ and ↓; eventually 67 mm Hg	40 mm Hg
		Longer time high; eventually 67 mm Hg	65
71	169	Sciatic nerve stimulation 89	Sciatic nerve stimulation 6
133	127–190	61	—
79	95–144	56	46

FIGURE 2-3. Localization of areas in the midbrain of rabbits that are involved in blood pressure control. Owsjannikow's data [1] established that medullary centers control the blood pressure. An anterior cut caused an *increase* in blood pressure, while a posterior cut elicited a substantial *decrease*. This and earlier work established the important principle that tonic discharge from the central nervous system regulates the peripheral blood pressure and that some inhibitory input maintains blood pressure at an intermediate level between what the blood pressure would have been without central nervous system input and the brain's maximal capacity to increase the blood pressure. There were only four rabbits in this study, and only the best of the rabbits' results were included. Despite this and the lack of statistical analysis, the author's theories were ultimately shown to be correct.

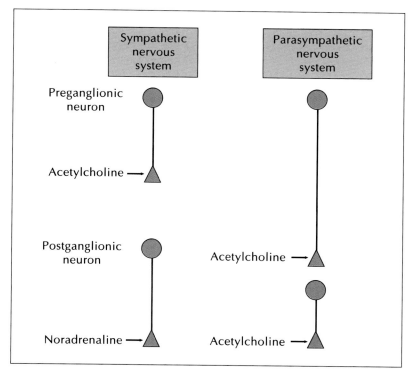

FIGURE 2-4. The neuronal organization of the autonomic nervous system. Neurons in the sympathetic nervous system emerge from the central nervous system (CNS) and run to sympathetic ganglia near the spinal cord. They synapse with postganglionic neurons, using acetylcholine as the neurotransmitter. Postganglionic neurons then run to the effector organ, where noradrenaline acts as the final neurotransmitter. In this system, there is a relatively short preganglionic neuron from the CNS and a long postganglionic neuron running from the ganglia to the periphery. The parasympathetic nervous system, which is craniolumbar in distribution, is organized so that a long neuron runs from the CNS to a ganglion located near the effector organ. In this ganglion, the preganglionic neuron synapses with a postganglionic neuron, which then innervates the target organ. In contrast to the sympathetic nervous system, acetylcholine is the neurotransmitter in parasympathetic ganglia and at the endplate [2]. (*Adapted from* Loewy [2].)

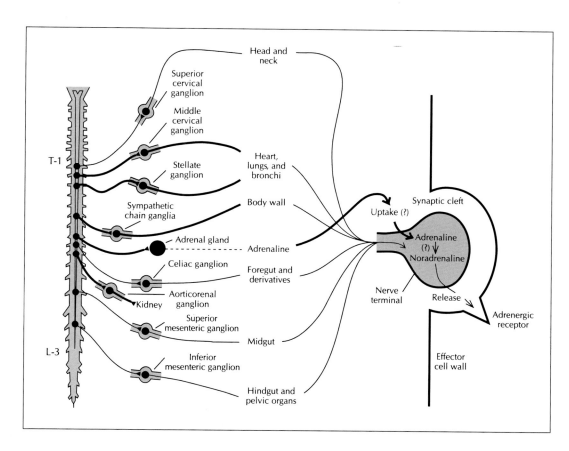

FIGURE 2-5. Structure and function of the sympathetic nervous system. Sympathetic tone in the end organs is controlled by regional sympathetic outflow. The final common pathway is the release of noradrenaline from the nerve terminal to stimulate adrenergic receptors. It has been hypothesized that circulating adrenaline (released from the adrenal gland) exerts its effect by being taken up rapidly by nerve terminals and converted to noradrenaline, in addition to acting directly on postsynaptic receptors [3]. (*Adapted from* Loewy [2].)

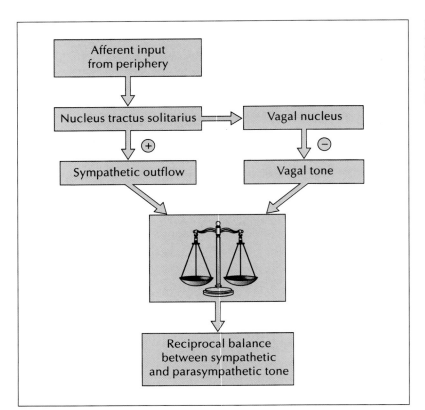

FIGURE 2-6. The balance between sympathetic and parasympathetic tone. The nucleus tractus solitarius in the brainstem is the switchboard that regulates autonomic tone. The nucleus receives and processes incoming signals from the periphery and modulates both the sympathetic and the parasympathetic outflow in an integrated and reciprocal manner.

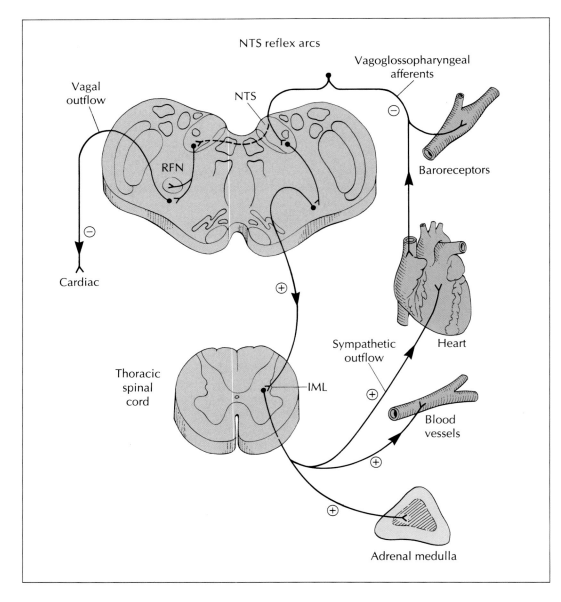

FIGURE 2-7. The central organization of the negative feedback loops in the autonomic nervous system. Inhibitory input from mechanoreceptors in the heart and aortic and carotid baroreceptors travels via afferent vagal fibers to the nucleus tractus solitarius (NTS). Sympathetic outflow is transmitted by efferent nerve fibers to the heart, blood vessels, and adrenal gland via the spinal cord. Cardiac parasympathetic tone originating from the vagal nuclei is modulated by the NTS in an integrated and reciprocal fashion. The resulting autonomic tone is determined by the balance between sympathetic and parasympathetic outflow [4]. IML—intermediolateral cell column; RFN—retrofacial nucleus. (*Adapted from* Spyer [3].)

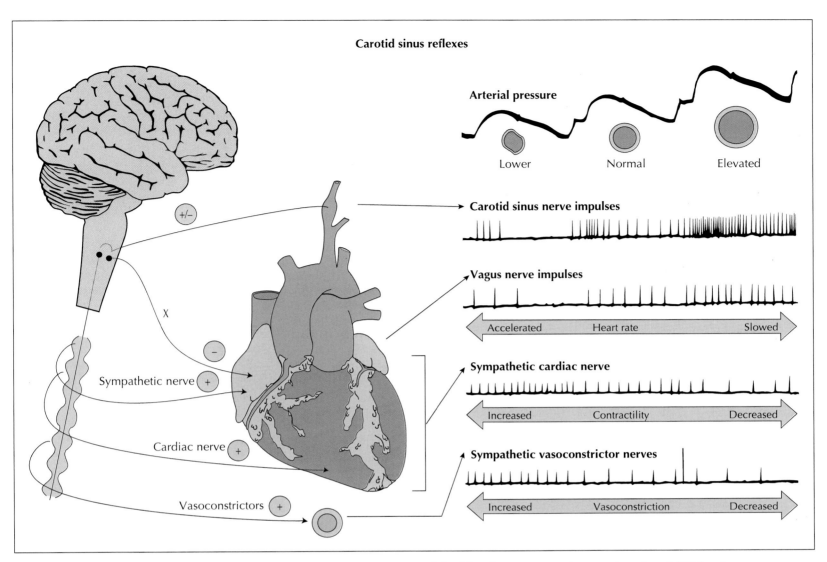

FIGURE 2-8. An example of a negative feedback loop in the autonomic nervous system. The aortic and carotid sinus mechanoreceptors are organized similarly. When blood pressure rises, more "stretch" is sensed by these mechanoreceptors. This results in an increase in discharge frequency from the receptors, which is then transmitted to the nucleus tractus solitarius (NTS) by vagal afferent fibers. In response, the NTS modulates a decrease in the sympathetic tone and a reciprocal increase in the vagal tone, which results in peripheral vasodilatation, slowing of the heart rate, and a reduction in cardiac output, leading to a return of the blood pressure to its previous level. If blood pressure falls, reflex changes in autonomic tone occur in the opposite direction (vasoconstriction and increased pulse rate and cardiac output) with the aim of restoring the blood pressure to its former level. Note that the negative feedback loops have different efferent pools of neurons to various organs. It is important to note that the efferent response is not always uniform; under some circumstances, the tone to one organ may be enhanced while the tone to other organs is not affected [3]. X—vagus. (*Adapted from* Spyer [3].)

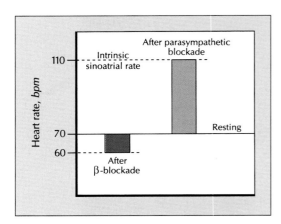

FIGURE 2-9. Dual autonomic control of the resting heart rate. Julius *et al.* [4] studied the relative influence of the sympathetic versus parasympathetic tone on heart rate. With the subject at rest, complete β-blockade causes the heart rate to fall to 60 beats per minute (bpm) (the change in heart rate represents the amount of resting sympathetic tone). With the subsequent abolition of the parasympathetic tone (with atropine) the heart rate increases to 110 bpm, the intrinsic discharge rate of the atrial pacemaker (sinoatrial node). The increase in heart rate with parasympathetic blockade is greater than the fall in heart rate with sympathetic blockade, demonstrating that parasympathetic inhibitory tone is the predominant factor in determining the resting heart rate.

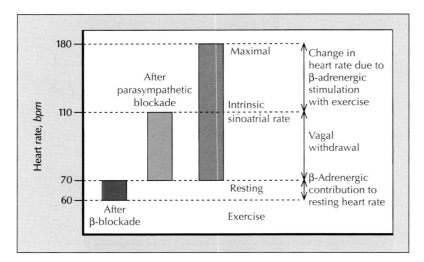

FIGURE 2-10. Dual control of the changes in heart rate with exercise. The resting heart rate is determined by the balance between sympathetic stimulation and parasympathetic inhibition of the sinoatrial node. The parasympathetic inhibitory tone generally predominates [4] (*see* Fig. 2-9); with vagal withdrawal the heart rate can increase to 110 beats per minute (bpm), which is the intrinsic pacemaker rate, even in the presence of β-blockade. However, with exercise, the heart rate can further increase to 180 bpm (or more), which is mediated by stimulation of β-adrenergic receptors.

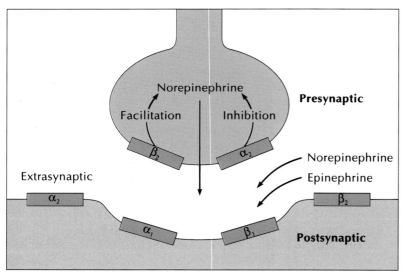

FIGURE 2-11. The pharmacologic and morphologic characteristics of peripheral adrenoreceptors. Nerve terminals within the autonomic nervous system are composed of several distinct receptor subtypes within and outside the synaptic cleft. These receptor subtypes have distinct and often opposing functional effects as well as different sensitivity to circulating catecholamines, depending on their site and affinity. Stimulation of vascular postsynaptic α_1-receptors is predominantly by norepinephrine released locally (from the nerve terminal) and causes vasoconstriction. Extrasynaptic α_2-receptors, which are abundant in blood vessels, also cause vasoconstriction but are more responsive to circulating catecholamines (epinephrine > norepinephrine) because of their extrasynaptic location. Presynaptic α_2-receptors are more sensitive to locally released norepinephrine but decrease vasoconstriction by inhibiting further release of norepinephrine from the nerve terminal. Postsynaptic β_1-receptors are abundant in the heart and control heart rate and contractility, while extrasynaptic β_2-receptors are predominantly located in resistance vessels in skeletal muscle and induce vasodilatation [5]. The overall physiologic effect of adrenergic receptor stimulation is determined by the degree of activation of the receptor subtypes and the balance between their opposing functional effects. (*Adapted from* Struyker Boudier [5].)

A. RELATIVE AFFINITY OF ADRENERGIC RECEPTOR AGONISTS

	α_1	α_2	β_1	β_2
Noradrenaline	+++	++	+++	++
Adrenaline	++	+++	++	+++
Isoprenaline	—	—	+++	+++
Phenylephrine	++	+	—	—
Azepexole	+	++	—	—
Dobutamine	+	—	++	+
Fenoterol	—	—	+	++

B. RELATIVE AFFINITY OF ADRENERGIC RECEPTOR ANTAGONISTS

	α_1	α_2	β_1	β_2
Phentolamine	++	++	—	—
Prazosin	++	+	—	—
Yohimbine	+	++	—	—
Propranolol	—	—	++	++
Metoprolol	—	—	++	+
ICI 118.551	—	—	+	++

FIGURE 2-12. The pharmacologic characterization of adrenergic receptor subtypes using agonists (**A**) and antagonists (**B**). Peripheral adrenergic receptors can be characterized into various subtypes by using natural and synthetic agonists and antagonists. It is important to realize that a difference in affinity does not necessarily mean a difference in function and that the total adrenergic tone at the endplate level is the summation of the effects of stimulation of the various receptor subtypes [5]. (*Adapted from* Struyker Boudier [5].)

DISTRIBUTION AND PHYSIOLOGIC EFFECTS OF DIFFERENT ADRENERGIC RECEPTORS

TISSUE	RECEPTOR TYPE	EFFECT
Blood vessels	α_1 and α_2	Constriction
	β_2	Dilatation
Heart	β_1	Tachycardia; increased contractility
	α_1	Increased contractility
Bronchi	β_2	Relaxation
Thrombocytes	α_2	Aggregation
Kidneys	α_1 and α_2	Vasoconstriction
	β_1 and β_2	Renin release; inhibition tubular sodium reabsorption
Adipocytes	α_2	Inhibition lipolysis
	β_1, β_2, and β_3 (?)	Lipolysis

FIGURE 2-13. Adrenergic receptor subtype characterization by distribution and physiologic function. Subtypes of adrenergic receptors can be characterized by their distribution and physiologic function [5]. Along with variation in the distribution between organs, there is variation in patterns of distribution within organs. For example, postsynaptic α_2-receptors are numerous in the peripheral vasculature but are present in greater numbers on the venous side of the circulation than on the arterial side. α-Receptors and β-receptors generally have opposite physiologic effects, but in some organs, *eg*, the heart, the effects are complementary. β_3-Receptors have been described recently in adipose tissue, but their physiologic role is uncertain, although a role in lipolysis has been postulated [6]. (*Adapted from* Struyker Boudier [5].)

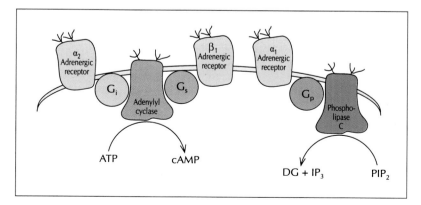

FIGURE 2-14. Types of adrenergic receptors and their functional relationship to G proteins. Adrenergic receptors are situated on the cellular membrane in close proximity to adenylyl cyclase (α_2 and β), phospholipase C (α_1), and the G protein subtypes G_i, G_s, and G_p, respectively [7]. Stimulation of β- or α_2-receptors leads to activation of G_s or G_i, which then act as transducers to activate (G_s) or inhibit (G_i) adenylyl cyclase. This results in increased or decreased production of cAMP from ATP. α_1-Receptors work through G_p, which activates phospholipase C to promote conversion of phosphatidylinositol bisphosphate (PIP_2) to diacylglycerol (DG) and inositol triphosphate (IP_3). (*Adapted from* Linden and Gilman [7].)

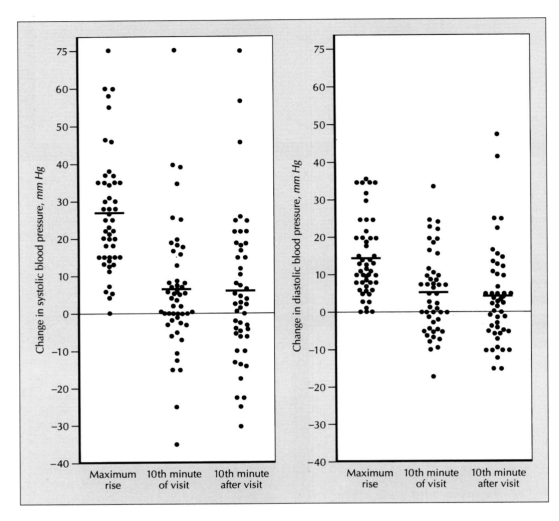

FIGURE 2-15. The acute effects of a physician visit on blood pressure as an example of cortical and emotional influences. Mancia *et al.* [8] elegantly demonstrated the effect of "mental stress" on blood pressure. Continuous intra-arterial blood pressure monitoring was performed on resting patients. When the physician entered the room, the blood pressure began to rise and continued to increase when he measured the blood pressure. There was a marked rise in systolic and diastolic blood pressure in both normotensive and hypertensive patients that was associated with an increase in pulse rate (but not to the same extent). The peak blood pressure elevation was recorded 4 minutes after the physician entered the room and slowly decreased over time, so that the blood pressure had almost completely returned to the baseline level after 10 minutes. (*Adapted from* Mancia *et al.* [8].)

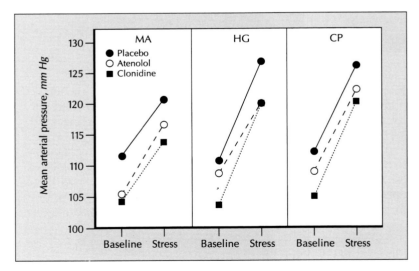

FIGURE 2-16. Reflex changes in blood pressure induced by mental arithmetic (MA), submaximal isometric handgrip (HG), and cold pressor testing (CP) in young men with borderline hypertension [8]. The rise in blood pressure produced by mental arithmetic represents a pure, centrally mediated response. Sustained handgrip and the cold pressor test cause a reflex rise in blood pressure by a combination of central and peripheral inputs to the nucleus tractus solitarius. The influence of the autonomic control of reflex blood pressure elevation is not affected by routine antihypertensive treatment. This illustration demonstrates that two agents, a β-blocker and an α_2-agonist, lower the resting blood pressure but do not affect the magnitude of the blood pressure response to these stimuli. (*Adapted from* Weder and Julius [9].)

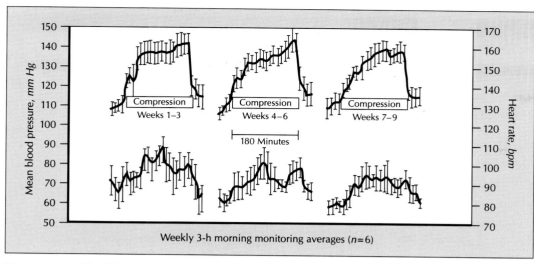

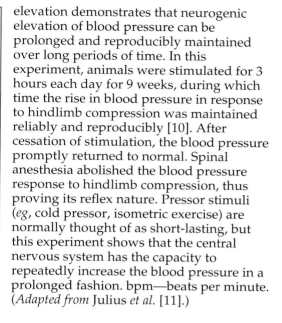

elevation demonstrates that neurogenic elevation of blood pressure can be prolonged and reproducibly maintained over long periods of time. In this experiment, animals were stimulated for 3 hours each day for 9 weeks, during which time the rise in blood pressure in response to hindlimb compression was maintained reliably and reproducibly [10]. After cessation of stimulation, the blood pressure promptly returned to normal. Spinal anesthesia abolished the blood pressure response to hindlimb compression, thus proving its reflex nature. Pressor stimuli (*eg*, cold pressor, isometric exercise) are normally thought of as short-lasting, but this experiment shows that the central nervous system has the capacity to repeatedly increase the blood pressure in a prolonged fashion. bpm—beats per minute. (*Adapted from* Julius *et al.* [11].)

FIGURE 2-17. The blood pressure response to hindquarter compression in conscious dogs. A sustained increase in blood pressure in conscious dogs can be induced by prolonged hindquarter compression with an inflatable suit. This type of reflex blood pressure

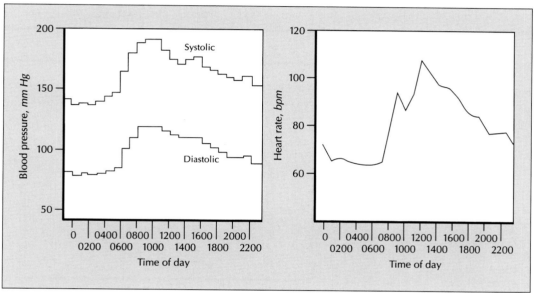

FIGURE 2-18. The circadian patterns of blood pressure and heart rate in humans are demonstrated on 24-hour ambulatory blood pressure monitoring in patients aged 34 to 72 years (*n* = 20). Large decreases in blood pressure and heart rate occur during the night when autonomic drive is at its lowest [11]. This is probably the best proof that the central nervous system has a substantial effect on the maintenance of blood pressure. bpm—beats per minute. (*Adapted from* Millar-Craig *et al.* [12].)

TESTING AUTONOMIC FUNCTION IN HUMANS

EFFECTS OF AUTONOMIC TONE ON CARDIOVASCULAR FUNCTION

Tone	**Organ status**
Inhibitory (parasympathetic)	Responsiveness
Stimulatory (sympathetic)	Structural factors
Receptor properties	**Feedback control**
Number	Baroreceptor properties
Sensitivity	
Affinity	

FIGURE 2-19. The effect of the autonomic nervous system on the circulation depends on a number of factors. It is not possible to assess total sympathetic function by measurement of one element alone, but unfortunately conclusions about overall autonomic function are drawn frequently from the assessment of only one component of the system, *eg*, catecholamine concentrations in plasma or urine. This section defines a range of factors that influence the circulating response to catecholamines. Figure 2-20 describes the multiple approaches that have been used effectively to assess autonomic function.

METHODS FOR ASSESSING SYMPATHETIC TONE

METHOD	ADVANTAGES	DISADVANTAGES
Urinary catecholamines	Measures integrated sympathetic function over 24 h	Very few released catecholamines are cleared in the urine; only a weak global measure of function
Plasma catecholamines	More sensitive than urinary catecholamines; can measure acute responses to stimuli	Very few released catecholamines are cleared in the plasma; very variable
Norepinephrine turnover tests	Studies true release	Complex technology
Regional norepinephrine studies	Gives specific organ information	Complex technology
Microneurography	"Direct" measurement	Complex technology
Spectral analysis of heart rate and blood pressure	"Naturalistic" observation; related to cardiovascular function	Relationship to other parameters of tone unknown; can be largely affected by organ responsiveness

FIGURE 2-20. Methods of assessing sympathetic tone. There are numerous methods of assessing sympathetic tone and function in humans. Each method has unique advantages and disadvantages, but measures only one component of a complex, integrated system.

ARTERIAL BARORECEPTORS

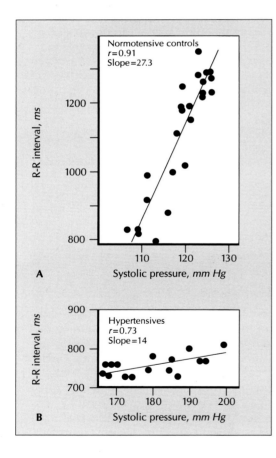

A

B

FIGURE 2-21. Testing baroreceptor function by the right atrial mean pressure method. Baroreceptor function in humans can be assessed by observing how heart rate changes in response to variation in blood pressure. Norepinephrine was injected into normotensive controls (**A**) and hypertensives (**B**), and the ensuing decrease in heart rate (beat to beat) in response to the rise in blood pressure was recorded on electrocardiogram [13]. The slope of the relationship between the decrease in heart rate and the increase in blood pressure is an index of the *sensitivity* of the baroreceptors.

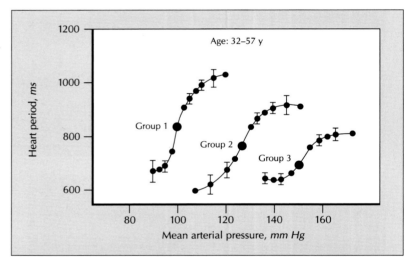

FIGURE 2-22. Testing baroreceptor function by the "steady state" method. In contrast to the right atrial mean pressure method, Korner's steady state method assesses both the slope and the set point of the baroreceptors. The set point of the baroreceptor reflex is that level of blood pressure at which an increase in blood pressure will decrease the sympathetic tone and produce bradycardia and a decrease in blood pressure will cause an increase in sympathetic tone, resulting in tachycardia. In both circumstances, the compensatory response tends to restore the blood pressure toward the desired set point. In Korner *et al.*'s [14] study, multiple doses of pressor and depressor substances were infused, and the steady state heart response evaluated. The heart rate is expressed as the heart period: a shorter period equals a faster heart rate. Note that the set point in hypertensive patients is shifted toward a higher blood pressure and that the slope (sensitivity) of the hypertensive baroreceptors is decreased. Note also that the operating range of the baroreceptors in hypertensive subjects is narrowed. Group 1 consisted of patients with a mean arterial pressure of 80 to 110 mm Hg; group 2, 117 to 136 mm Hg; and group 3, 143 to 163 mm Hg. (*Adapted from* Korner *et al.* [14].)

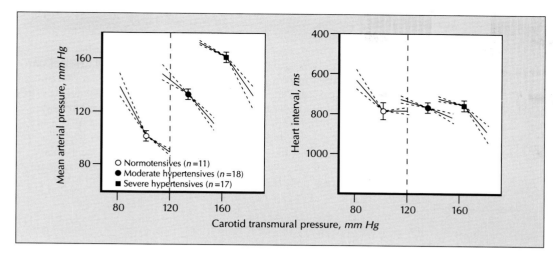

FIGURE 2-23. Testing baroreceptor function by the variable neck pressure chamber method. The function of the carotid sinus baroreceptors can be changed by either decreasing or increasing the pressure in a sealed neck chamber. The chamber pressure is transmitted to the carotid artery and the degree of stretch of the arterial wall is altered in a direction opposite the pressure in the chamber. Mancia *et al.* [15] investigated the baroreceptor function in normotensive and hypertensive patients

and documented that the mean operating pressure (the baseline blood pressure) is shifted toward much higher pressures in hypertension. Physiologically, this means that the arterial baroreceptors tend to restore normal blood pressure in normotensive patients and elevate blood pressure in hypertensive patients. For example, a mean transmural pressure of 120 mm Hg elicits a decrease in the mean blood pressure in normotensive patients, but in hypertensive patients the response is an increase in blood pressure. The normotensive patient reads this transmural pressure as *excessive*, and the compensatory response tends to lower the blood pressure toward the normal mean. In hypertensive patients, this transmural pressure is read as *too low*, so that the compensatory response is an increase in blood pressure back toward its higher set point. *T bars* indicate ± SEM. (*Adapted from* Mancia *et al.* [15].)

ORGAN AND RECEPTOR RESPONSIVENESS

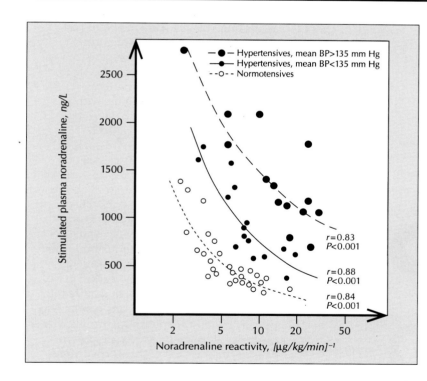

FIGURE 2-24. Testing adrenergic responsiveness with a systemic (intravenous) infusion of an adrenergic agonist. It is tempting to evaluate the adrenergic responsiveness by measuring the blood pressure (BP) response to an infusion of norepinephrine. However, Philipp *et al.* [16] have shown that the response is affected by both the endogenous level of norepinephrine and the baseline BP. In these experiments, stimulated endogenous norepinephrine is the plasma norepinephrine level during exercise. After exercise and an appropriate rest period, norepinephrine was infused in increasing doses, and the BP response evaluated. The "noradrenaline reactivity" is given as the reciprocal of the noradrenaline dose. Note that within each group, there is a negative relationship between the endogenous level and the noradrenergic activity. However, the higher the mean BP, the more reactivity is shifted toward the right, *eg*, to increased reactivity. Consequently, both the endogenous noradrenaline levels and the underlying blood pressure affect the reactivity to norepinephrine, with higher BPs associated with increased noradrenaline reactivity. (*Adapted from* Philipp *et al.* [16].)

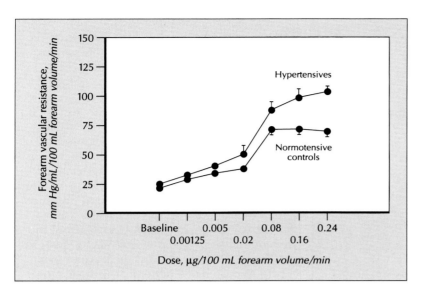

FIGURE 2-25. Regional testing of the α-adrenergic responsiveness. Response to systemic infusion of norepinephrine is complex and affected by endogenous levels of norepinephrine, the state of the vasculature (blood pressure level), and the competence of arterial baroreceptors. Direct infusion into the brachial artery gives more relevant information because the doses are small and have no systemic effects. In this example, norepinephrine infusion into the brachial artery demonstrated that patients with hypertension show an increased vascular reactivity compared with normotensive subjects [17]. However, these results still do not permit any conclusions about the α-adrenergic receptor properties (*see* Fig. 2-23). *T bars* indicate ± SEM. (*Adapted from* Egan *et al.* [17].)

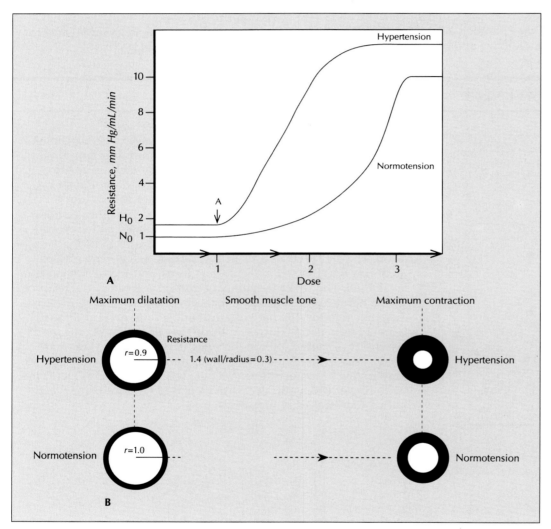

FIGURE 2-26. Assessment of vascular responses to intra-arterial norepinephrine infusion. **A,** Points H_0 and N_0 refer to the vascular resistance at maximal dilatation in this schematic illustration of the response of resistance vessels to agonist in hypertensive and normotensive subjects. The higher minimal resistance in the hypertensive vessel at the point of maximal dilatation (when the muscle is deprived of all intrinsic tone) suggests that there is a decrease in luminal size due to encroachment on the lumen by a thicker vessel wall. The arrow at *A* denotes the threshold response to an agonist. Note that the threshold is the same for hypertensive and normotensive vessels but that the response to agonist is exaggerated in the hypertensive vessel. The steeper curve in the hypertensive vessels could result from structural or receptor properties.

Hypertensive and normotensive vessels show the same threshold to agonists; if there were true receptor hyper-responsiveness in hypertension, the threshold to agonists would be lower in these vessels. The higher achieved vascular resistance in hypertensive vessels in response to agonist and the elevated minimal vascular resistance at maximal dilatation are therefore best explained by vascular "restructuring," rather than receptor hyper-responsiveness. **B,** Demonstration of Folkow's theory of structural adaptation to hypertension [18]. An increase in medial thickness with a decrease in wall-lumen ratio develops in resistance vessels with sustained hypertension because of remodeling, or hypertrophy, of smooth muscle cells, or both [19]. This results in increased vascular resistance in vessels of hypertensive patients that persists even at maximal dilatation. Arteries that have undergone structural adaptation have been shown to be hyper-responsive to adrenergic stimulation. The thicker wall of hypertrophic vessels encroaches on the lumen more so than in normal vessels. Because the resistance is the fourth power of the radius, any contraction of a structurally adapted hypertrophic vessel produces a relatively greater increase in resistance compared with a normal vessel. Thus for the same level of sympathetic vasoconstrictor tone, the vascular resistance will be much greater in the hypertensive patient whose resistance vessels have undergone structural adaptation than in normotensive subjects whose vessels have normal architecture [20]. Because the hyper-responsiveness of hypertensive vessels is caused by structural changes, *all* vasoconstrictive agonists will cause an excessive response (nonspecific hyper-responsiveness). (*Adapted from* Wikstrand [20].)

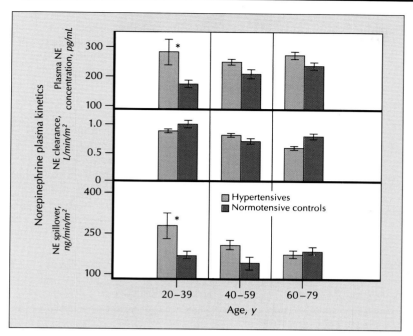

FIGURE 2-27. Norepinephrine (NE) turnover studies. Plasma NE values will be elevated if the spillover from nerve endings is normal but the clearance from plasma is decreased. In that case, the NE level would not reflect the sympathetic tone at the nerve endings. Esler *et al.* [21] developed a method using tritiated NE to measure true NE spillover from the nerve endings. In this study, elevated plasma NE values in younger patients with hypertension reflected an increased spillover, suggesting that these patients exhibit a true increase in sympathetic tone. Asterisks indicate $P < 0.05$; *t bars* indicate ± SE. (*Adapted from* Esler *et al.* [21].)

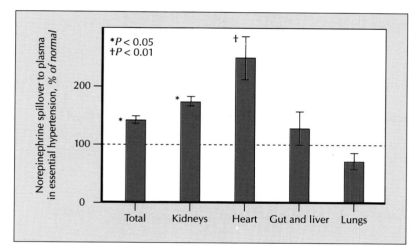

FIGURE 2-28. Regional norepinephrine sampling. The sympathetic discharge from the central nervous system is not uniform; pools of neurons to one organ may be activated, whereas the other pools may not be affected or even show decreased activity. In this example, Esler *et al.* [22] performed regional catheterization of arteries and veins to various organs and measured regional flow rates and norepinephrine concentrations. From these data, organ-specific spillover rates adjusted for differences in flow were calculated. A selective excess activation of the heart and kidney compared with other organs was found in patients with hypertension. *T bars* indicate ± SE.

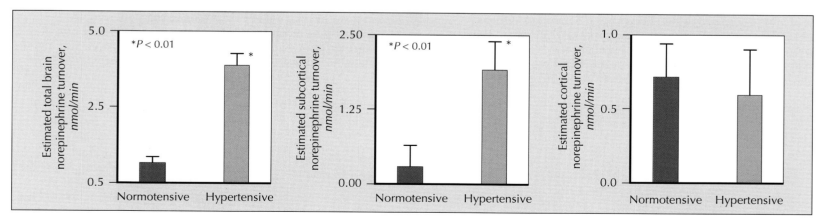

FIGURE 2-29. Central norepinephrine turnover. Lambert *et al.* [23] recently demonstrated that there is an increase in central norepinephrine turnover in hypertensive patients and that this increase originates in the subcortical regions, rather than in the cortex. This finding was still present after blockade with trimethaphan, suggesting that the increased norepinephrine turnover was from the brain, rather than from central sympathetic ganglia. The increased subcortical norepinephrine turnover correlated with total body norepinephrine spillover, heart rate, and mean arterial pressure, supporting the case for the role of excess central sympathetic nervous tone in the genesis of hypertension. (*Adapted from* Lambert *et al.* [23].)

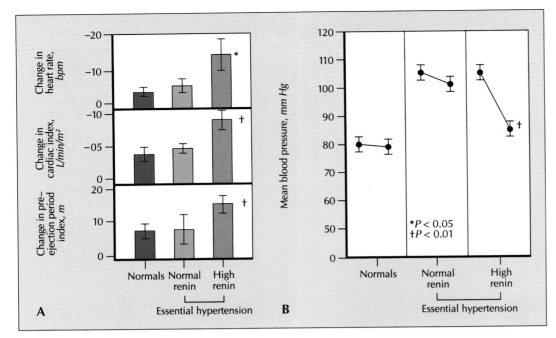

FIGURE 2-30. Use of adrenergic receptor blockade to assess sympathetic function. In this study, Esler *et al.* [24] first infused blocking doses of propranolol to assess β-adrenergic function in patients with mild hypertension. The β-adrenergic drive in one group of patients (high renin) was excessive; they responded with a greater change in cardiac output, heart rate, and pre-ejection period (**A**). The investigators then proceeded to block the α-adrenergic drive with intravenous phentolamine (**B**). Again patients with high renin values responded with a larger decrease in blood pressure (to near-normal values), suggesting an excessive α-adrenergic drive in these patients. *T bars* indicate ± SE. bpm—beats per minute. (*Adapted from* Esler *et al.* [24].)

MICRONEUROGRAPHY AND SPECTRAL ANALYSIS OF HEART RATE

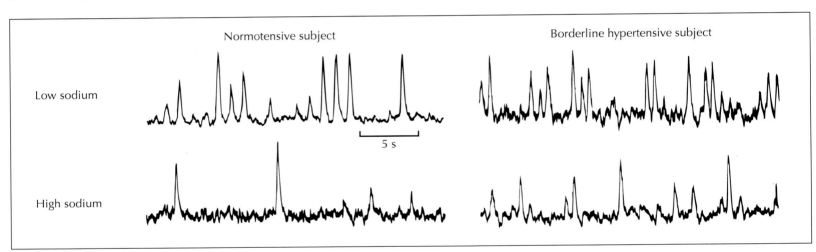

FIGURE 2-31. Microneurographic recordings in a normotensive and a borderline hypertensive subject. Microneurography permits recording of the rate of sympathetic bursts in the peroneal nerve. This method is excellent for evaluation of reflex responses within the same individual and it has been recognized recently to be a sufficiently sensitive and reproducible technique to allow comparison between groups. These recordings show increased rates of sympathetic bursts in the patient with borderline hypertension [25]. They also show a higher rate of discharge on a low-sodium diet in both normotensive and hypertensive subjects. (*Adapted from* Anderson *et al.* [25].)

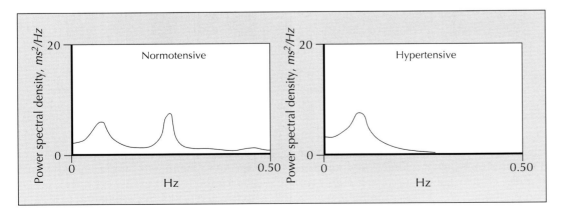

FIGURE 2-32. Comparison of sympathetic and parasympathetic activity by spectral analysis of the heart rate variability. After collection of beat-to-beat heart rate variability over a prolonged time period the data were subjected to a spectral autoregression analysis to yield components of the spectrum. The low-frequency component relates to sympathetic activity and the higher-frequency component to parasympathetic activity. Note that the patients with hypertension had an increased sympathetic and a decreased parasympathetic component compared with normotensive subjects. (*Adapted from* Guzzetti *et al.* [26].)

EVIDENCE

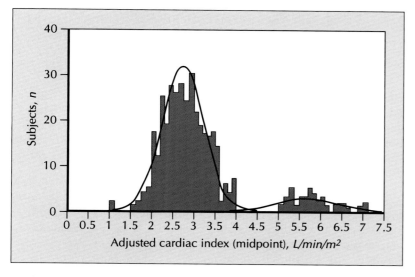

FIGURE 2-33. The distribution of cardiac index in the Tecumseh Study [27] is bimodal with a distinct population of subjects characterized by an increased cardiac index. Thirty-seven percent of all subjects with borderline hypertension were found to have this elevation in cardiac index and an elevated heart rate (which also had a bimodal distribution). This constellation of high blood pressure, fast heart rate, and high cardiac index, usually called *hyperkinetic borderline hypertension*, has been described in numerous studies from all over the world (United States, the former Czechoslovakia, Argentina, Sweden, Norway, Japan, and France). For a more complete review *see* Julius and Jamerson [27].

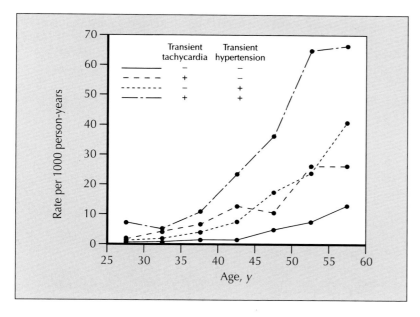

FIGURE 2-34. Heart rate as a predictor of future hypertension. In this study, US Army personnel of various ages were followed up for 5 years and new cases of sustained hypertension were recorded [28]. Note that transient tachycardia independently predicts more hypertension at all ages, and that when tachycardia is associated with borderline hypertension, the incidence of future hypertension is three to six times higher than in normotensive subjects. (*Adapted from* Levy *et al.* [28].)

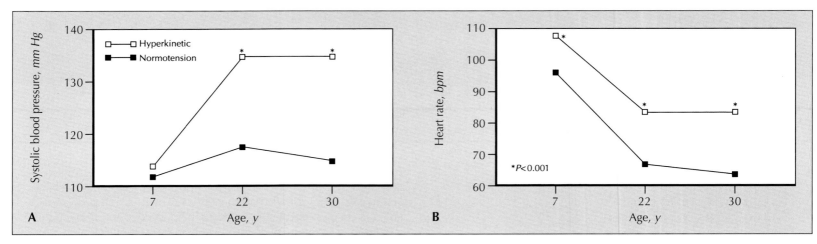

FIGURE 2-35. Early elevation of the heart rate in future hypertensive subjects. The elevation of heart rate is an early childhood characteristic of individuals destined to develop hypertension as adults. In Tecumseh, Michigan, hemodynamic measurements were performed when the subjects were an average of 30 years of age [27]. At that point, based on their blood pressure (**A**) and heart rate (**B**), they were classified as normotensive ($n = 787$) or hyperkinetic (fast heart rate and increased cardiac output) borderline hypertensive ($n=24$). Their childhood blood pressures and heart rates retrieved from the records of the Tecumseh study illustrate that tachycardia was present first, and that they later developed hypertension as young adults. bpm—beats per minute. (*Adapted from* Julius and Jamerson [27].)

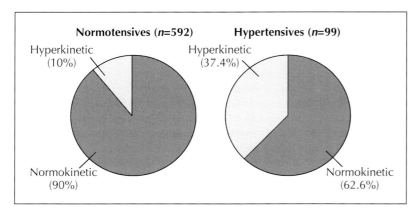

FIGURE 2-36. A large proportion of subjects with mild hypertension exhibit a hyperkinetic state. All studies of the hyperkinetic state have been hospital-based and performed on selected patients. The question therefore arose as to whether the percentage of such patients is over-represented in hospital populations. The Tecumseh study [29] investigated healthy, untreated, and unselected subjects in Tecumseh, Michigan, and found that the hyperkinetic state was present in 37% of all subjects with elevated blood pressure readings. These subjects also had significantly elevated plasma norepinephrine values. (*Adapted from* Julius and Jamerson [27].)

OTHER EVIDENCE OF INCREASED SYMPATHETIC TONE			
STUDY	METHOD	RESULT	CORRESPONDING FIGURE
Esler *et al.* [22]	Autonomic blockade with atropine, propranolol, and Regitine (phentolamine mesylate)	After a complete autonomic blockade the blood pressure fell into a normal range in 30% of patients with mild hypertension; these patients with "neurogenic" borderline hypertension characteristically have faster heart rates, elevated plasma norepinephrine, and higher plasma renin values	Fig. 2-28
Esler *et al.* [21]	Norepinephrine spillover by a radioactive tracer	Norepinephrine spillover increased in young patients with hypertension	Fig. 2-27
Esler *et al.* [24]	Norepinephrine spillover by a radioactive tracer	Spillover increased predominantly in the heart and kidneys	Fig. 2-30
Guzzetti *et al.* [26]	Spectral analysis of the heart rate interval	Low-frequency wave (sympathetic activity) increased	Fig. 2-32
Anderson *et al.* [25]	Microneurography	Rate of sympathetic bursts in the peroneal nerve increased in borderline hypertension	Fig. 2-31

FIGURE 2-37. Other evidence of an increased sympathetic tone in borderline hypertension. This table lists other studies that have examined different components of the autonomic nervous system using various methods [21,24–26]. The combined results support the theory that there is an increase in sympathetic activity in borderline hypertension. In most studies, only one method of assessment of autonomic function has been used. Consequently, data on concordance of findings with different methods in the same subjects are not available. However, the populations studied in these various papers have similar characteristics (young, male, borderline hypertensive, hyperkinetic), suggesting that sympathetic overactivity in such populations can be reproducibly found regardless of the method used.

OBESITY, HYPERTENSION, AND THE SYMPATHETIC NERVOUS SYSTEM

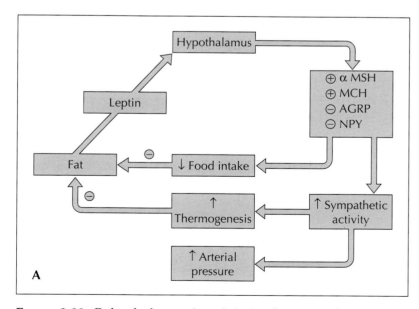

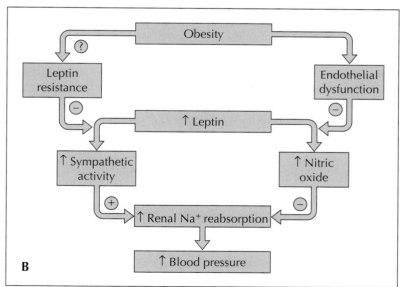

FIGURE 2-38. Role of adrenergic activity in chronic cardiovascular and renal action of leptin. **A,** There is increasing evidence that the hypertension associated with obesity is mediated through the sympathetic nervous system. **B,** Leptin resistance in obese patients raises plasma leptin levels, which affect the hypothalamic output of neurohormones influencing appetite and sympathetic activity. These changes result in increased appetite and inhibition of thermogenesis, which compound further weight gain. Activation of the sympathetic nervous system by increased levels of leptin may result in increased vasoconstrictor tone and renal retention of sodium, producing an elevation of blood pressure. (*Adapted from* Carlyle [30].)

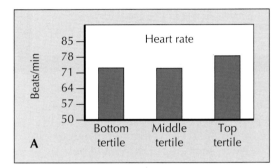

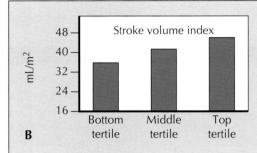

FIGURE 2-39. Regional noradrenaline spillover rates for the kidneys (A) and heart (B) in lean and obese subjects, who either are normotensive (NS) or have essential hypertension

(EH). In obese patients with hypertension, there is increased renal sympathetic activity compared with lean normotensive patients. In obese hypertensive patients, the adaptive suppression of cardiac sympathetic outflow seen in normotensive obese patients is absent, which suggests that this excess of cardiac sympathetic tone may contribute to the development of hypertension in this population. It is tempting to speculate that this failure of suppression of excess cardiac sympathetic tone in obese hypertensives is mediated directly or indirectly by leptin, but this has not been demonstrated to date. BMI—body mass index. (*Adapted from* Esler [31].)

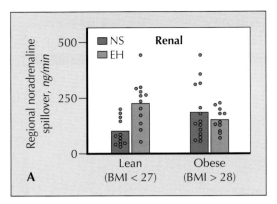

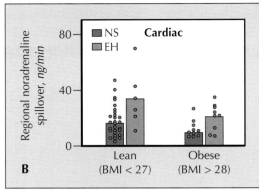

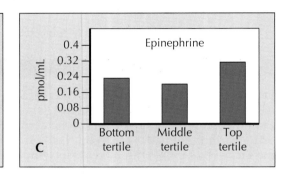

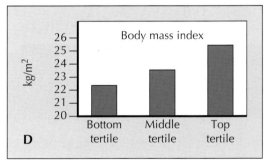

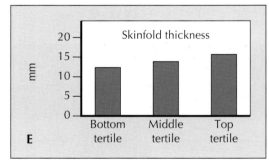

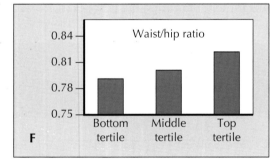

FIGURE 2-40. Data from the Tecumseh Offspring Study. Offspring were divided into tertiles according to the cardiac index of their parents (as an indicator of the hyperkinetic state). Those in the upper tertile had increased indices of sympathetic tone (heart rate, epinephrine, and stroke volume) as well as increased adiposity as measured by skin-fold thickness, body mass index, and waist-to-hip ratio. Prolonged excess sympathetic tone may cause selective functional downregulation of β-adrenergic receptors with decreased thermogenesis and predisposition to the development

of obesity. The increased sympathetic tone in obesity may be mediated by leptin, as described in Figure 2-38 [29].

Patients were grouped into tertiles of cardiac index. Data were adjusted for age and gender. For each variable, significant differences were found between tertiles. **A,** Clinical heart rate ($P = 0.001$). **B,** Stroke volume index ($P = 0.0001$). **C,** Plasma epinephrine level ($P = 0.02$). **D,** Body mass index ($P = 0.001$). **E,** Skinfold thickness ($P = 0.008$). **F,** Waist-to-hip ratio ($P = 0.02$). (*Adapted from* Palatini *et al.* [32].)

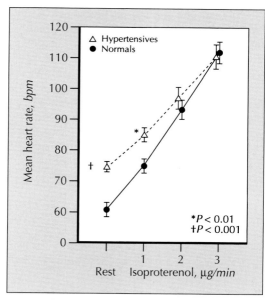

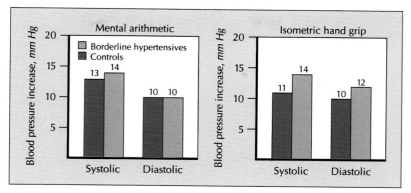

FIGURE 2-41. Decreased β-adrenergic responsiveness in borderline hypertension. The elevation of cardiac output and heart rate in hyperkinetic borderline hypertension could reflect increased β-adrenergic responsiveness. The data in Figure 2-40, however, show that the β-adrenergic responsiveness in borderline hypertension is decreased [33]. After an infusion of increasing doses of isoproterenol, hypertensive patients (n = 9) showed a lesser increase of heart rate than did normotensive subjects (n = 20). T bars indicate ± SE. bpm—beats per minute. (*Adapted from* Julius [33].)

FIGURE 2-42. Response to mental and physical stressors in the setting of an epidemiologic study. It has been reported frequently that patients with borderline hypertension are hyper-reactors to mental and physical stresses. All such studies are hospital-based, and the patients reported in them are not necessarily representative of the population at large. In this study, performed in Tecumseh, Michigan, 250 normotensive and 37 borderline hypertensive subjects who were unaware of their blood pressure were tested [34]. One or more resting office blood pressure measurements greater than 140/90 mm Hg were defined as borderline hypertension. Subjects with borderline hypertension showed blood pressure responses similar to those of normotensive subjects. In the entire population, there was a negative correlation between the blood pressure level and the blood pressure response to the stress. Mental arithmetic and isometric exercise are standard stressors for investigating blood pressure reactivity. Apparently in the general population, as opposed to hospital-based populations, there is no evidence of excessive blood pressure responsiveness in hypertensive subjects. (*Adapted from* Julius *et al.* [34].)

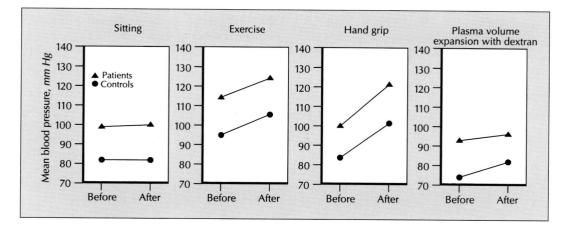

FIGURE 2-43. Blood pressure response of patients and control subjects to various stimuli. This illustration was compiled from various experiments performed in our laboratory at the University of Michigan [35,36]. Patients and controls were age- and gender-matched. There were at least 12 patients and 18 control subjects in each experiment. Note that by and large patients' blood pressure responses to various types of stimuli were not different from those of the control subjects, but the patients' blood pressures were consistently higher. Consequently, in hypertension there is no evidence of blood pressure hyperactivity. The blood pressure is set at a higher level but is regulated in a normal fashion from that level.

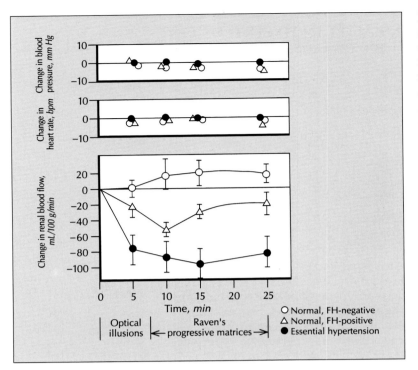

FIGURE 2-44. Renal hemodynamic responses to mild psychologic stimuli in hypertensive patients. Hollenberg *et al.* [37] demonstrated different patterns of regional blood flow in normotensive subjects (*n* = 24) and hypertensive patients (*n* = 15) in response to a nonverbal IQ test. The changes in blood pressure and heart rate induced by the stimulus were similar in both groups. However, there was a sustained reduction in renal blood flow associated with an increase in plasma renin activity and aldosterone in hypertensive subjects, whereas renal blood flow increased and plasma renin activity and aldosterone levels decreased in normotensive subjects. These results corroborate Esler *et al.*'s [24] findings and are another demonstration of the differences in regional sympathetic responses that can be produced by central nervous system control of blood flow in hypertension. bpm—beats per minute; FH—family history. (*Adapted from* Hollenberg *et al.* [37].)

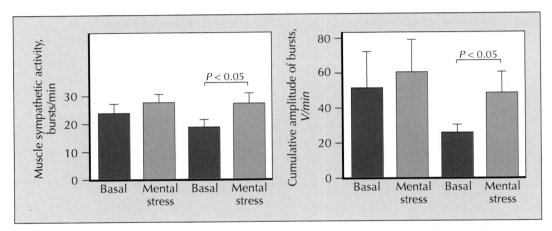

FIGURE 2-45. Excessive sympathetic nervous activity in normotensive subjects with a family history of hypertension. This study [38] shows that normotensive subjects with a family history of hypertension had an excess of sympathetic discharge in response to mental stress compared with normotensive subjects without a family history of

hypertension. The increased rate of discharge in the peroneal nerve as recorded by microneurography was associated with a significant increase in plasma norepi-nephrine and a significant increase in systolic and diastolic blood pressure in the group with positive family history. There was also an increase in plasma endothelin with mental stress in this group, which raises the intriguing possibility that the propensity for increased central sympathetic nervous discharge is inherited, and that the effects on blood pressure may be mediated by endothelin. *Dark bars* indicate the offspring of normotensive subjects (*n* = 8); *light bars* indicate the offspring of hypertensive subjects (*n* = 10). Data are mean ± SEM. (*Adapted from* Noll *et al.* [38].)

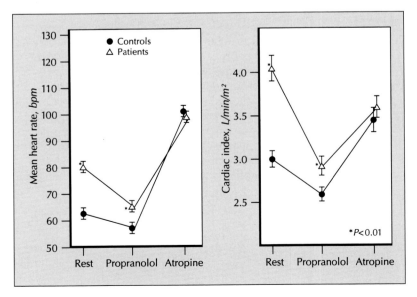

FIGURE 2-46. Both the sympathetic and parasympathetic systems play a role in the neurogenic elevation of the heart rate and cardiac output in borderline hypertension. In this experiment [4], blocking doses of propranolol (0.2 mg/kg) and atropine (0.04 mg/kg) were given intravenously and the mean heart rate and cardiac output responses were recorded. When the effect of β-adrenergic sympa-thetic drive to the heart was abolished by propranolol, heart rate and cardiac output in the patient group did not decrease into the normal range. However, after additional parasympathetic blockade with atropine, heart rate and cardiac output levels in this group became comparable to the values in control subjects. Consequently, the elevation of cardiac output and heart rate was maintained by both branches of the autonomic nervous system. After receiving propranolol, the heart rate and cardiac output of the patients decreased more than those of controls, demonstrating that an excessive β-adrenergic drive has been present in these individuals. Conversely, after atropine the heart rate and cardiac output increased less in this group, a sign of decreased para-sympathetic inhibition. *T bars* indicate ± SE. bpm—beats per minute.

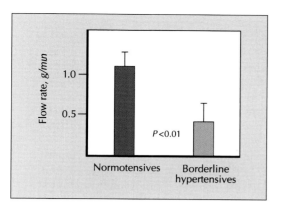

FIGURE 2-47. The documented reduction in parasympathetic inhibitory tone in hypertension (*see* Fig. 2-44) is not limited to the cardiovascular system. Böhm *et al.* [39] demonstrated that salivary flow is decreased at rest (shown) and when stimulated by neostigmine (not shown) in hypertensive patients compared with normotensive subjects. *T bars* indicate ± SEM. (*Adapted from* Böhm *et al.* [39].)

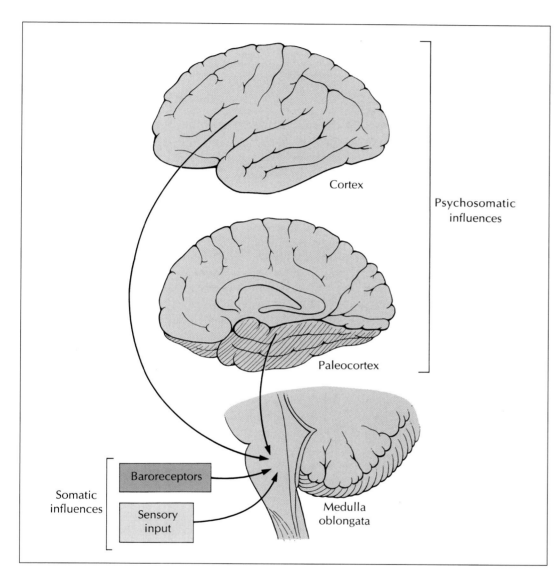

FIGURE 2-48. Factors that could affect the integration of the sympathetic tone in the medulla oblongata. The relationship between the sympathetic and the parasympathetic tones is integrated in the medulla oblongata in a reciprocal fashion: an increase in one of the components is associated with a decrease in tone in the other branch of the autonomic nervous system. Consequently, the reciprocal change in the autonomic tone in borderline hypertension—more sympathetic and less parasympathetic tone than in normals—suggests that the abnormality is of central nervous system origin and emanates from the medulla oblongata. A number of inputs converge on the medulla oblongata and conceivably could cause the observed abnormalities in borderline hypertension. These inputs can be investigated by different methods.

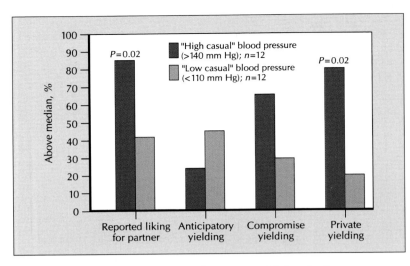

FIGURE 2-49. Personality traits of patients with borderline hypertension. The possibility that borderline hypertension is a

psychosomatic disease has been investigated using personality inventories. Major findings are that patients are submissive [40,41] and prone to holding anger in without expressing it [41]. In this study [40], an experimental protocol was designed to test whether the borderline hypertensive patients are actually submissive. Using a seven-point scale, the subjects indicated their attitudes about some important topics (*ie*, capital punishment). They were later matched into pairs in which maximal disagreement existed on most of the six topics, and were asked to arrive, through discussion, at a compromise and indicate the point of agreement on the scale. Patients with borderline hypertension anticipated they would not yield but in fact did. Furthermore, they indicated they "yielded privately," *ie*, they not only compromised but also actually changed their opinion. They also expressed a great degree of liking for the dominant partner who influenced them to change their opinion. This experiment confirmed that borderline hypertensive patients are indeed submissive. These same findings hold for the total group when divided at the median systolic level. (*Adapted from* Harburg *et al.* [40].)

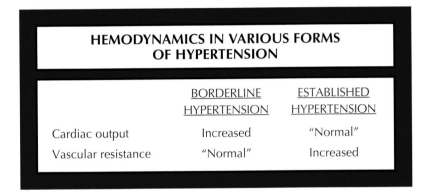

FIGURE 2-50. Hemodynamically essential hypertension is very different from borderline hypertension. Because the hyperkinetic state predicts the development of future established hypertension (*see* Fig. 2-34), apparently in the course of hypertension there is a transition from a high cardiac output state to a high resistance state. The question therefore arises as to what mechanisms could lead to such a hemodynamic transition. Note the quotation marks on normal values. The vascular resistance in borderline hypertension is not elevated numerically. However, because of the increased cardiac output the resistance is *relatively* elevated, since the normal response to a higher cardiac output is a decrease in vascular resistance. Similarly, the cardiac output in established hypertension is only normal numerically, but such patients have a decreased stroke volume and maintain the normal output by a faster heart rate.

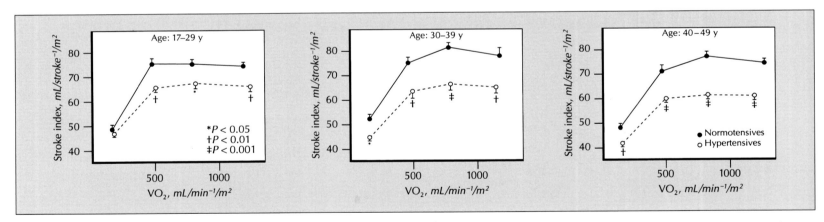

FIGURE 2-51. The effect of mild hypertension on stroke volume in Lund-Johansen's cross-sectional study [39]. The graphs start with resting values and show the response to three increasing levels of exercise. Note that the youngest patients had a normal resting stroke volume but that physical exercise uncovered an underlying inability to increase the stroke volume adequately. In older patients, who presumably had a longer duration of mild blood pressure elevation, the stroke volume is already decreased at rest and continues to be depressed during exercise. *T bars* indicate ± SEM.

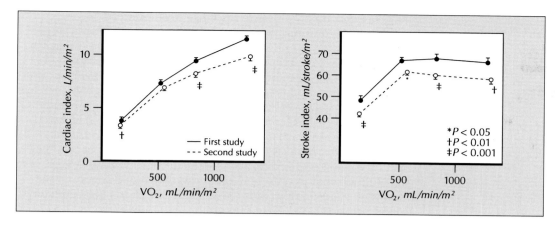

FIGURE 2-52. The hemodynamic transition in hypertension. Lund-Johansen [42] followed up on patients ranging in age from 17 to 29 years. The studies were repeated after 10 years, during which the subjects ($n = 15$) did not receive antihypertensive

treatment. The graphs start with resting values and show the response to three increasing levels of exercise. Note the substantial decrease of the cardiac index and stroke volume both at rest and during exercise with the passing of time. At 10-year follow-up these patients had not yet developed treatment-requiring hypertension. *Open circles* represent hypertensive patients; *closed circles*, normotensive patients. However, in a later report Lund-Johansen [43] found that after 20 years the blood pressure had risen in all patients to hypertensive levels and that this was associated with a further decrease of stroke volume and a large increase in vascular resistance. *T bars* indicate ± SEM.

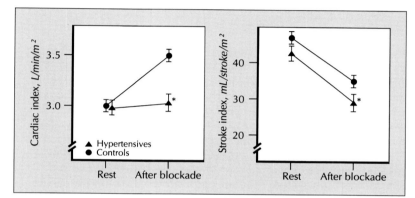

FIGURE 2-53. Autonomic blockade demonstrates an underlying cardiac abnormality in patients with borderline hypertension with normal cardiac output. In this study [44], patients with borderline hypertension with a normal cardiac output were given an autonomic blockade with intravenous propranolol and atropine. It was assumed, but not documented, that such patients may have undergone a phase of increased cardiac output in the past. The patients had a significantly elevated heart rate prior to blockade (> 10 beats per minute above controls; $P < 0.001$). When the difference in the heart rate between the two groups was removed with autonomic blockade, the patients' cardiac output fell to values significantly lower than those in control subjects. A pharmacologically denervated heart devoid of autonomic control operates as a Starling preparation: the stroke volume is related to end-diastolic distention. Because indices of venous filling after blockade in both groups were similar but the patients had decreased stroke volume, the data suggest that the patients' hearts may have been less compliant, thereby resulting in less end-diastolic distention. The corollary of these observations is that an increased autonomic nervous drive at rest was needed to maintain patients' cardiac output in the normal range. *T bars* indicate ± SEM; *asterisks* indicate $P < 0.01$.

Organ		Time, y →	Mechanism
Heart	β-Adrenergic responses		Receptor downregulation **A**
	Stroke volume		Decreased cardiac compliance **B**
	Cardiac output		Combination of **A** and **B**
Arterioles	Vascular resistance		Increased vascular reactivity secondary to hypertrophy of the resistance vessels (thicker walls)
			Possibly endothelial dysfunction

FIGURE 2-54. The proposed mechanism of hemodynamic transition in hypertension, showing the effects of decreased β-adrenergic responsiveness (*see* Fig. 2-39) and decreased cardiac compliance/low stroke volume (*see* Fig. 2-51) on the cardiac output. The cardiac output first decreases and then levels off. Later, if the patient develops congestive heart failure, the resting cardiac output decreases further. The process of structural amplification as a result of the hypertrophy of the arteriolar wall (*see* Fig. 2-26) supports the increase in vascular resistance. With time the hemodynamics of hypertension change from an increase in cardiac output to an increase in vascular resistance.

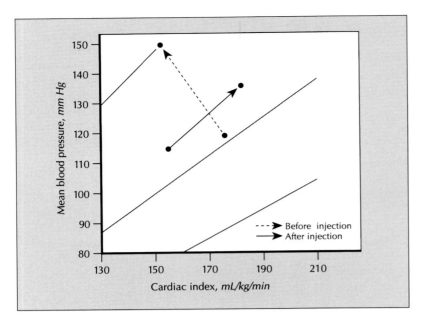

FIGURE 2-55. Blood pressure response to 60 minutes of hindquarter compression in eight chloralose-anesthetized dogs before and after administration of phenoxybenzamine, 1 mg/kg intravenously [45]. Hindquarter compression in dogs causes a potent reflex increase in blood pressure [10]. The normal response to this stimulus is an increase in blood pressure through an increase in vascular resistance, but when the vasoconstriction is prevented by α-adrenergic blockade the blood pressure increase is achieved by an increase in cardiac output. It appears that the *central nervous system regulates the blood pressure* and uses the accessible hemodynamic response to achieve the desired blood pressure. It also follows that in order to closely regulate blood pressure, the central nervous system must be able to *sense* (read) the achieved blood pressure level. *Diagonals* are lines of isoresistance.

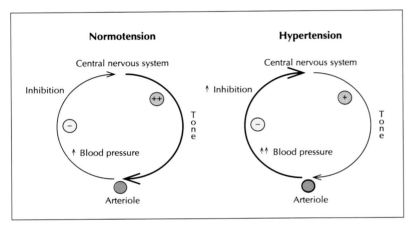

FIGURE 2-56. Under a number of circumstances, the brain preserves the pressure response while permitting a wide variation in the cardiac output and vascular resistance (*see* Figs. 2-53 to 2-55). In all of these circumstances, the brain appears to "seek" a predetermined pressure. To achieve the same pressure always and to stabilize the response at that level, the brain must be able to sense the achieved pressure. Long-standing hypertension eventually causes arteriolar hypertrophy. The thickened wall of arterioles enhances arteriolar responsiveness to vasoconstrictive stimuli (*see* Fig. 2-27). In the presence of hypertrophic vessels, a smaller stimulus causes a larger blood pressure increase. If the central nervous system regulates and senses the blood pressure when the blood vessels are hyper-responsive, less sympathetic tone is needed to achieve the same blood pressure level. The hypothesis of the "blood pressure seeking property of the brain" [46] predicts a resetting of the sympathetic tone toward lower values in patients with hyper-responsive arterioles, and thus explains why measures of sympathetic tone are "normal" in established hypertension.

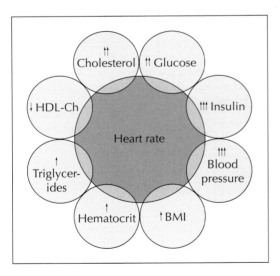

FIGURE 2-57. The clinical significance of increased heart rate as a marker of elevated sympathetic tone. In 434 men in the Tecumseh study [47] there is a strong correlation between heart rate and atherogenic risk factors, which has also been documented in other population-based studies. These relationships may help to explain the increased risk of cardiovascular disease in patients with hypertension. *One arrow* indicates $P < 0.05$; *two arrows* indicate $P < 0.01$; *three arrows* indicate $P < 0.0001$. BMI—body mass index; HDL-Ch—high-density lipoprotein cholesterol. (*Adapted from* Palatini and Julius [48].)

1. Owsjannikow PH: Die tonische und reflectorische centren de gefassnervum. *Verh K Sachs Ges Wisse* 1871, 23:134.

2. Loewy AD: Anatomy of the autonomic nervous system. In *Central Regulation of Autonomic Functions*. Edited by Loewy AD, Spyer KM. New York: Oxford University Press; 1990:3–16.

3. Spyer KM: CNS organization of reflex circulatory control. In *Central Regulation of Autonomic Functions*. Edited by Loewy AD, Spyer KM. New York: Oxford University Press; 1990:168–188.

4. Julius S, Pascual A, London R: Role of parasympathetic inhibition in the hyperkinetic type of borderline hypertension. *Circulation* 1971, 44:413–418.

5. Struyker Boudier HAJ: Adrenergic mechanisms and pharmacotherapy of hypertension. In *Adrenergic Blood Pressure Regulation: Proceedings of a Symposium*. Edited by Birkenhäger WH, Folkow B, Struyker Boudier HAJ. Amsterdam, The Netherlands: Excerpta Medica; 1985:114–123.

6. Krief S, Lonnqvist F, Raimbaults, *et al.*: Tissue distribution of the β-3 receptor m-RNA in man. *J Clin Invest* 1993, 91:344–349.

7. Linden ME, Gilman AG: G proteins. *Sci Am* 1992, 267:56–91.

8. Mancia G, Grasso G, Bertinieri G, *et al.*: Effects of blood pressure measurement by the doctor on the patient's blood pressure and heart rate. *Lancet* 1983, 2:695–698.

9. Weder AB, Julius S: Behavior, blood pressure variability and hypertension. *Psychosomatics* 1985, 47:406–414.

10. Osterziel KJ, Julius S, Brant D: Blood pressure elevation during hindquarter compression in dogs is neurogenic. *J Hypertens* 1984, 4:411–417.

11. Julius S, Sanches R, Malayen S, *et al.*: Sustained blood pressure elevation to lower body compression in pigs and dogs. *Hypertension* 1982, 4:782–788.

12. Millar-Craig MW, Bishop CN, Raftery EB: Circadian variation of blood-pressure. *Lancet* 1978, 1(8068):795–797.

13. Bristow JD, Honour AJ, Pickering GW, *et al.*: Diminished baroreceptor sensitivity in high blood pressure. *Circulation* 1969, 39:48–54.

14. Korner PI, West MJ, Shaw J, *et al.*: "Steady state" properties of the baroreceptor-heart rate reflex in essential hypertension in man. *Clin Exp Pharmacol Physiol* 1974, 1:65–76.

15. Mancia G, Ludbrook J, Ferrari A, *et al.*: Baroreceptor reflexes in human hypertension. *Circ Res* 1978, 43:170–177.

16. Philipp T, Distler A, Cordes U: Sympathetic nervous system and blood pressure control in essential hypertension. *Lancet* 1978, 2(8097):959–963.

17. Egan BM, Panis R, Hinderliter A, *et al.*: Mechanism of increased α-adrenergic vasoconstriction in human hypertension. *J Clin Invest* 1987, 80:812–817.

18. Folkow B, Grumby G, Thulesius O: Adaptive structural changes of the vascular wall in hypertension and their relationship to control of the peripheral resistance. *Acta Physiol Scand* 1958, 44:255.

19. Korsgaard K, Aalkjaer C, Heagerty G, *et al.*: Histology of subcutaneous small arteries from patients with essential hypertension. *Hypertension* 1993, 22:523–526.

20. Wikstrand J: Cardiovascular function during long term antihypertensive adrenergic blockade. In *Adrenergic Blood Pressure Regulation: Proceedings of a Symposium*. Edited by Birkenhäger WH, Folkow B, Struyker Boudier HAJ. Amsterdam, The Netherlands: Excerpta Medica; 1985:125–137.

21. Esler M, Jennings G, Lambert G: Noradrenaline release and the pathophysiology of primary human hypertension. *Am J Hypertens* 1989, 2:140S–146S.

22. Esler M, Lambert G, Jennings G: Regional norepinephrine turnover in human hypertension. *Clin Exp Theory Pract* 1989, A11(suppl 1):75–89.

23. Lambert GW, Ferrier C, Kaye D, *et al.*: Central nervous system norephinephrine turnover in essential hypertension. *Ann N Y Acad Sci* 1995, 763:679–694.

24. Esler M, Julius S, Zweifler A, *et al.*: Mild high renin essential hypertension: neurogenic human hypertension. *N Engl J Med* 1977, 296:405–411.

25. Anderson EA, Sinkey CA, Lawton WJ, Mark AL: Elevated sympathetic nerve activity in borderline hypertensive humans: evidence from direct intra-neural recordings. *Hypertension* 1989, 14:177–183.

26. Guzzetti S, Piccaluga E, Casati R, *et al.*: Sympathetic predominance in essential hypertension: a study employing spectral analysis of heart rate variability. *J Hypertens* 1988, 6:711–717.

27. Julius S, Jamerson K: Sympathetics, insulin resistance and coronary risk in hypertension: the chicken-and-egg question. *J Hypertens* 1994, 12:495–502.

28. Levy RL, White PD, Stroud WD, *et al.*: Transient tachycardia: prognostic significance alone and in association with transient hypertension. *JAMA* 1945, 129:585–588.

29. Julius S, Krause L, Schork N, *et al.*: Hyperkinetic borderline hypertension in Tecumseh, Michigan. *J Hypertens* 1991, 9:77–84.

30. Carlyle M, Jones OB, Kuo JJ, Hall JE: Chronic cardiovascular and renal actions of leptin: role of adrenergic activity. *Hypertension* 2002, 39 (2 Pt 2):496–501.

31. Esler M: The sympathetic nervous system and hypertension. *Am J Hypertens* 2000, 13 (6 Pt 2)99S–105S.

32. Palatini P, Vriz O, Nesbitt S, *et al.*: Parental hyperdynamic circulation predicts insulin resistance in offspring: the Tecumseh Offspring Study. *Hypertension* 1999, 33:769–774.

33. Julius S: Neurogenic component in borderline hypertension. In *The Nervous System in Arterial Hypertension*. Edited by Julius S, Esler MD. Springfield, IL: Charles C. Thomas; 1976:301–330.

34. Julius S, Schork N, Johnson E, *et al.*:Independence of pressure reactivity from blood pressure levels in Tecumseh, Michigan. *Hypertension* 1991, 17:13–19.

35. Julius S, Pascual A, Sannerstedt R, *et al.*: Relationship between cardiac output and peripheral resistance in borderline hypertension. *Circulation* 1971, 43:382–390.

36. Sannerstedt R, Julius S: Systemic haemodynamics in borderline arterial hypertension: responses to static exercise before and under the influence of propranolol. *Cardiovasc Res* 1972, 6:398–403.

37. Hollenberg NK, Williams GH, Adams DF: Essential hypertension: abnormal renal vascular and endocrine responses to a mild psychological stimulus. *Hypertension* 1981, 3:11–17.

38. Noll G, Wenzel R, Schneider M, *et al.*: Increased activation of sympathetic nervous system and endothelin by mental stress in normotensive offspring of hypertensive parents. *Circulation* 1996, 93:866–869.

39. Böhm R, van Baak M, van Hooff M, *et al.*: Salivary flow in borderline hypertension. *Klin Wochenschr* 1985, 63:154–156.

40. Harburg E, Julius S, McGinn NF, *et al.*: Personality traits and behavioral patterns associated with systolic blood pressure levels in college males. *J Chronic Dis* 1964, 17:405–414.

41. Esler M, Julius S, Zweifler A, *et al.*: Mild high-renin essential hypertension: neurogenic human hypertension? *N Engl J Med* 1977, 296:405–411.

42. Lund-Johansen P: Hemodynamic patterns of untreated hypertensive disease. In *Hypertension: Pathophysiology, Diagnosis, and Management.* Edited by Laragh JH, Brenner BM. New York: Raven Press; 1990:305–327.

43. Lund-Johansen P: Central haemodynamics in essential hypertension at rest and during exercise: a 20-year follow-up study. *J Hypertens* 1989, 7(suppl 6):52–55.

44. Julius S, Randall OS, Esler MD, *et al.*: Altered cardiac responsiveness and regulation in the normal cardiac output type of borderline hypertension. *Circ Res* 1975, 36–37(suppl I):199–207.

45. Julius S, Sanchez R, Brant D: Pressure increase to external hindquarter compression in dogs: a facultative regulatory response. *J Hypertens* 1986, 4(suppl 6):54–56.

46. Julius S: Editorial review: the blood pressure seeking properties of the central nervous system. *J Hypertens* 1988, 6:177–185.

47. Julius S, Jamerson K, Mejia A, *et al.*: The association of borderline hypertension with target organ changes and higher coronary risk. Tecumseh Blood Pressure study. *JAMA* 1990, 264:354–358.

48. Palatini P, Julius S: Heart rate and the cardiovascular risk. *J Hypertens* 1997, 15:3–17.

KIDNEY, SODIUM, AND THE RENIN-ANGIOTENSIN SYSTEM

Helmy M. Siragy and Robert M. Carey

The renin-angiotensin system is a coordinated hormonal cascade in the control of renal function, fluid and electrolyte balance, and blood pressure. Although the existence of the renin-angiotensin system has been known for over two decades, recent advances in cell and molecular biology as well as renal physiology have opened the doors for a greater understanding of the role of this system in normal and disease states. Exciting new concepts, such as molecular cloning of genes for renin, angiotensinogen, angiotensin-converting enzyme, and the angiotensin AT_1 receptor, have been derived from recent studies. New angiotensin peptides with unique actions have been identified, and the role of angiotensins as cell-to-cell mediators (*ie*, paracrine substances) in the kidney has recently been appreciated.

Renin, a glycoprotein enzyme, is synthesized in, stored in, and released from the renal juxta-glomerular cells of the afferent arteriole. Renin is released in response to individual nephron signals, whole-kidney modulating signals, and several local effectors. Renin acts on angiotensinogen, a high molecular weight protein that is synthesized by the liver and kidney tubules, to form an inactive decapeptide, angiotensin I. Angiotensin I is converted by angiotensin-converting enzyme to the octapeptide, angiotensin II, which is a potent effector of renal vasoconstriction and sodium resorption. Other potential renal angiotensin agonists include the angiotensin II metabolites, angiotensin III, angiotensin IV, and angiotensin (1-7) (*see* Fig. 3-17). In the kidney, angiotensins act at the AT_1 receptor in renal blood vessels, glomerular mesangium, and proximal tubules. Angiotensin II action in the kidney is mediated by phospholipase C and D and is associated with decreased adenylyl cyclase activity.

Intrarenal blockade of the renin-angiotensin system leads to renal vasodilation, natriuresis, and diuresis, suggesting that the angiotensin II found in the kidney serves as a paracrine substance in the control of renal function. Angiotensin II may regulate renal function through a variety of mechanisms, including angiotensin peptide formation, transport, and action in the renal interstitial compartment.

Plasma renin activity is a useful measure of renin secretion in humans. Renin activity measurements ideally should be indexed against 24-hour urinary sodium excretion, because there is an inverse hyperbolic relationship between renin activity and sodium excretion. Approximately 15% of patients with essential hypertension have high plasma renin activity, 25%

have low plasma renin activity, and the remaining 60% have normal plasma renin activity when indexed against 24-hour urinary sodium excretion values. Such studies can help classify the renin status of patients with hypertension but are not recommended in the routine work-up of hypertension.

Renovascular hypertension serves as a model of a disease process whose cause is linked to the renin-angiotensin system. Renovascular hypertension is usually caused by athero-sclerosis or fibromuscular dysplasia of renal arteries. Several clinical clues are usually associated with renovascular hypertension. Peripheral plasma renin activity or a captopril test (*see* Figs. 3-36 and 3-37) can be used as a screening device in suspected cases. A definitive anatomic diagnosis can be established only by selective renal arteriography. The functional significance of stenotic lesions can be determined by measurement of renal vein renin activity.

ANATOMY AND PHYSIOLOGY

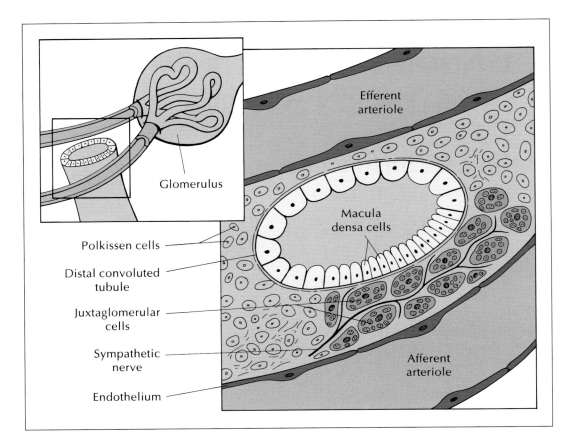

FIGURE 3-1. The juxtaglomerular apparatus, illustrating tubular and vascular components. The tubular component consists of 1) a specialized region of the distal convoluted tubule, which bends between the afferent and efferent arterioles, and 2) the macula densa, which contains cells that are sensitive to sodium chloride flux and control renin secretion. The macula densa cells can be identified by the proximity of their nuclei to each other. The vascular component consists of the afferent and efferent arterioles as well as the extraglomerular mesangium. The extra-glomerular mesangium is a collection of small cells with pale nuclei, called Polkissen cells, the function of which is unknown. The juxtaglomerular cells, in which renin is synthesized and stored, and from which it is secreted, are vascular smooth muscle cells modified by the presence of secretory and lysosomal granules; juxtaglomerular cells are absent from the efferent arteriole. The macula densa cells have no basement membrane, allowing intimate contact of the juxta-glomerular cells with tubular cells. Renin is stored in and secreted from the granules of the juxtaglomerular cells. The vascular and tubular components are innervated by sympathetic nerves. Renal nerve stimulation increases renin secretion by norepinephrine-induced stimulation of β-adrenergic receptors. Juxtaglomerular cells also have angiotensin II receptors, the stimulation of which leads to inhibition of renin secretion.

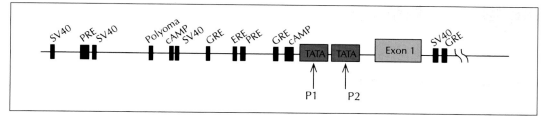

FIGURE 3-2. The 5' flanking region of the human renin gene. Genomic analysis of this gene has shown that it is encoded by a 12.5-kb DNA sequence. A single locus is found in the human gene, which contains 10 exons and nine introns. Its 5' flanking region contains several identifiable promoter (P) and enhancer regions as well as regulatory elements that combine to regulate tissue-specific biologic expression of the gene. Promoter regions are specific sites on the DNA template where RNA polymerase binds and initiates transcription of messenger RNA. Enhancers are sequences that increase promoter activity by elevating the binding affinity of RNA polymerase for the promoter renin. In the renin gene, there are two promoters; these promoters are TATA boxes, which are designated P1 and P2. Only the P2 box appears to act as a transcriptional start site. The function of P1 is unknown. A cAMP-response element and glucocorticoid (GRE)-, estrogen (ERE)-, and progesterone (PRE)-response elements have been observed in the sequences of the 5' region. Sequences homologous to the core sequences of the polyoma and SV40 viral enhancers are also present. (*Adapted from* Griendling *et al.* [1].)

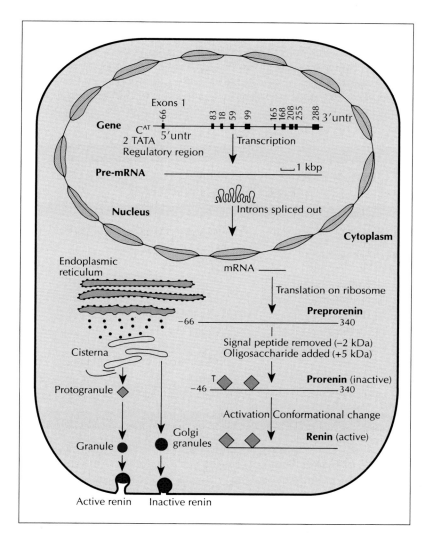

FIGURE 3-3. Biosynthetic pathway of active renin in the juxtaglomerular cell from its gene to release into the circulation. Renin is encoded by a single gene (*top*). Renin mRNA is formed from prerenin mRNA after intron splicing in the nucleus. The mRNA of the renin gene is translated into the protein preprorenin, which consists of 401 amino acid residues. In the endoplasmic reticulum, a 20-amino-acid signal peptide is cleaved from preprorenin, thereby leaving prorenin, a glycoprotein of 381 amino acids. Prorenin, which is enzymatically inactive, is packaged into secretory granules at the Golgi apparatus, where it is further processed into active renin by cleavage of a 46-amino-acid peptide from the *N*-terminus of the molecule. Mature, active renin is a glycosylated carboxypeptidase with a molecular weight of approximately 44 kD. Two major forms of renin granules originate from the Golgi apparatus. The first is a classic secretory granule from which active renin is released by exocytosis. The second is a lysosome-like granule, which remains in the cytoplasm and catalyzes autolytic processes. Active renin is released by an exocytic process involving stimulus-secretion coupling. Inactive prorenin is released largely by an uncontrolled constitutive process across the cell membrane. *Diamonds* represent glycosylation sites. kbp—kilobase pair; TATA—two promoters in the renin gene, P1 and P2; untr—untranslated.

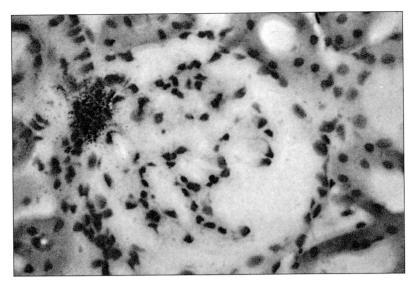

FIGURE 3-4. In situ hybridization histochemistry of a section of rat kidney showing renin mRNA accumulation in the juxtaglomerular cells of an afferent arteriole. The mRNA is depicted by the black grains at the glomerular pole. Accumulation of mRNA is a measure of renin gene expression; in the normal adult rat kidney, renin gene expression is confined to the immediate juxtaglomerular location.

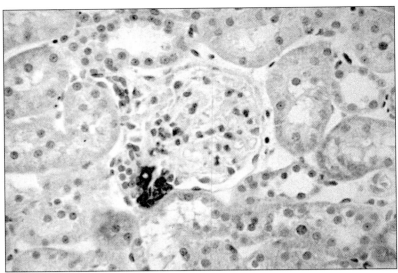

FIGURE 3-5. Immunohistochemistry of a section of rat kidney showing renin protein in the juxtaglomerular cells of the afferent arteriole. Specific renin immunoreactivity is indicated by the dark brown staining. In the normal adult rat kidney, renin protein expression, like gene expression, is confined to the immediate juxtaglomerular location.

MAJOR MECHANISMS OF RENIN RELEASE

Individual nephron signals
  Low macula densa sodium chloride (stimulates)
  Decreased afferent arteriolar pressure (stimulates)
Whole kidney modulating signals
  Angiotensin II negative feedback (inhibits)
  β-1 receptor stimulation (stimulates)
  Other humoral factors
    Vasopressin (inhibits)
    Atrial natriuretic peptide (inhibits)
    Dopamine DA-1 receptor (stimulates)
Local effectors
  Prostaglandins (stimulate)
  Nitric oxide (inhibits)
  Adenosine (inhibits)
  Kinins (stimulate)

FIGURE 3-6. Major mechanisms of renin release. Three major mechanisms are thought to govern renin release: 1) signals at the individual nephron, 2) signals involving the entire kidney, and 3) local effectors. Individual nephron signals include decreased sodium chloride load at the macula densa, which is the specialized group of distal tubular cells in approximation to the juxtaglomerular apparatus, and decreased afferent arteriolar pressure, which is probably mediated by a cellular stretch mechanism. Whole kidney signals include negative-feedback inhibition by angiotensin II at the juxtaglomerular cell, β_1-adrenergic receptor stimulation at the juxtaglomerular cell, and other hormonal factors. Local effectors include the prostaglandins E_2 and I_2, nitric oxide, adenosine, dopamine, and arginine vasopressin. The angiotensin II inhibitory feedback loop is thought to be the predominant and overriding mechanism that controls renin release in humans.

PHYSIOLOGIC AND PHARMACOLOGIC FACTORS AFFECTING RENIN RELEASE

PHYSIOLOGY	PHARMACOLOGY
Blood pressure	Antihypertensive agents
Fluid volume	Stimulators
Sodium intake	Renin-angiotensin blockade
Hydration	Diuretics
Diuretics	Vasodilators
Menstrual cycle	Suppressors
Diurnal changes	β-Adrenergic blockers
Posture	Central α_2-adrenergic agonists
Potassium intake	Neutral
Protein intake	Calcium antagonists

FIGURE 3-7. Physiologic stimulation of renin release occurs in the presence of hypotension, decreased sodium intake, dehydration, and upright posture as well as with changes in the time of day (morning) or the menstrual cycle. Increased potassium intake or serum potassium concentration can also stimulate renin release. Nearly all diuretics and antihypertensive agents affect renin release; if the renin-angiotensin system is to be clinically evaluated, these agents should be tapered and discontinued 3 weeks before evaluation, if possible.

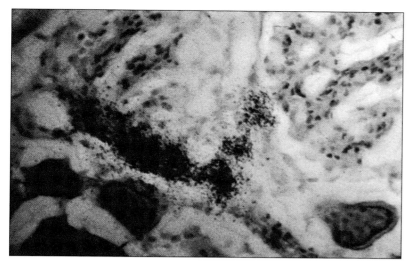

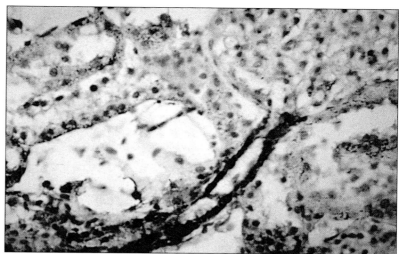

FIGURE 3-8. In situ hybridization histochemistry of a section of rat kidney showing renin mRNA accumulation along the afferent arteriole and interlobular artery. The animal had been treated with the angiotensin-converting enzyme (ACE) inhibitor enalapril to block the angiotensin II inhibitory feedback loop on renin secretion. Fetal rat kidneys as well as kidneys of animals treated with ACE inhibitor show expression of the renin gene throughout the renal vasculature. Interruption of angiotensin II feedback inhibition increases renin gene expression, renin protein accumulation, and renin release into the circulation and causes reversion of renin to the fetal pattern of expression.

FIGURE 3-9. Immunohistochemistry of a section of rat kidney. Renin accumulation is indicated by the brown staining along the length of the afferent arteriole. The animal had been treated with the angiotensin-converting enzyme (ACE) inhibitor enalapril. The same widespread pattern of renin distribution is present throughout the renal vasculature of the fetus. Thus, ACE inhibition increases the capacity of renovascular smooth muscle cells to synthesize and store renin. These observations indicate that renin may be important in the ontologic development of kidney vasculature as well as in response to stress in the adult kidney.

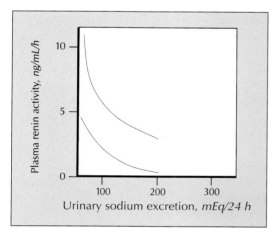

FIGURE 3-10. Relationship of plasma renin activity in ambulatory human subjects to the concurrent daily rate of urinary sodium excretion. The hyperbolic curves define the normal range. Approximately 25% of patients with untreated essential hypertension have low renin profiles, whereas approximately 15% have high renin profiles. Only 50% to 80% of patients with renovascular hypertension have elevated plasma renin activity. (*Adapted from* Brunner *et al.* [2].)

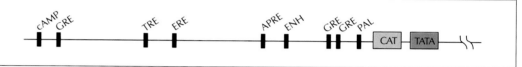

FIGURE 3-11. Analysis of human genomic DNA indicates that there is a single gene for angiotensinogen. The gene is composed of five exons and four introns and encompasses approximately 13 kb of genomic sequences. Glucocorticoid, estrogen, and thyroid hormones increase angiotensinogen mRNA. Analysis of the 5′ flanking region of the angiotensin gene has shown consensus sequences for three glucocorticoid-responsive elements (GRE), a thyroid hormone–responsive element (TRE), and an estrogen-responsive element (ERE). In addition, a virus-enhancer element sequence (ENH) is present in the midrange of this region of the gene and two promoter sequences, a TATA box and a catalytic element (CAT), have been identified near the transcriptional start site. Finally, the angiotensinogen gene contains an acute-phase response element (APRE). PAL—palindromic sequence. (*Adapted from* Griendling *et al.* [1].)

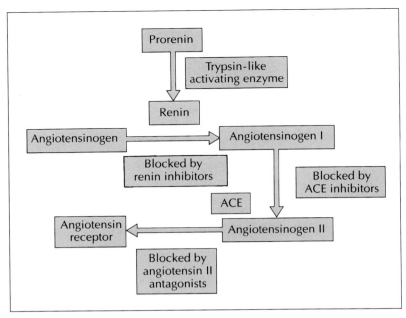

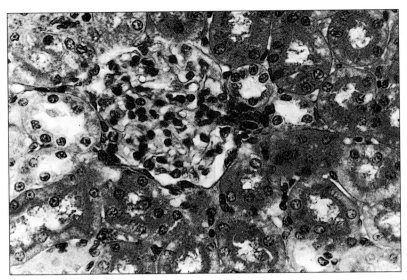

FIGURE 3-13. Immunohistochemistry of a section of rat kidney showing angiotensinogen in the proximal tubular cells. Angiotensinogen is synthesized, stored, and released constitutively in the kidney by these cells. Angiotensinogen is also synthesized in the liver (and in several other tissues) and is the only known substrate for the formation of angiotensin I. Angiotensinogen synthesized in the kidney is probably available for intrarenal generation of the components of the angiotensin cascade; such components can serve as cell-to-cell mediators that regulate renal function.

FIGURE 3-12. The renin-angiotensin system. Prorenin is converted to active renin by a trypsin-like activating enzyme. Renin enzymatically cleaves angiotensinogen to form the decapeptide angiotensin I; this step can be blocked by renin inhibitors. Angiotensin I is hydrolyzed to the octapeptide angiotensin II by angiotensin-converting enzyme (ACE); this step is blocked by ACE inhibitors. Angiotensin II acts at a specific receptor, and this interaction can be blocked by a variety of peptide or nonpeptide angiotensin II antagonists. Blockade of the renin-angiotensin system at each step results in an increase in the components proximal to the indicated step. For example, renin inhibitors, which block enzymatic cleavage of angiotensinogen to angiotensin I, increase the formation and release of renin; however, renin *activity* (ie, generation of angiotensin I) is decreased. ACE inhibition decreases angiotensin II and increases plasma renin activity and angiotensin I. Blockade of angiotensin receptors increases plasma renin activity as well as concentrations of angiotensins I and II.

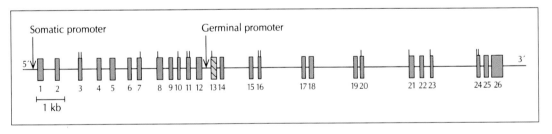

FIGURE 3-14. The human angiotensin-converting enzyme (ACE) gene containing 26 exons. Several studies have demonstrated the presence of two alternate promoters in the ACE gene: the somatic promoter, which is located on the 5' side of the first exon of the gene, and the germinal promoter, which is located on the 5' side of the specific 5' end of germinal ACE mRNA. The somatic ACE mRNA is transcribed from exon 1 to exon 26, but exon 13 is spliced during maturation of the somatic ACE transcript. The germinal mRNA is transcribed from exon 13 to exon 26. Exon 13 is specific to testicular ACE mRNA. The *vertical lines* above the exon boxes indicate the location of the cysteine residues. (*Adapted from* Soubrier *et al.* [3].)

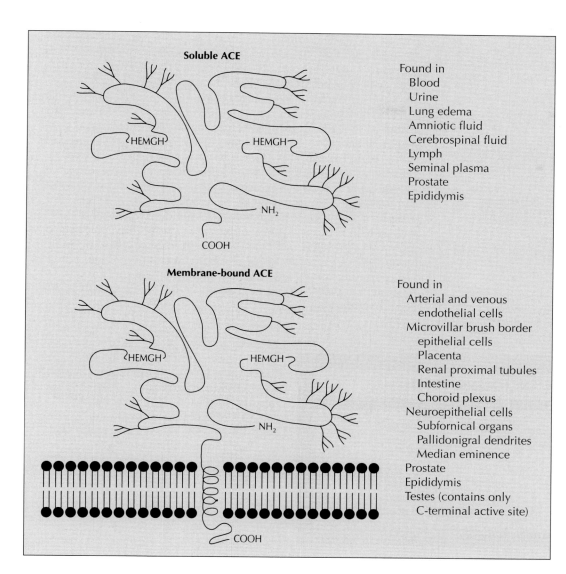

Soluble ACE

Found in
Blood
Urine
Lung edema
Amniotic fluid
Cerebrospinal fluid
Lymph
Seminal plasma
Prostate
Epididymis

Membrane-bound ACE

Found in
Arterial and venous
    endothelial cells
Microvillar brush border
    epithelial cells
    Placenta
    Renal proximal tubules
    Intestine
    Choroid plexus
Neuroepithelial cells
    Subfornical organs
    Pallidonigral dendrites
    Median eminence
Prostate
Epididymis
Testes (contains only
    C-terminal active site)

FIGURE 3-15. Angiotensin-converting enzyme (ACE) is a glycoprotein with a molecular weight of 150 to 180 kD that hydrolyzes inactive angiotensin I to active angiotensin II. The HEMGH (His-Glu-Met-Gly-His) sequence represents the zinc-binding motif in the two active site domains of ACE, and the branched structures denote potential glycosylation sites. The enzyme has been shown to exist in two forms: soluble and membrane-bound. Most ACE is membrane-bound and is found on the plasma membrane of various cell types. Membrane-bound ACE is inserted into the membrane by a 17-amino-acid hydrophobic region near the carboxy terminus. ACE is released from the plasma membrane by proteolytic cleavage near the carboxy terminus. In vascular beds, ACE is bound to the plasma membranes of endothelial cells. Testicular ACE has a different molecular structure different from that of ACE from other tissues and contains only one active carboxy terminal site, whereas ACE from other tissues contains two active carboxy terminal sites. (*Adapted from* Skidgel and Erdos [4].)

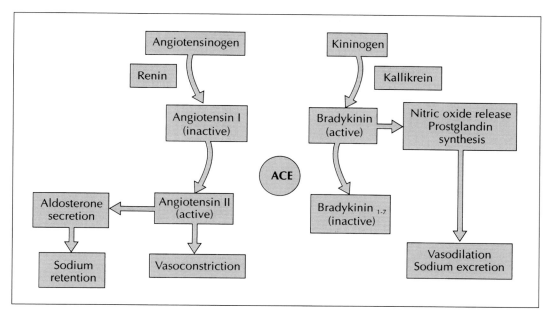

FIGURE 3-16. The actions of angiotensin-converting enzyme (ACE). The *left side* of the figure demonstrates how the enzyme converts inactive angiotensin I to active angiotensin II. The *right side* depicts how ACE metabolizes bradykinin, an active vasodilator and natriuretic substance, to bradykinin$_{1-7}$, an inactive metabolite. ACE therefore increases production of a potent vasoconstrictor, angiotensin II, while promoting the degradation of a vasodilator, bradykinin. Both actions of ACE increase vasoconstriction, and inhibition of ACE leads to vasodilation and natriuresis. Bradykinin is formed by the action of the enzyme kallikrein on substrate kininogen. Bradykinin acts as a vasodilator and natriuretic substance by releasing nitric oxide (an endothelium-derived relaxing factor) and stimulating formation of prostaglandins E_2 and I_2.

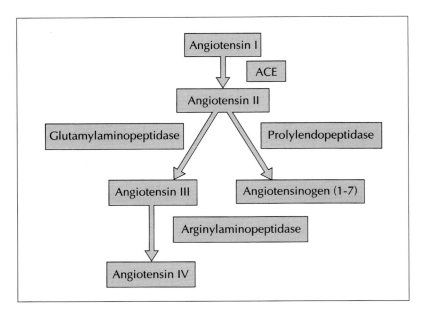

FIGURE 3-17. Metabolism of the angiotensin peptides. Angiotensin I is a decapeptide. Amino acids are numbered sequentially from the amino terminus. Angiotensin converting-enzyme (ACE) cleaves two carboxy terminal amino acids (9 and 10) of angiotensin I to form the octapeptide angiotensin II. Angiotensin I can also be processed by a family of endopeptidases to remove amino acids 8 through 10, thereby forming angiotensin (1-7). Angiotensin (1-7) is a biologically active peptide that stimulates vasopressin release, acts as a neurotransmitter, and increases synthesis and secretion of vasodilator prostaglandins. Angiotensin II can be converted to the heptapeptide angiotensin III by glutamylaminopeptidase or to angiotensin (1-7) by prolylendopeptidase. Angiotensin III generally is less potent than angiotensin II but is equally potent as a stimulator of aldosterone secretion. Angiotensin III can be metabolized to a hexapeptide (angiotensin$_{3-8}$) fragment by an arginylaminopeptidase. This hexapeptide is being assigned the name *angiotensin IV*. Angiotensin IV is currently being studied as a biologically active peptide with potential physiologic significance.

METABOLISM OF THE RENIN-ANGIOTENSIN SYSTEM

COMPONENT	HALF-LIFE IN CIRCULATION	DEGRADING ENZYME(S)
Renin	15–20 min	—
Angiotensinogen	4–16 h	Renin
Angiotensin I	1–2 min	Angiotensin-converting enzyme
Angiotensin II	Seconds	Aminopeptidase A, endopeptidase, prolylcarboxypeptidase

FIGURE 3-18. Renin has a relatively long half-life in the circulation compared with the angiotensin peptides, which are rapidly degraded by angiotensin-converting enzyme and various angiotensinases. Angiotensinogen also has a long half-life in plasma.

ANGIOTENSIN PEPTIDES AND THE RECEPTOR SUBTYPES THAT INTERACT WITH EACH PEPTIDE

RECEPTOR	ANGIOTENSIN
None	Angiotensinogen
	Asp-Arg-Val-Tyr-Ile-His-Pro-Phe-His-Leu-Val-Ile-His-Asn-Glu
	↓ Renin
None	Angiotensin I
	NH2-Asp-Arg-Val-Tyr-Ile-His-Pro-Phe-His-Leu-COOH
	↓ Angiotensin-converting enzyme
AT$_1$, AT$_2$	Angiotensin II
	Asp-Arg-Val-Tyr-Ile-His-Pro-Phe
	↓ Angiotensinases
AT$_1$, AT$_2$	Angiotensin III
	Arg-Val-Tyr-Ile-His-Pro-Phe
	↓ Angiotensinases
Unknown	Angiotensin (1-7)
	Asp-Arg-Val-Tyr-Ile-His-Pro
	↓ Angiotensinases
AT$_4$	Angiotensin (3-7)
	Val-Tyr-Ile-His-Pro

FIGURE 3-19. Angiotensin (AT) peptides and the receptor subtypes that interact with each peptide [5]. The proteolytic enzyme renin splits angiotensinogen between amino acid 10, leucine, and amino acid 11, valine, in the N terminal to produce the decapeptide angiotensin I. Angiotensin I is further degraded to the active octapeptide, angiotensin II, by cleavage of the C-terminal decapeptide His-Leu by angiotensin-converting enzyme. Angiotensin II is further degraded by peptidases, collectively termed *angiotensinases*, at different sites to form different angiotensin fragments, mainly angiotensin III, angiotensin (1-7), and angiotensin (3-7).

CLASSIFICATION CRITERIA OF ANGIOTENSIN RECEPTOR SUBTYPES

	AT_1	AT_2
Potency order	Angiotensin II > angiotensin III	Angiotensin II = angiotensin III
Selective antagonistsl	Losartan	PD 123177 (Parke-Davis, Morris Plains, NJ)
		PD 123319 (Parke-Davis)
	Valsartan	CGP 42112A (Novartis, Basel, Switzerland)
	Eprosartan	
	Zolarsartan	
	Irbesartan	
	Candesartan	
	Telmisartan	
	Tasosartan	
Effector pathways	↑ Phospholipase C	↓ Guanylate cyclase
	↑ Phospholipase D	
	↓ Adenylate cyclase	
Sensitivity to dithiothreitol (sulfhydryl-reducing agents)	↓ Binding	↑ Binding
Effect of GppNHp	↓ Affinity	No change
	↑ Hill coefficient to no change ~1	

FIGURE 3-20. Pharmacologic and biologic evidence suggests the existence of heterogeneity in the angiotensin (AT) II receptor population. AT_1 receptors are those selectively blocked by biphenylimidazoles, such as the compound losartan (DuP 753), whereas AT_2 binding sites are blocked by tetrahydroimidazopyridines, typified by PD 123177. AT_1 receptors are more responsive to angiotensin II than to angiotensin III, are positively coupled to phospholipase C, and may be negatively coupled to adenylyl cyclase. AT_2 binding sites may be involved in modulation of the intracellular content of cGMP. Angiotensin II and angiotensin III are equally potent in binding to AT_2 receptors. AT_1 receptors mediate vascular smooth muscle contraction, aldosterone secretion, pressor and tachycardic responses, angiotensin II–induced water consumption, and hypertension in cases of renal artery stenosis. The physiologic effects of AT_2 receptor activation are unknown. GppNH—guanylyl-imidodiphosphate. (*Adapted from* Griendling *et al.* [1].)

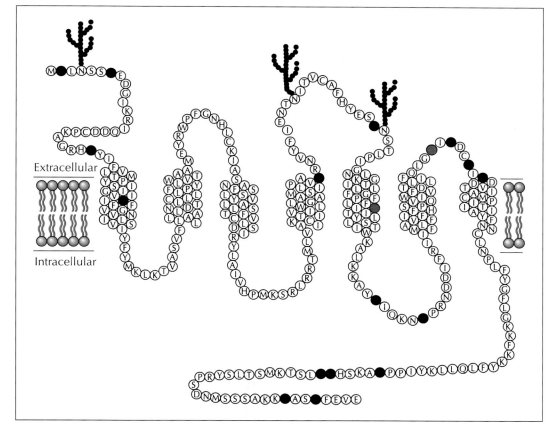

FIGURE 3-21. The AT_1 receptor is a member of the superfamily of G-protein–coupled receptors that have seven transmembrane regions. The cDNA for this receptor encodes a 359-amino-acid protein with a molecular weight of 41 kD. The protein contains three potential consensus sites for *N*-glycosylation on the putative extracellular domains. Each of the four extracellular domains also contains a cysteine residue, which may be responsible for the sensitivity of angiotensin II binding to sulfhydryl reagents. Subtypes of the AT_1 receptor are found in rats and mice. The vascular receptor is denoted as AT_{1A}, and the adrenal receptor is classified as AT_{1B}. Divergence between the AT_{1A} and the AT_{1B} receptors is indicated by *black circles*, representing nonconservative changes, and *red circles*, representing conservative changes. Potential glycosylation sites are depicted by *branched structures*, representing sugar molecules.

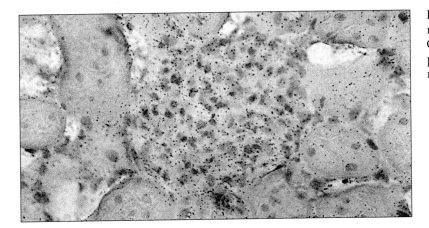

FIGURE 3-22. In situ hybridization histochemistry of a section of rat kidney showing the mRNA for the angiotensin AT$_1$ receptor. Grains representing accumulation of AT$_1$ receptor mRNA are present in the afferent and efferent arterioles, the glomerular mesangium, and the proximal tubular cells.

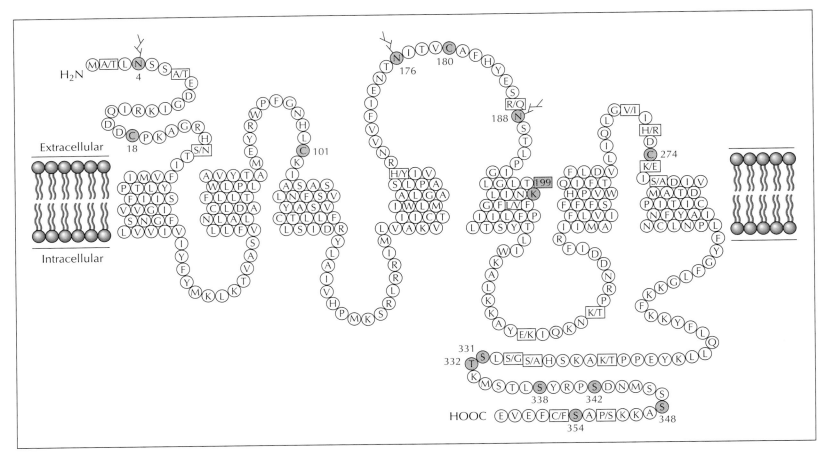

FIGURE 3-23. The angiotensin subtype-2 (AT$_2$) receptor is a G-protein–coupled receptor that has seven transmembrane-spanning regions. The cDNA for this receptor encodes a 363-amino-acid protein with a molecular weight of 44 kD. There are five potential *N*-glycosylation sites in the extracellular *N*-terminus. The AT$_2$ receptor displays a structure-activity relationship similar to that observed for the AT$_1$ receptor on the *C*-terminal position of the peptide hormone.

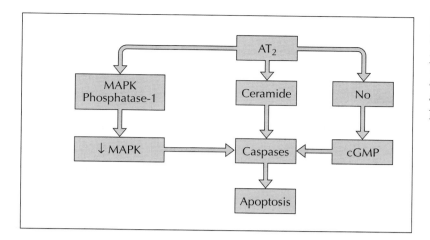

FIGURE 3-24. The signal transduction mechanisms for the AT_2 receptor are still not well defined. The growth-inhibitory and apoptosis effects of the AT_2 receptor are at least partially mediated by the activation of phosphotyrosine phosphatase, resulting in the activation of mitogen-activated protein phosphatase-1 and through a ceramide-dependent pathway. MAPK—mitogen-activated protein kinase.

RENAL EFFECTS OF ANGIOTENSIN SUBTYPE-2 RECEPTOR

Release of bradykinin, nitric oxide, and cGMP
Cell differentiation
Antiproliferation
Apoptosis
Vasodilation

FIGURE 3-25. Activation of renin-angiotensin system during sodium depletion or administration of angiotensin II increases renal bradykinin, nitric oxide, and cGMP production through stimulation at the AT_2 receptor [6–11]. Additionally, the AT_2 receptor contributes to cell differentiation, antiproliferation, stimulation of apoptosis, and vasodilation.

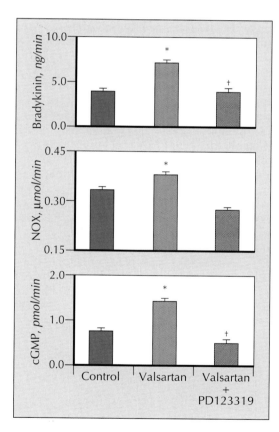

FIGURE 3-26. Blocking the AT_1 receptor with valsartan enhances angiotensin II formation that in turn stimulates the AT_2 receptor to increase tissue levels of bradykinin, nitric oxide (NOX), and cGMP. The AT_2 receptor blocker PD123319 prevents the increase in bradykinin, NOX, and cGMP and indicates that AT_2 receptor mediates release of these factors. The responses associated with AT_1 receptor blockade are partially mediated by the AT_2 receptor. *Asterisk* indicates $P < 0.01$ from control. *Dagger* indicates $P < 0.01$ from valsartan.

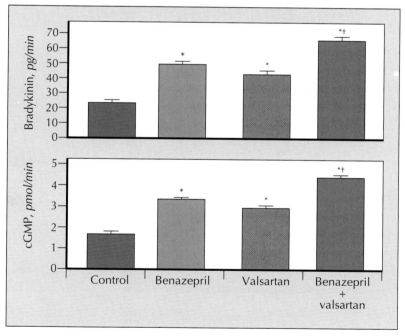

FIGURE 3-27. The angiotensin-converting enzyme (ACE) inhibitor benazepril and the AT_1 receptor blocker (ARB) valsartan potentiate each other and lead to further generation of bradykinin and cGMP. The combination of an ACE inhibitor and ARB could be beneficial in clinical states marked by angiotensin II elevation. *Asterisk* indicates $P < 0.01$ from control. *Dagger* indicates $P < 0.01$ from benazepril and valsartan.

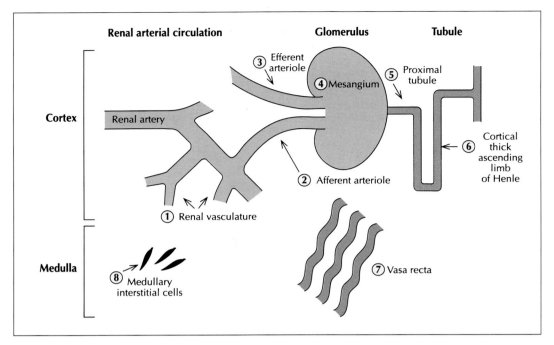

FIGURE 3-28. The renal tissue localization of angiotensin II receptors and the physiologic action stimulated by these receptors. Vasoconstriction occurs when angiotensin II acts at receptors in the arcuate and interlobular arteries, the afferent and efferent arterioles, and the medullary vasa recta. Angiotensin II preferentially constricts the efferent arteriole, thereby increasing glomerular filtration pressure; however, angiotensin II also acts on mesangial cell receptors to produce cellular contraction and reduce glomerular filtration. Angiotensin II receptors also are localized to the proximal tubule and the cortical thick ascending loop of Henle cells, which cause sodium resorption. Angiotensin II receptors recently have been found on renomedullary interstitial cell membranes, but the physiologic significance of these receptors is still unknown. 1—vasoconstriction; 2—limited vasoconstriction, and inhibition of renin synthesis and release; 3—preferential vasoconstriction; 4—contraction; 5 and 6—sodium reabsorption; 7—vasoconstriction; 8—unknown action.

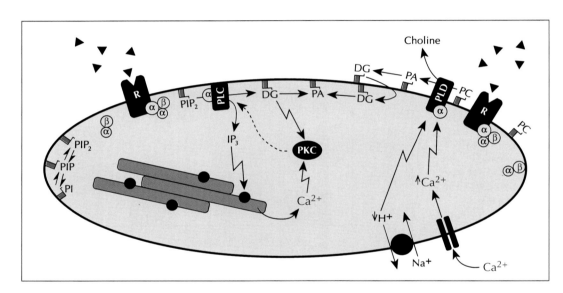

FIGURE 3-29. Cellular action of angiotensin II (ATII). When ATII activates AT_1 receptors in vascular cells, the peptide initiates a biphasic signaling response. The initial phase comprises phospholipase C (PLC)–mediated breakdown of the inositol polyphospholipids to generate inositol triphosphate (IP_3) and diacylglycerol (DG) as well as to mobilize intracellular calcium. The second phase is characterized by a sustained accumulation of diacylglycerol, activation of protein kinase C (PKC), hydrolysis of phosphatidylcholine (PC) mediated by phospholipase D (PLD), and intracellular alkalinization. Early signaling events are independent of calcium and are attenuated by PKC. The sustained response is independent of PKC and depends on intracellular alkalinization and continuing calcium influx as well as cellular processing or internalization of the ATII receptor (R) complex. PA—phosphatidic acid; PI—phosphatidylinositol; PIP—PI 4-phosphate; PIP_2—PI 4,5 biphosphonate. (*Adapted from* Griendling *et al.* [1].)

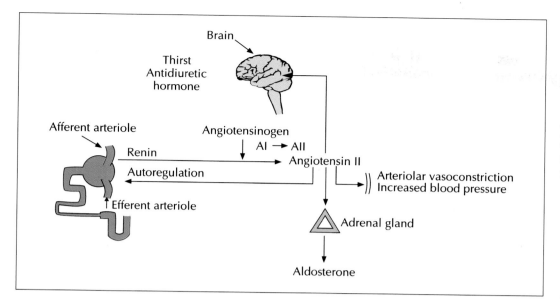

FIGURE 3-30. Angiotension II effects. Angiotensin II has three major effects: 1) arteriolar vasoconstriction; 2) renal sodium retention; and 3) increased aldosterone biosynthesis, all of which result in sodium retention [12,13]. These effects work together to maintain arterial blood pressure and blood volume. Angiotensin II also stimulates the sympathetic nervous system, particularly the thirst center in the hypothalamus.

RENAL EFFECTS OF ANGIOTENSIN II

Decreased renal blood flow

Proportionately increased efferent arteriolar resistance → increased glomerular capillary hydrostatic pressure → increased filtration

Glomerular mesangial cell contraction → decreased glomerular capillary surface area available for filtration → decreased filtration (offsets above effect)

Decreased medullary blood flow

Increased tubular sodium reabsorption → sodium retention

FIGURE 3-31. Renal effects of angiotensin II. The major hemodynamic action of angiotensin II in the kidney is vasoconstriction, which results in decreased blood flow in the renal cortex and medulla. Angiotensin II also reduces the glomerular filtration rate. The predominant renal tubular effect of angiotensin II is increased sodium reabsorption, which results in antinatriuresis. Blockade of intrarenal angiotensin II results in increased renal blood flow, increased glomerular filtration rate, and sodium and water excretion, thereby indicating that angiotensin II formed in the kidney acts as a cell-to-cell mediator (ie, paracrine substance) in the control of renal function [13].

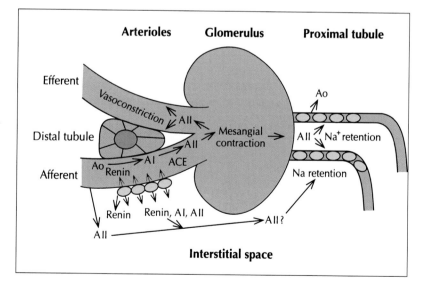

FIGURE 3-32. The cell-to-cell (ie, paracrine) effects of angiotensin II in the kidney. Angiotensinogen (Ao) either circulates to the kidney from the site of production in the liver or is synthesized in proximal tubular cells in the kidney. It is likely that renal interstitial angiotensinogen is derived predominantly from proximal tubular synthesis. Renin is synthesized in and released from the juxtaglomerular cells into the afferent arteriolar lumen or into the renal interstitium. Angiotensin I (AI) is generated in the afferent arteriole and is converted to angiotensin II (AII) by angiotensin-converting enzyme (ACE). AII can cause mesangial cell contraction or efferent arteriolar constriction. AII can also be filtered at the glomerulus and may subsequently act at the proximal tubular cells to increase sodium reabsorption. In the renal interstitium, renin can cleave angiotensinogen to produce angiotensin peptides; these peptides may act at vascular and tubular structures. Angiotensin peptides may also be synthesized in and released from renal juxtaglomerular cells. Alternatively, the peptides may be taken up by renal cells from either interstitial fluid or the renal circulation.

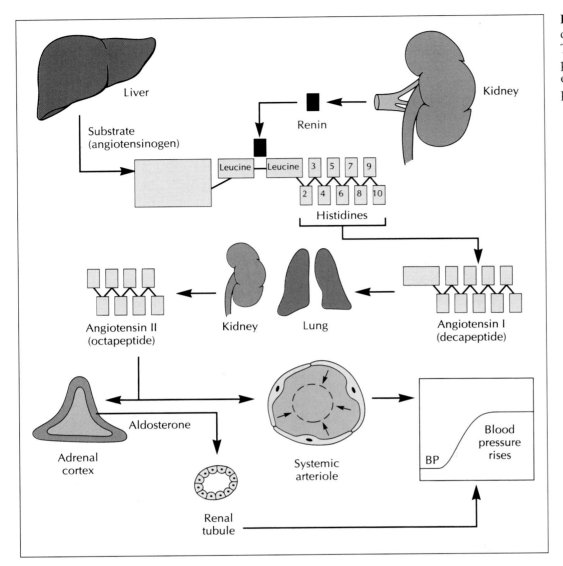

FIGURE 3-33. The circulating components of the renin-angiotensin system [14,15]. The circulating renin-angiotensin system plays a role in body fluid regulation, electrolyte homeostasis, and blood pressure control.

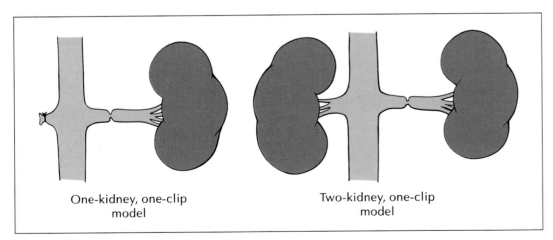

FIGURE 3-34. To understand the mechanisms involved in renovascular hypertension, two experimental animal models were developed by Goldblatt *et al.* [16]. In the first model, one renal artery is clipped (partially occluded) and the other kidney is removed; this is known as the *one-kidney, one-clip* model. In the other model, one renal artery is clipped and the other kidney is left in place; this is known as the *two-kidney, one-clip* model. These models differ in a fundamental way: the two-kidney, one-clip model leaves an intact kidney for regulation of extracellular fluid volume, whereas the one-kidney, one-clip model leaves all available renal tissue distal to and directly influenced by the reduction in pressure. (*Adapted from* Laragh *et al.* [17].)

Pathophysiology of renovascular hypertension

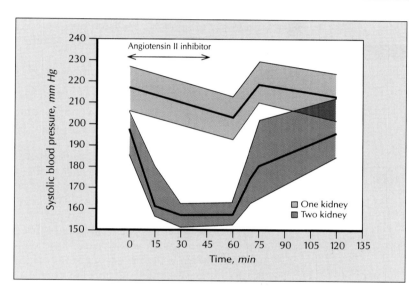

		Decreases on contralateral side	Increases on stenotic side
Renin content of kidney	No change	Decreases on contralateral side	Increases on stenotic side
Blood pressure	Significantly increases	Significantly increases	
Plasma renin activity	No change or decreases	Significantly increases	
Plasma volume	Increases	No change	
Blood pressure after block of angiotensin II	No change	Decreases	

FIGURE 3-35. Pathophysiology of renovascular hypertension. Although hypertension is equally present in both models, the one-kidney model demonstrates normal to low plasma renin activity, low renin content in the kidney, and increased plasma volume; the two-kidney model demonstrates increased renin in the plasma and clipped kidney as well as reduced or absent renin in the unclipped kidney. The hypertension of the two-kidney model can be normalized with an angiotensin II antagonist; however, the hypertension of the one-kidney model does not respond to such treatment. (*Adapted from* Laragh *et al.* [17].)

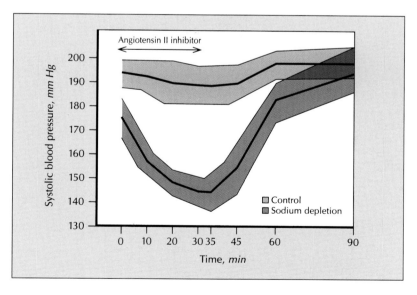

FIGURE 3-36. Renin-angiotensin dependency in the two-kidney, one-clip model. Although administration of an angiotensin II inhibitor does not affect blood pressure in the one-kidney, one-clip model, it does lower blood pressure in the two-kidney, one-clip model. The fact that the hypertension demonstrated in the two-kidney, one-clip model is renin-angiotensin–dependent is thus indicated. The presence of the normal kidney prevents volume expansion by allowing a response to the increased pressure with pressure-induced natriuresis. (*Adapted from* Brunner *et al.* [18].)

FIGURE 3-37. Sodium dependency in the one-kidney, one-clip model. Here, hypertension usually does not respond to angiotensin II inhibition, suggesting that increased intravascular volume is a major pathophysiologic mechanism in cases of hypertension. Because there is no normal kidney to respond to the increased blood pressure of pressure-induced natriuresis, sodium and fluid retention occur and extracellular fluid volume expands. The hypertension then becomes volume-dependent, rather than angiotensin-dependent. Salt depletion in this model significantly increases plasma renin activity, causing the hypertension to become more responsive to inhibition of angiotensin II [19,20]. (*Adapted from* Gavras *et al.* [19].)

CLINICAL CLUES SUGGESTING RENOVASCULAR HYPERTENSION

Systolic/diastolic epigastric, subcostal, or flank bruit
Accelerated or malignant hypertension
Unilateral small kidney discovered by any clinical study
Severe hypertension in child or young adult, or after age 50 y
Sudden development or worsening of hypertension at any age
Hypertension and unexplained impairment of renal function
Sudden worsening of renal function in hypertensive patient
Hypertension refractory to appropriate three-drug regimen
Impairment in renal function in response to ACE inhibitor
Extensive occlusive disease in coronary, cerebral, and peripheral circulation

FIGURE 3-38. Causes of renal artery stenosis. Lesions of the renal arteries associated with hypertension can be divided into several categories. Atherosclerosis, which tends to occur in older individuals, and fibromuscular hyperplasia, which tends to occur in young women, are the most common causes of significant renal artery stenosis. Other causes are uncommon. Renal artery stenosis occurs in the absence of hypertension and may be present in a hypertensive patient without being the cause of the hypertension. Therefore, the functional significance of the renal artery lesion as a cause of hypertension must be validated by appropriate tests. The clinical characteristics listed here should raise the index of clinical suspicion for renovascular hypertension. ACE—angiotensin-converting enzyme.

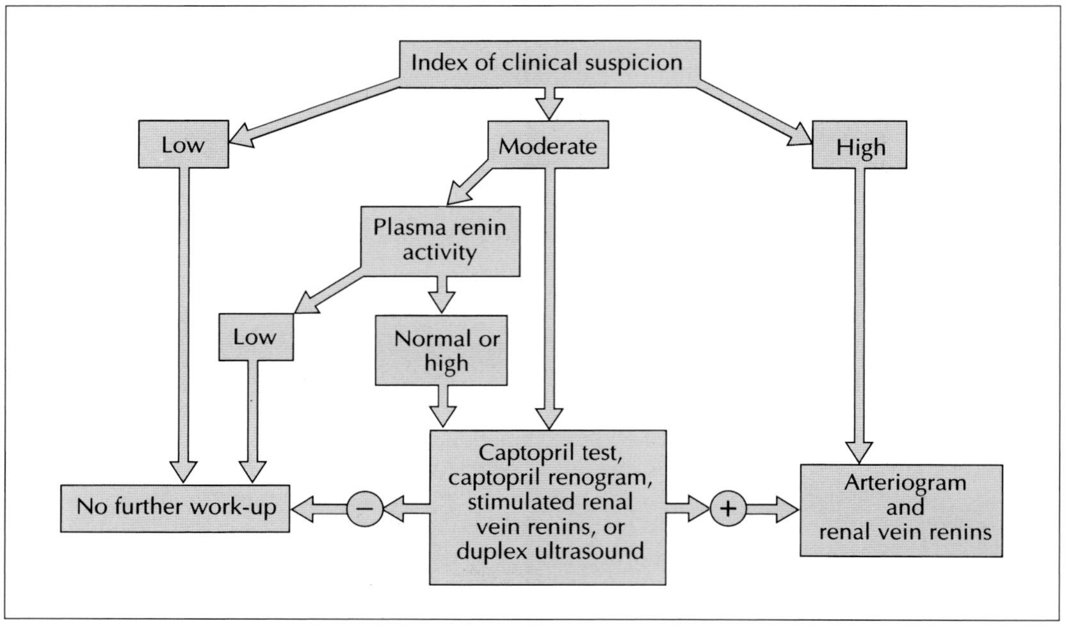

FIGURE 3-39. The work-up for renovascular hypertension depends on the index of clinical suspicion. In the absence of suggestive signs, it is likely that test results would be inconclusive; in such cases, no work-up is recommended. Patients with suggestive clinical clues (*see* Fig. 3-35) have a 5% to 15% likelihood of having renovascular hypertension. Such patients can be screened with noninvasive studies and, if results are positive, confirmation of the diagnosis can be accomplished with renal arteriography and sampling of renin in the renal vein. If renovascular hypertension is strongly suggested, renal arteriography and sampling of renin in the renal vein are recommended, regardless of the results of noninvasive tests.

DIAGNOSTIC STUDIES FOR RENOVASCULAR HYPERTENSION

	SENSITIVITY, %	SPECIFICITY, %
Rapid sequence IVP	74	86
Isotope renography with ACE inhibition test	93	95
Peripheral vein PRA with ACE inhibition test (captopril test)	74	89
Renal vein ratio of PRA test (stenotic/contralateral):		
>1.3	85	40
>1.9	78	60
Peripheral vein PRA	92	96
Intravenous digital subtraction angiography	88	89
Doppler ultrasonography	86	93
MRI	97	95
Renal artery angiography	100	100

FIGURE 3-40. Diagnostic studies for renovascular hypertension. Three indicators have been defined and evaluated for their ability to identify curable renovascular hypertension: 1) elevation of peripheral plasma renin activity (PRA) when considered in relation to 24-hour urinary sodium excretion; 2) suppression of renin secretion from the contralateral uninvolved kidney; and 3) abnormally increased renin in the renal vein as compared with renin in the artery of the suspect kidney—this relationship has been shown to provide an index for the degree of ischemia in the suspect kidney. The sensitivity and selectivity of various tests are shown. ACE—angiotensin-converting enzyme; IVP—intravenous pyelography.

CRITERIA FOR RENOVASCULAR HYPERTENSION

Stimulated PRA of ≥12 ng/mL/h
Absolute increase in PRA of ≥10 ng/mL/h
Increase in plasma renin activity PRA of ≥150% or ≥400% if baseline PRA is < 3 ng/mL/h

FIGURE 3-41. The criteria for distinguishing renovascular hypertension from essential hypertension by the captopril test. The captopril test is used to identify patients with renovascular hypertension. The patient should consume a normal amount of salt and receive no diuretics. If possible, all antihypertensive medications should be withdrawn 3 weeks before the test. The patient should be seated for at least 3 minutes. Blood pressure should be measured at 20, 25, and 30 minutes, and the three readings averaged for a baseline. A blood sample is then drawn from a vein for measurement of baseline plasma renin activity (PRA). Captopril (50 mg diluted in 10 mL of water immediately before the test) is administered orally. Blood pressure is measured 15, 30, 40, 45, 50, 55, and 60 minutes after administration of captopril; at 60 minutes, a blood sample is drawn from a vein for measurement of stimulated PRA. Three variables define the renin secretory response: 1) stimulated renin level, 60 minutes after captopril administration; 2) the absolute increase in PRA; and 3) the percent increase in PRA after captopril administration.

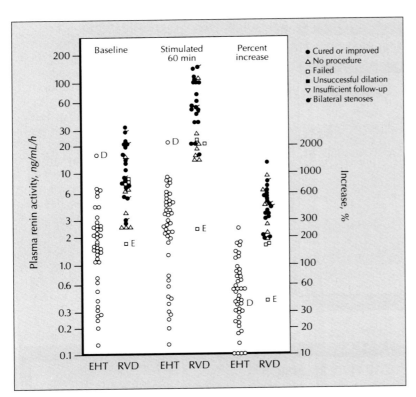

FIGURE 3-42. Plasma renin response to captopril. Although the baseline renin value does not discriminate between patients with renovascular disease (RVD) and essential hypertension (EHT), the stimulated plasma renin activity measured 60 minutes after oral captopril does discriminate between these two groups. Patient D, with EHT, had a stimulated renin value in the same range as that found in patients with RVD. However, this patient had the highest baseline plasma renin value and had only a 37% increase in renin. Conversely, patient E had arteriographic evidence of a significant renovascular lesion but his stimulated renin value was only 2.4 ng/mL/h, well below that of the other patients with RVD. (*Adapted from* Muller *et al.* [21].)

OUTCOME AFTER ANGIOPLASTY OR SURGERY FOR RENAL ARTERY STENOSIS

ETIOLOGY	ATHEROMA		FIBROMUSCULAR DYSPLASIA	
Treatment	Angioplasty	Surgery	Angioplasty	Surgery
Patients, n	391	1310	175	486
Blood pressure response, n				
Cured	19	45	50	64 (range, 56–81)
Improved	52	29	42	23 (range, 5–40)
Failed	30	24	9	11 (range, 0–25)

FIGURE 3-43. Summary of the outcome of angioplasty compared with surgery for renal artery stenosis. The major objectives in the management of renovascular hypertension are to prevent complications of hypertension by controlling blood pressure and to prevent or slow the loss of renal function. Management of renovascular hypertension can be achieved by angioplasty, surgery, or medical treatment. Surgery is favored over other forms of treatment in cases of hypertension that are refractory to medication, in young people, and if renal function is threatened by progressive renal artery disease. Percutaneous transluminal renal angioplasty provides a nonsurgical but invasive method of treating renal artery stenosis. This procedure offers the advantages of local anesthesia, minimal morbidity, a short hospital stay, and relatively low cost. In cases of fibromuscular hyperplasia, the restenosis rate is less than 5%; in atherosclerotic disease, restenosis occurs in 20% to 30% in response to percutaneous transluminal angioplasty.

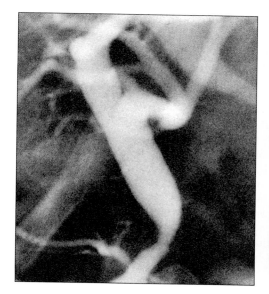

FIGURE 3-44. Selective renal arteriogram of a 43-year-old, nonsmoking, white man with a 2-year history of hypertension. The arteriogram shows 80% stenosis of the left renal artery with poststenotic dilatation caused by atherosclerotic vascular disease. Transluminal angioplasty or surgery can be successful in opening the artery and abrogating or curing the hypertension.

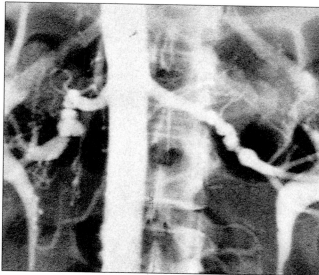

FIGURE 3-45. Selective renal arteriogram of a 31-year-old, white woman with a 13-year history of hypertension. The arteriogram shows bilateral medial-type fibromuscular hyperplasia of the renal arteries.

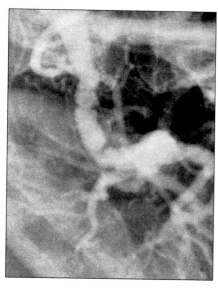

FIGURE 3-46. Renal arteriogram of a 31-year-old, white woman with poorly controlled hypertension. The arteriogram shows that the right renal artery was beaded and narrow and had 90% stenosis. The left renal artery was normal.

FIGURE 3-47. Renal causes of hypertension. The frequency of renal causes among patients with hypertension is less than 5%.

RENAL CAUSES OF HYPERTENSION

RENAL PARENCHYMAL

Acute and chronic glomerulonephritis; pyelonephritis; nephrocalcinosis; neoplasms; glomerulosclerosis; interstitial, hereditary, or radiation nephritis

Obstructive uropathies and hydronephrosis

Renin-secreting renal tumors

Renal trauma

RENOVASCULAR

Renal arterial lesions; occlusions; stenosis; aneurysms; thrombosis; vasculitis

Connective tissue or autoimmune disease with renal vasculitis or glomerulitis

Coarctation of the aorta with renal ischemia

Aortitis with renal ischemia

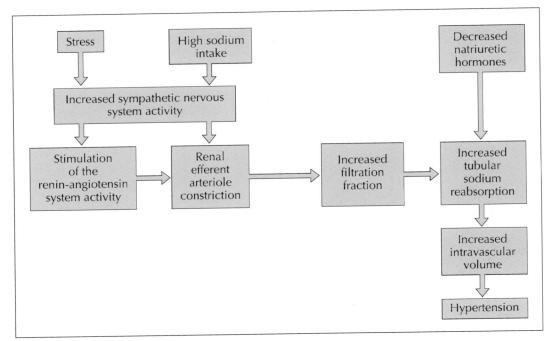

Figure 3-48. Mechanisms that can influence the kidney and lead to development of hypertension. The combination of physical or emotional stress and high sodium intake, especially in the absence of a natriuretic hormone, increases sympathetic nervous system activity. As a result, either directly or through stimulation of the renin-angiotensin system, renal efferent arterioles are constricted, causing fluid retention and development of hypertension. Natriuretic hormone deficiency or increased activity of the sympathetic nervous system or the renin-angiotensin system can increase sodium resorption and expand extracellular fluid volume, leading to hypertension. (*Adapted from* Kaplan [22].)

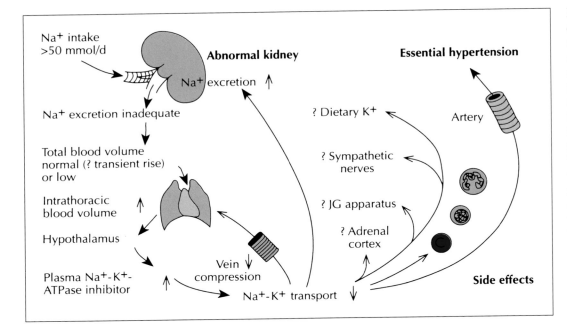

Figure 3-49. Hypothetical sequence of events demonstrating the role of sodium retention in cases of hypertension. An underlying genetic lesion may be expressed as a deficiency of sodium excretion, which becomes more apparent as sodium intake increases. The reduction in sodium excretion may initially cause a transient increase in total blood volume and a rise in intrathoracic blood volume. This change stimulates the hypothalamus to secrete a circulating sodium transport inhibitor, which adjusts renal sodium excretion, returning the sodium balance to normal. This balance is sustained only by a continuously high level of circulating sodium transport inhibitor, which raises the tone and reactivity of vascular smooth muscle. As a result, arterial pressure rises and venous compliance diminishes. Increased venous tone shifts blood from the periphery to the central vascular bed and thus raises intrathoracic pressure and perpetuates the stimulus for greater secretion of the sodium transport inhibitor. Total blood volume may be normal or low. (*Adapted from* de Wardener and MacGregor [23].)

REFERENCES

1. Griendling KK, Murphy TJ, Alexander RW: Molecular biology of the renin-angiotensin system. *Circulation* 1993, 87:1816–1828.

2. Brunner HR, Laragh JH, Baer L, *et al.*: Essential hypertension: renin and aldosterone, heart attack and stroke. *N Engl J Med* 1972, 286:441–449.

3. Soubrier F, Hubert C, Testut P, *et al.*: Molecular biology of the angiotensin I converting enzyme: 1. Biochemistry and structure of the gene. *J Hypertens* 1993, 11:471–476.

4. Skidgel RA, Erdos E: Angiotensin I-converting enzyme. In *Hypertension Primer*. Edited by Izzo J, Black HR. Dallas: American Heart Association; 1993:12.

5. Unger T, Chung O, Csikos T, *et al.*: Angiotensin receptors. *J Hypertens* 1996, 14(suppl 5):95–103.

6. Siragy HM, Carey RM: The subtype-2 (AT2) angiotensin receptor regulates renal cyclic guanosine 3', 5'-monophophate and AT1 receptor-mediated prostaglandin E2 production in conscious rats. *J Clin Invest* 1996, 97:1978–1982.

7. Siragy HM, Carey RM: The subtype 2 (AT2) angiotensin receptor mediates renal production of nitric oxide in conscious rats. *J Clin Invest* 1997, 100:264–269.

8. Siragy HM, Carey RM: Protective role of the angiotensin AT2 receptor in a renal wrap hypertension model. *Hypertension* 1999, 33:1237–1242.

9. Siragy HM, de Gasparo M, Carey RM: Angiotensin type 2 receptor mediates valsartan-induced hypotension in conscious rats. *Hypertension* 2000, 35:1074–1077.

10. Siragy HM, de Gasparo M, El-Kersh M, Carey RM: Angiotensin-converting enzyme inhibition potentiates angiotensin II type 1 receptor effects on renal bradykinin and cGMP. *Hypertension* 2001, 38:183–186.

11. Carey RM, Howell NL, Jin XH, Siragy HM: Angiotensin type 2 receptor-mediated hypotension in angiotensin type-1 receptor-blocked rats. *Hypertension* 2001, 38:1272–1277.

12. Burnier M, Brunner HR: Renal effects of angiotensin II receptor blockade and angiotensin-converting enzyme inhibition in healthy subjects. *Exp Nephrol* 1996, 4(suppl 1):41–46.

13. Harris RC, Cheng HF: The intrarenal renin-angiotensin system: a paracrine system for the local control of renal function separate from the systemic axis. *Exp Nephrol* 1996, 4(suppl 1):2–8.

14. Chobanian AV: Hypertension. *CIBA Found Symp* 1982, 34:3–32.

15. Hall JE, Brands MW, Shek ED: Central role of the kidney and abnormal fluid volume in hypertension. *J Hum Hypertens* 1996, 10:633–639.

16. Goldblatt H, Lynch J, Hunzal RF, *et al.*: Studies in experimental hypertension: I. The production of persistent elevation of systolic blood pressure by means of renal ischemia. J Exp Med 1934, 59: 347–379.

17. Laragh JH, Sealey JE, Buhler FR, *et al.*: The renin axis and vaso-constriction volume analysis for understanding and treating renovascular and renal hypertension. *Am J Med* 1975, 58:4–13.

18. Brunner HR, Kirschman JD, Sealey JE, *et al.*: Hypertension of renal origin: evidence for two different mechanisms. *Science* 1971, 174:1344–1346.

19. Gavras H, Brunner HR, Vaughan ED, Jr, *et al.*: Angiotensin-sodium interaction in blood pressure maintenance of renal hypertensive and normotensive rats. *Science* 1973, 180:1369–1371.

20. Romero JC, Feldstein AE, Rodriguez-Porcel MG, *et al.*: New insights into the pathophysiology of renovascular hypertension. *Mayo Clin Proc* 1997, 72:251–260.

21. Muller SB, Sealey JE, Case DB, *et al.*: The captopril test for identifying renovascular disease in hypertensive patients. *Am J Med* 1986, 80:633–644.

22. Kaplan NM: Systemic hypertension: mechanisms and diagnosis. In *Heart Disease*. Edited by Braunwald E. Philadelphia: WB Saunders; 1988:819–883.

23. de Wardener HE, MacGregor GA: Natriuretic hormone and essential hypertension as an endocrine disease. In *Essential Hypertension as an Endocrine Disease*. Edited by Edwards CRW, Carey RM. London: Butterworths; 1985:132–157.

CHAPTER 4

PATHOGENESIS OF HYPERTENSION: VASCULAR MECHANISMS

R. Wayne Alexander, Randolph A. Hennigar, and Kathy K. Griendling

The mechanisms involved in the pathogenesis of hypertension are increasingly well understood. The focus classically has been on neural and humoral stimuli of vascular constriction and on endocrine and renal stimuli that control blood volume. It has become clear that strong environmental and genetic influences converge to result in the hypertensive phenotype [1]. With the development of the science of vascular biology in recent years there has been increasing focus on the blood vessel wall itself in the pathogenesis of hypertension. The current view is that the resistance arteriole may be involved in the pathogenesis of the disease, both primarily and secondarily. Hemodynamic, neural, and humoral factors or mechanisms intrinsic to the vessel wall itself may initiate contractile or structural changes that result in initial increases in pressure. The adaptive changes in the arteriole in response to an elevated intravascular pressure perpetuate and probably worsen the hypertension. Significant new insights have been developed into both functional and structural changes that may contribute to the initiation and/or progression of this condition.

The arterial wall in hypertension is characterized by thickening or remodeling of the media. The mechanisms that underlie the increase in smooth muscle mass have received a great deal of attention. There may be either proliferation of vascular smooth muscle cells or an increase in cell size associated with endoreplication of the DNA [2]. This latter event creates polyploid cells, suggesting that there is an incomplete growth stimulus in which cell division does not occur. The increase in medial mass is also due in part to increased synthesis of connective tissue, which has the added effect of decreasing arteriolar distensibility [2].

The structural consequence of medial thickening or remodeling is narrowing of the luminal diameter. This luminal narrowing causes increased resistance in the basal state and also provides a mechanical advantage in the response to vasoconstrictors, since the same extent of contraction in a vessel with a narrowed lumen (as opposed to one with a normal-sized lumen) may result in marked enhancement of resistance [3]. An additional mechanism for increased arterial resistance is rarefaction or loss of arterioles, which decreases total arteriolar cross-sectional area [4].

Although most of the histopathologic photomicrographs in this chapter depict renovascular damage secondary to hypertension, it is not our intent to suggest that such changes are limited only to the kidney. Indeed, the arterial systems of other organs, particularly those of the brain, spinal cord, retina, heart, and lung, may show similar vascular damage in the setting of hypertension. As in the kidney, these structural and functional changes represent primary adaptive changes that can cause progressive increases in resistance.

The structural changes in the arterial wall that lead to arteriolar thickening can be reflected in functional changes. In human hypertensives, there is apparent increased sensitivity to vasoconstrictors in the resistance circulation. Controversy exists as to whether this apparent increased contractile sensitivity reflects true increased sensitivity to the agonist or is the result of the increased mechanical advantage mentioned previously.

The endothelium probably plays a fundamental role in the pathogenesis of hypertension [5]. Endothelium-derived dilator factors are critically important in the control of vascular tone. The endothelium produces several potent vasodilator substances, including the prostaglandins, undefined dilator factors, and nitric oxide. The latter is perhaps the most important intrinsic dilator system in the vessel wall [6]. In normal vessels, it is produced predominantly by the endothelium. Endothelium-dependent vasodilatation is impaired in the coronary vascular bed in human hypertension [7]. One major cause of impaired relaxation is the inactivation of nitric oxide by superoxide [8]. Compelling clinical evidence is now available that activation of the renin-angiotensin system (renal artery stenosis) leads to excessive production of reactive oxygen species that is associated with endothelial dysfunction [9].

Excessive production of endothelium-derived vasoconstrictor factors has been demonstrated in animal models of hypertension [5]. Distinctive morphologic changes in the endothelium have also been described [10].

Finally, considerable progress has been made in understanding the intrinsic abnormalities in the vessel wall that may account for hypertension. It is not clear whether the associated endothelial defects are primary or secondary. There is, however, compelling evidence for abnormalities in vascular smooth muscle that may be primary. In human hypertensive patients, defects have been observed in membrane ion transporters that may have specific effects in increasing both contractile and growth responses. These primary abnormalities also contribute to an increase in intracellular calcium and an increase in the activity of the sodium/hydrogen antiporter. Because classic vasoconstrictor agonists and conventional growth factors share many of the same signaling pathways, ionic abnormalities may contribute generally to the hypertensive phenotype.

IDENTIFICATION OF THE PROBLEM

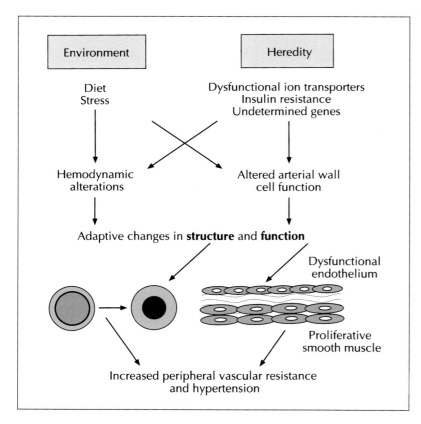

FIGURE 4-1. Development of structural and functional alterations in the hypertensive vessel wall. Both environmental and hereditary factors contribute to the development of hypertension. Hemodynamic changes and altered function of arterial wall cells cause adaptive or maladaptive changes, which may be progressive, in both structure and function of blood vessels. Decreased luminal diameter due to thickening of the arterial wall resulting from remodeling and smooth muscle cell hypertrophy or hyperplasia, as well as deposition of connective tissue, leads to increased peripheral vascular resistance and hypertension [1]. Another cardinal feature of hypertensive arteries is a dysfunctional endothelium [7,10], which contributes to abnormal vasoconstriction and growth by creating an imbalance between the release of vasoconstricting and vasorelaxing factors or growth-promoting and growth-inhibiting substances.

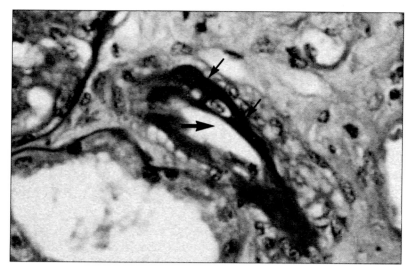

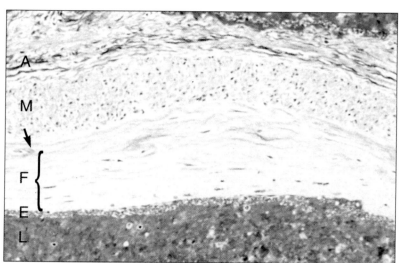

FIGURE 4-2. Hyaline arteriolosclerosis in essential hypertension. This micrograph depicts hyaline arteriosclerosis in a 60-year-old man who developed benign nephrosclerosis after longstanding essential hypertension. The primary histologic lesion of benign nephrosclerosis is hyaline arteriolosclerosis, shown here as pink, amorphous, glassy-appearing material accumulating beneath the vascular endothelium (*thin arrows*). The thickened, hyalinized vascular wall partially obliterates the lumen (*thick arrow*). Periodic acid–Schiff stain, original magnification, × 400.

FIGURE 4-3. Vascular changes in benign nephrosclerosis in a 61-year-old woman. This image shows arterial thickening caused by fibrointimal proliferation (F) with heavy deposition of collagen and by medial smooth muscle cell hypertrophy. The patient suffered from longstanding essential hypertension and developed endstage renal disease secondary to severe benign nephrosclerosis. Hypertension accelerates vascular intimal thickening, manifested here as fibrointimal proliferation in the renal arcuate artery. In cross-section the intima is markedly thickened, primarily by collagenization. In addition, there is mild smooth muscle hypertrophy of the medial wall (M). *Arrow* indicates the internal elastic intima. A—adventitia; E—endothelium; L—arterial lumen. Masson's trichrome stain, original magnification, × 400.

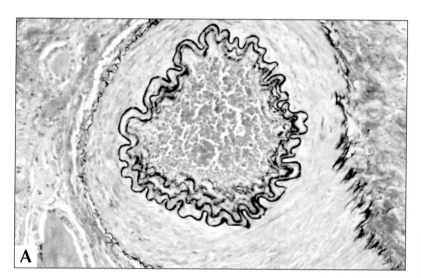

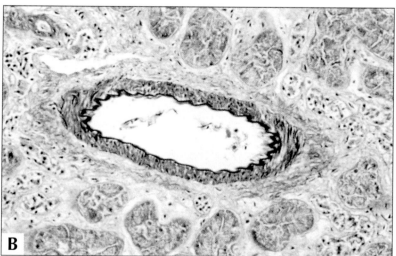

FIGURE 4-4. Fibroelastic hyperplasia in hypertension. **A,** Fibroelastic hyperplasia in a proximal renal interlobular artery from the same patient presented in Figure 4-3. As a consequence of ongoing benign essential hypertension, there is marked reduplication (splitting) of the internal elastic lamina (*stained black*), marked smooth muscle hypertrophy of the media, mild medial fibrosis, and intimal thickening (compare with **B**). Original magnification, × 200. **B,** Normal proximal interlobular artery at same magnification as artery in **A.** Verhoeff–van Gieson stain for elastic tissue, original magnification, × 200.

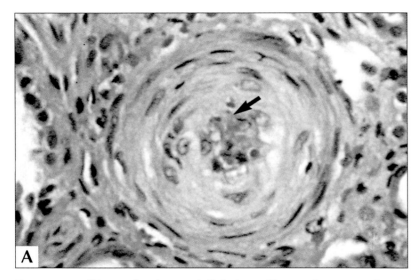

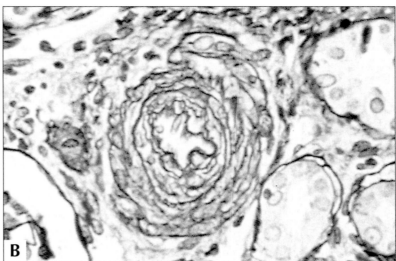

A

B

FIGURE 4-5. Hyperplastic arteriolitis in malignant hypertension. **A,** Early hyperplastic arteriolitis "onion-skinning" in a 48-year-old patient in the malignant phase of hypertension. A distal renal interlobular artery exhibits luminal reduction and intimal thickening secondary to myointimal cell proliferation, early fibrosis, and accumulation of basophilic mucinous material (primarily proteoglycans). These alterations are accompanied by concentric collagenization of the smooth muscle and adventitia.

In addition, fragmented erythrocytes (*arrow*) have deposited in the intima, consistent with this patient's history of helmet and burr cells on peripheral smear. Original magnification, × 400. **B,** Hyperplastic arteriolitis in a kidney blood vessel stained with Jones' methenamine silver. Silver stains accentuate the concentric layers of fibrosis in this early example of onion-skinning. Original magnification, × 400.

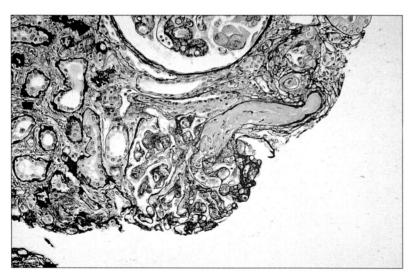

FIGURE 4-6. Necrotizing arteriolitis in malignant hypertension. This 46-year-old patient with malignant hypertension experienced acute renal failure. A kidney biopsy was performed and revealed obliteration of several glomerular arterioles (one of which is shown here) by acute necrosis with accumulation of pink fibrinoid material, or so-called *fibrinoid* necrosis. Necrotizing arteriolitis is a consequence of acutely and markedly elevated blood pressure and is most often encountered in the renal and gastrointestinal vasculature of patients suffering from malignant hypertension. Although not shown here, this lesion is usually superimposed on hyperplastic arteriosclerosis (*see* Fig. 4-5). Jones' methenamine silver stain with periodic acid–Schiff counterstain, original magnification, × 200.

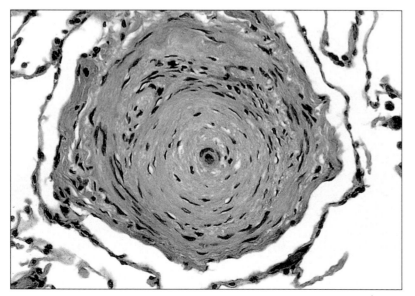

FIGURE 4-7. Arterial thickening secondary to severe fibrointimal fibrosis in pulmonary hypertension. Arterial changes in the lungs of a 35-year-old patient with longstanding pulmonary hypertension of unknown etiology. The lumen of the pulmonary artery is virtually obliterated by extensive concentric laminar fibrointimal proliferation. Some adventitial fibrosis and mild medial hypertrophy are also present. This figure illustrates the generality of the fibrointimal proliferative response to increased pressure in arteries in any vascular bed. The encroachment on the lumen causes a progressive increase in resistance. Original magnification, × 400. (*Courtesy of* Dr. Anthony Gal, Emory University Hospital, Atlanta, GA.)

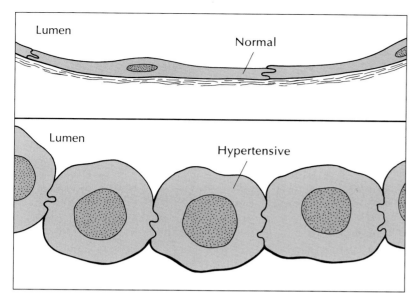

FIGURE 4-8. Morphologic abnormalities of the endothelium of hypertensive animals. This figure illustrates the structural alteration of the endothelium in hypertension. The volume of the cells increases and the surface configuration becomes more globular, so that the cells protrude into the lumen of the vessel. In addition, the endothelial cells develop prominent cytoplasmic bundles of actin microfilaments. The alterations in surface configuration increase permeability, thus altering one important endothelial cell function. The structural alterations may also reflect other functional alterations of the endothelium. (*Adapted from* Hüttner and Gabbiani [6].)

MECHANISMS UNDERLYING STRUCTURAL CHANGES

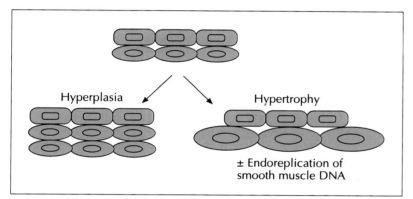

FIGURE 4-9. Smooth muscle changes in hypertensive vessels. The smooth muscle content of arteries can be augmented by either an increase in cell number (hyperplasia) or an increase in cell mass (hypertrophy) [2]. In large vessels of hypertensive animals, there is good evidence that changes in smooth muscle mass are caused by hypertrophy. Very often this hypertrophy is accompanied by endoreplication of DNA, so that the ploidy (or DNA content) of individual cells is greater than the normal diploid content of DNA [11]. In contrast, in arterioles the increase in smooth muscle cell mass appears to be caused by a true increase in cell number [12].

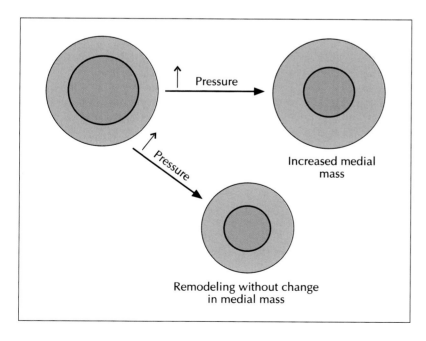

FIGURE 4-10. Structural responses to increased pressure loading that decrease luminal diameter. Two major mechanisms have been described that decrease the diameter of the lumen in resistance arteries. The first involves a pressure-induced increase in medial mass associated with increased smooth muscle cell growth or hypertrophy, together with increased connective tissue. Second, remodeling of the vessel wall causes a decrease in luminal diameter that is unassociated with growth of cellular or connective tissue elements. Rarefaction (or dropout) of these vessels is an additional mechanism that may decrease the total cross-sectional area of resistance arterioles in hypertension.

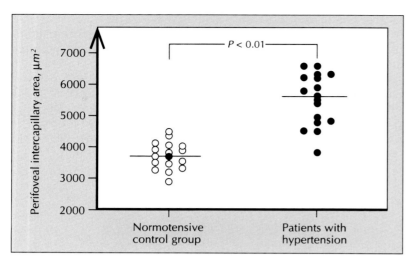

FIGURE 4-11. Capillary rarefaction in essential hypertension. As noted in Figure 4-10, rarefaction (reduction in capillary density) is an additional mechanism that contributes to increased peripheral resistance in hypertension. Such changes have been measured in human skin and conjunctiva [13,14]. This figure shows the *inter*capillary density in the retinas near the foveae of control and hypertensive patients. The mean area between capillaries is significantly higher in hypertensive patients, indicating global capillary loss. (*Adapted from* Wolf *et al.* [15].)

FUNCTIONAL ALTERATIONS IN HYPERTENSION

EFFECT OF STRUCTURAL ALTERATIONS ON RESISTANCE

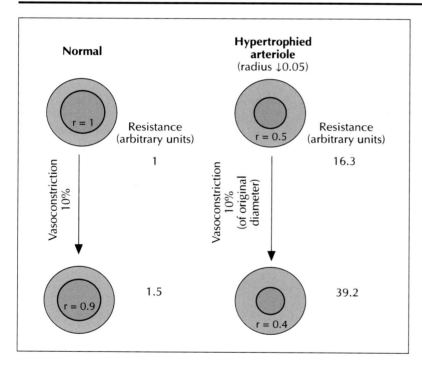

FIGURE 4-12. Linkage between structural and functional changes. Structural alterations that decrease luminal diameter increase vascular resistance. Hypertrophy of the arteriolar wall that encroaches on the luminal diameter has significant functional implications. A 0.1 (10% constriction) decrease in radius (from 1 to 0.9) leads to an increase in resistance of 50%. Hypertrophy of the vessel media that decreases the radius by 50% (from 1 to 0.5) increases the resistance 16.3-fold. The same constriction (0.1 of the radius of the original normal vessel; from 0.5 to 0.4) now would cause a 2.4-fold increase in resistance from the new baseline. Thus, the same stimulus response that caused a 50% increase in resistance in a normal vessel is associated with a 39-fold increase in resistance in the hypertrophied vessel. Therefore, structural alterations in the vessel wall can have important functional implications. r—radius.

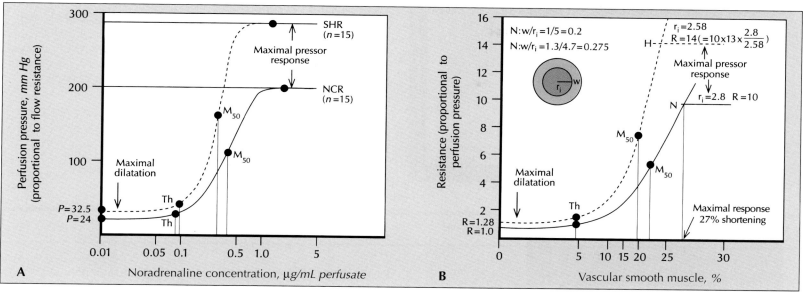

FIGURE 4-13. Influence of organic vascular changes on vascular reactivity. Folkow *et al.* [3] elucidated the role of structural changes in vascular reactivity. Their laboratory compared actual measurements of resistance changes in spontaneously hypertensive (SHR) and normotensive Wistar control (NCR) rats with mathematically calculated resistance curves in which the only difference between hypertensive and normotensive vessels was a 30% increase in medial encroachment on the lumen of the diseased vessel at maximal relaxation. As shown, there is very little difference in the threshold (maximal dilatation) between hypertensive and normotensive vessels, but the enhanced reactivity (increased resistance) is expressed as an increase in slope. Their interpretation of these curves is that the determinants of the threshold response (*eg*, receptor number, second messenger activation, contractile protein sensitivity) are unchanged in hypertension, and the increased resistance that occurs when contraction develops is in fact due to the structural change in the vessel wall (in this case a change in medial thickness). Comparison shows that actual (**A**) and hypothetical (**B**) resistances agree well, suggesting that the structural factor is sufficient to explain at least some types of increased hypertensive vascular resistance. H—hypertensive resistance vessel with a 30% increase in medial thickness; M_{50}—50% of the maximal pressor (resistance) response; N—normotensive resistance vessel; R—resistance; r_i—internal radius; Th—threshold; w—medial thickness. (*Adapted from* Folkow *et al.* [3].)

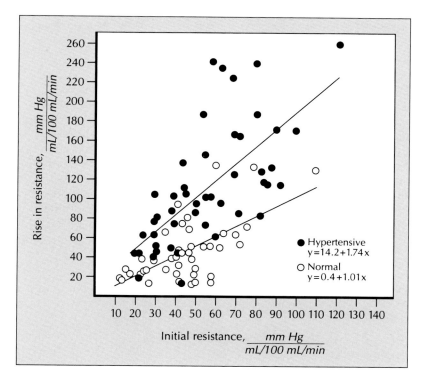

FIGURE 4-14. Increased sensitivity to vasoconstrictors in essential hypertension. These data from patients with essential hypertension illustrate apparent increased sensitivity to forearm infusion of norepinephrine (0.40 µg/min) as reflected in the extent of the increase in resistance. Such observations can be explained on the basis of mechanical effects of wall thickening and luminal encroachment, as shown in Figures 4-12 and 4-13. An increase in sensitivity to the effects of α-adrenergic agonists cannot be excluded by these data. (*Adapted from* Doyle and Fraser [16].)

POSSIBLE MECHANISMS OF APPARENT INCREASED SENSITIVITY TO VASOCONSTRICTORS

True increased sensitivity to vasoconstrictors
  Increased receptor sensitivity
  Increased activation of second messengers or ion channels

Apparent increased sensitivity due to effects of structure or function to increase resistance
  Hypertrophy or hyperplasia
  Rarefaction with loss of resistance vasculature
  Decreased endothelial-dependent vasodilator mechanisms

FIGURE 4-15. Possible mechanisms of apparent increased sensitivity to vasoconstrictors. Increased sensitivity to vasoconstrictors is a well-established observation in hypertensive patients and animal models. This table summarizes some of the possible mechanisms responsible for the apparent increased sensitivity. There may be a true increased sensitivity to vasoconstrictors (*see* Fig. 4-14), based on a change in receptor number or coupling to intracellular second messengers. Alternatively, the apparent increase in sensitivity may be due to structural or functional changes in the artery, resulting in greater force generation for a given concentration of vasoconstrictor. This is illustrated in Figure 4-13.

ENDOTHELIAL DYSFUNCTION

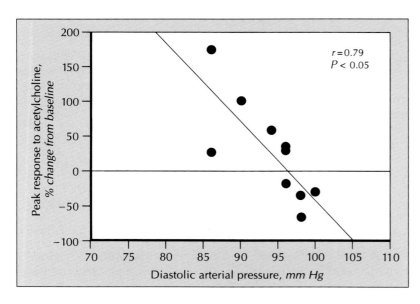

FIGURE 4-16. Evidence for defective endothelium-dependent relaxation in the coronary arteries of hypertensive subjects. Infusion of acetylcholine into the left anterior descending coronary artery of normal subjects leads to a dose-related increase in flow. The mechanism is presumably through the increased release of nitric oxide in the resistance circulation. In contrast, the increase in flow in response to acetylcholine infusion is markedly impaired in hypertensive subjects with ventricular hypertrophy. Maximal dilator capacity in response to nonendothelium-dependent dilators is not different between the two groups. The loss of this endothelial vasodilator mechanism probably contributes to disordered coronary flow regulation. Loss of endothelial-dependent vasodilator mechanisms could be associated more generally with the increase in vascular resistance in hypertension. M—molar. (*Adapted from* Treasure *et al.* [7].)

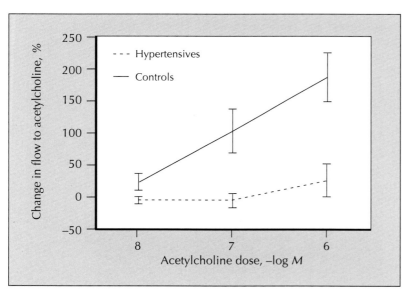

FIGURE 4-17. Correlation of peak coronary flow response to acetylcholine with diastolic arterial pressure in hypertensive patients. Diastolic blood pressure is correlated with endothelium-dependent relaxation. As diastolic arterial pressure increases, the ability of acetylcholine to increase flow decreases, so that at high pressure all vasodilator effects are lost and the arterial smooth muscle actually contracts. The relationship between diastolic pressure and the peak flow response to acetylcholine suggests that hypertension itself is sufficient to cause endothelial dysfunction in resistance arteries. (*Adapted from* Treasure *et al.* [7].)

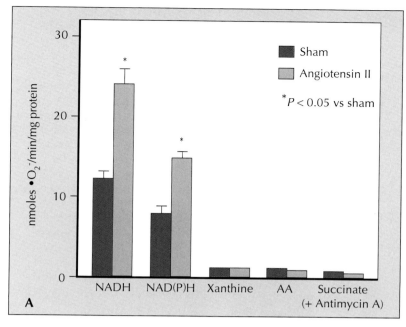

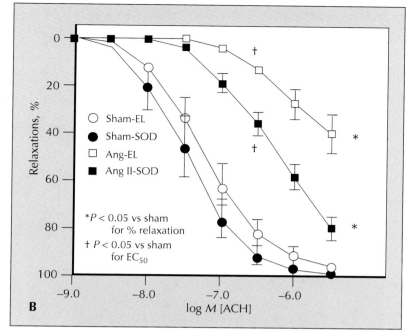

FIGURE 4-18. Role of oxidative stress in high angiotensin II models of hypertension. **A,** When hypertension is accompanied by or induced with high circulating angiotensin II, a superoxide anion ($\bullet O_2^-$)-producing NAD(P)H oxidase is activated in the vessel wall. In these experiments, rats were infused with angiotensin II (0.7 mg/kg/d), and the activity of various oxidases was measured in vessel homogenates. Only NADH- and NAD(P)H-dependent $\bullet O_2^-$ production was increased [17]. **B,** The local production of $\bullet O_2^-$ has profound effects on endothelium-dependent relaxation, as demonstrated by diminished relaxation of rat aortic rings in response to acetylcholine (compare sham and Ang-EL). Impaired endothelial function can be corrected by administration of superoxide dismutase (SOD), demonstrating the involvement of $\bullet O_2^-$ in the functional lesion in this model of hypertension. AA—arachidonic acid; ACH—acetylcholine; Ang-EL—angiotensin II–infused rats that received empty liposomes; Ang II-SOD—angiotensin II–infused rats treated with liposomal SOD; NADH—reduced nicotinamide adenine dinucleotide; NAD(P)H—reduced nicotinamide adenine dinucleotide phosphate; Sham-EL—sham rats that received empty liposomes; Sham-SOD—sham rats treated with liposomal SOD. (*Adapted from* Rajagopalan *et al.* [18].)

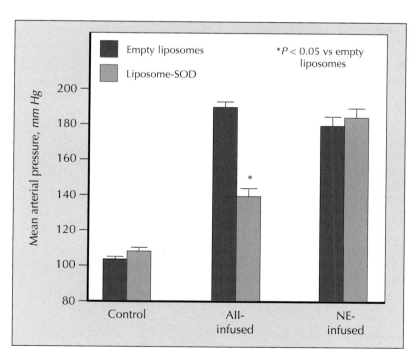

FIGURE 4-19. Correction of hypertension with superoxide dismutase (SOD). The role of $\bullet O_2^-$ in hypertension extends beyond endothelial dysfunction. In both spontaneously hypertensive rats and in rats made hypertensive by angiotensin II (AII) infusion, administration of SOD corrects the elevated blood pressure [19,20]. In rats infused with angiotensin II, administration of either heparin-binding SOD [19] or liposomal-entrapped SOD counteracts the increase in blood pressure, suggesting that vascular oxidative stress also occurs in the resistance vessels [21]. Similar results have been found in spontaneously hypertensive rats [20]. However, if animals are made hypertensive by infusion of norepinephrine (NE), SOD has no effect on blood pressure. These studies suggest that in some forms of hypertension, vascular oxidative stress also occurs in the resistance vessels, and that it contributes to the development of high blood pressure. Additional evidence that oxidative stress is a cause or consequence of hypertension comes from observations that both antioxidant defenses and lipid peroxidation products are increased in patients with essential hypertension [22]. (*Adapted from* Bech-Laursen *et al.* [19].)

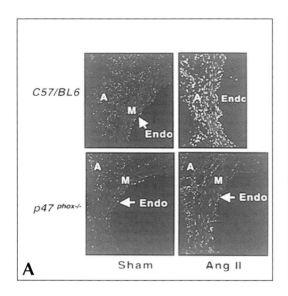

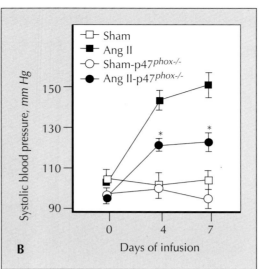

B

FIGURE 4-20. The role of NAD(P)H oxidase in angiotensin II–induced hypertension. **A**, Recently, transgenic mice deficient in p47phox, a critical component of the vascular NAD(P)H oxidase, have been used to unequivocally implicate this enzyme and the subsequent production of superoxide anion ($\bullet O_2^-$) in the development of angiotensin II–induced hypertension. The increase in aortic $\bullet O_2^-$ that results from angiotensin II infusion (0.7 mg/kg/d) is abolished in mice lacking the p47phox gene. **B**, The p47phox-deficient mice develop significantly less hypertension over a period of 7 days. This supports the pharmacologic experiments with superoxide dismutase (SOD) (*see* Fig. 4-19) and establishes the underlying source of the $\bullet O_2^-$ as the NAD(P)H oxidase. A—adventitia; Endo—endothelium; M—media. (**A** *adapted from* Landmesser *et al.* [23].)

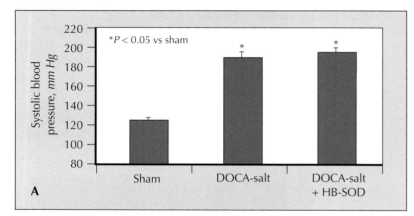

A

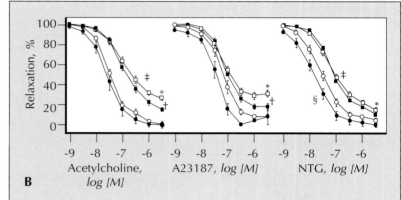

B

FIGURE 4-21. **A** and **B**, The role of superoxide in chronic, low-renin hypertension. The studies shown in Figures 4-19 and 4-20 implicate reactive oxygen species in the development of acute hypertension, but do not provide insight into whether this mechanism is extant in longer term hypertension, especially if antioxidant expression is increased in compensation. Using a deoxycorticosterone acetate–salt (DOCA-salt) model in which hypertension develops over a period of 3 weeks, Somers *et al.* [24] showed that superoxide anion ($\bullet O_2^-$) is increased in the aortas of these rats, and that impaired endothelium-dependent relaxation in response to acetylcholine or the calcium ionophore A23187 can be partially corrected by administration of heparin-binding superoxide dismutase (HB-SOD). In contrast, endothelium-independent relaxation in response to nitroglycerin is unaffected

by SOD. Of interest, in contrast to angiotensin II–induced hypertension, SOD treatment did not correct the blood pressure effects of DOCA-salt, perhaps because hypertension in this model is largely mediated by increased intravascular volume and circulating catecholamines. Nonetheless, these studies clearly implicate reactive oxygen species in the pathologic manifestations of chronic hypertension. *P* values are defined as follows: *asterisk* indicates $P < 0.05$ peak relaxations for sham versus DOCA-salt; *dagger* indicates $P < 0.05$ peak relaxations for HB-SOD versus no HB-SOD; *double dagger* indicates $P < 0.05$ for ED_{50} for sham versus DOCA-salt; *section symbol* indicates $P < 0.05$ for ED_{50} for HB-SOD versus no HB-SOD. NTG—nitroglycerin. (*Adapted from* Somers *et al.* [24].)

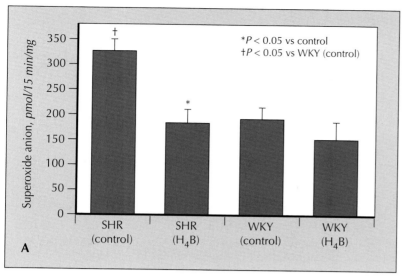

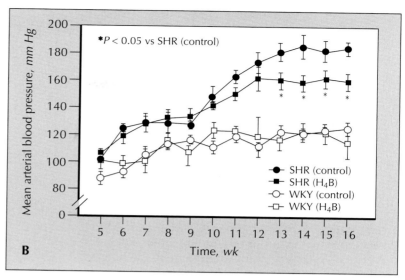

FIGURE 4-22. Tetrahydrobiopterin treatment suppresses the development of hypertension. Recent work has shown that another important source of superoxide anion ($\bullet O_2^-$) in the vessel wall is uncoupled endothelial nitric oxide synthase (eNOS) [25]. Uncoupling of eNOS appears to be related to oxidation of its essential cofactor tetrahydrobiopterin (H_4B). Intraperitoneal replacement of H_4B reduces vascular $\bullet O_2^-$ production (**A**) and suppresses the development of hypertension in spontaneously hypertensive rats (**B**), while having no effect on these parameters in Wistar-Kyoto rats. These results thus suggest an additional mechanism whereby eNOS contributes to blood pressure regulation in hypertension. (*Adapted from* Hong *et al.* [26].)

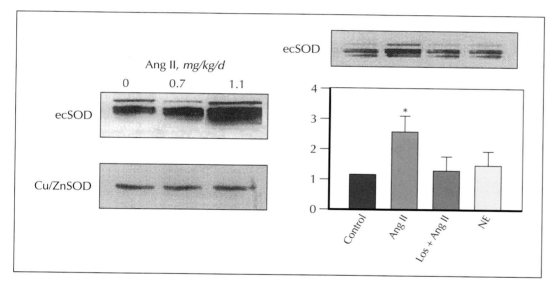

FIGURE 4-23. Upregulation of extracellular superoxide dismutase (ecSOD) by angiotensin II infusion. Not only can external administration of SOD correct the oxidative stress imposed on the vessel by angiotensin II, but angiotensin II itself may upregulate antioxidant defense mechanisms such as ecSOD to partially correct the oxidative insult. Ang II—angiotensin II; Los—losartan. (*Adapted from* Fukai *et al.* [27].)

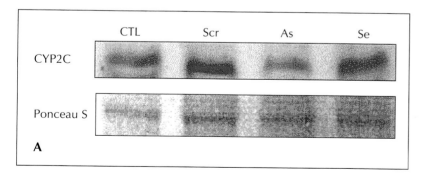

FIGURE 4-24. The "other" endothelial-relaxing factor: endothelium-derived hyperpolarizing factor (EDHF). The identity of EDHF has been elusive, but recent work strongly suggests that epoxyeicosatrienoic acids (EETs), products of cytochrome P450 epoxygenase (CYP), are potent endothelial-relaxing factors that induce hyperpolarization. Selective CYP inhibitors have been shown to abolish nitric oxide and prostaglandin I_2 (PGI_2)-independent vasodilation [28], and EETs have been shown to hyperpolarize cells by activating calcium-dependent K^+ channels as well as the Na^+,K^+-ATPase [29]. More importantly, administration of antisense oligonucleotides against CYP2C8/34 (an isoform of CYP expressed in endothelial cells) attenuates relaxation to EDHF [30]. **A,** Western blot of porcine coronary arteries treated with scrambled (Scr), antisense (As), or sense (Se) CYP2C8/34 oligonucleotides. The As but not Se or Scr oligonucleotides decreased CYP2C expression but did not affect expression of unrelated proteins as assessed by Ponceau S staining.

Continued on next page

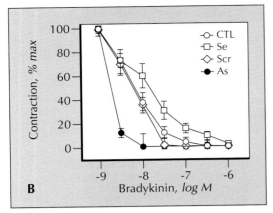
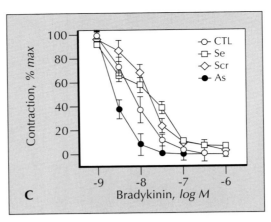
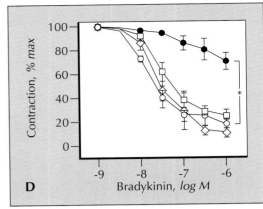

FIGURE 4-24. *(Continued)* Inhibitors were then used to block specific vasodilatory pathways (while leaving others intact) in the presence of these treatments to determine the functional implications of reducing CYP2C expression. Treated vessels were examined for their ability to relax to bradykinin after precontraction with U46619. **B,** Relaxations measured in the presence of diclofenac (cyclooxygenase inhibitor that prevents PGI_2 formation) and sulfaphenazole (CYP inhibitor), representing NO-dependent relaxations. Attenuation of CYP2C expression had no effect on NO responses. **C,** Relaxations measured in the presence of diclofenac alone, representing NO- and EDHF-mediated

relaxations. Here, the NO effects predominate, because reduction of CYP2C by AS oligonucleotides did not impair relaxations. **D,** Relaxations measured in the presence of diclofenac and N^{ω}nitro-L-arginine (NO synthase inhibitor), representing EDHF-mediated vasodilation. When EDHF-mediated responses are examined independently of PGI_2 and NO, it becomes clear that blocking CYP2C dramatically attenuates relaxation. These findings strongly support the concept that cytochrome p450 metabolites function as EDHF and, as such, may play an important role in hypertension. *(Adapted from* Fisslthaler *et al.* [30].)

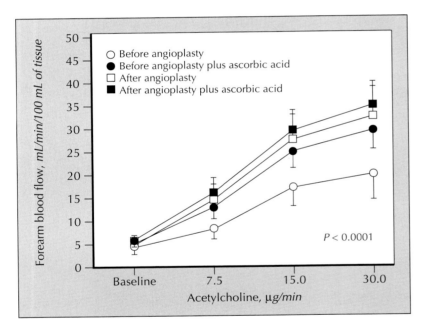

FIGURE 4-25. Endothelial-dependent vasodilation assessment. Higashi *et al.* [9] have provided compelling clinical evidence for the role of reactive oxygen species in endothelial dysfunction in human hypertension due to renal artery stenosis in which the renin-angiotensin system was activated. Endothelial-dependent vasodilation was assessed by measuring forearm blood flow basally and with three doses of acetylcholine infused into the brachial artery before and after angioplasty. Endothelial-dependent increases in forearm flow were diminished in the hypertensive subjects relative to controls. As shown here, endothelial function *before* angioplasty was strikingly improved by infusion of the antioxidant ascorbic acid. After angioplasty of the renal artery lesion, endothelial-dependent forearm blood flow improved significantly and was not affected by ascorbic acid. Renal artery angioplasty was also associated with decreases in systemic markers of oxidative stress. These results are consistent with animal models in which angiotensin II–dependent hypertension is associated with increased endothelial production of NAD(P)H-derived reactive oxygen species that degrade NO, resulting in impaired endothelium-mediated vasodilation. This mechanism may contribute importantly to the sustained elevation of blood pressure [9].

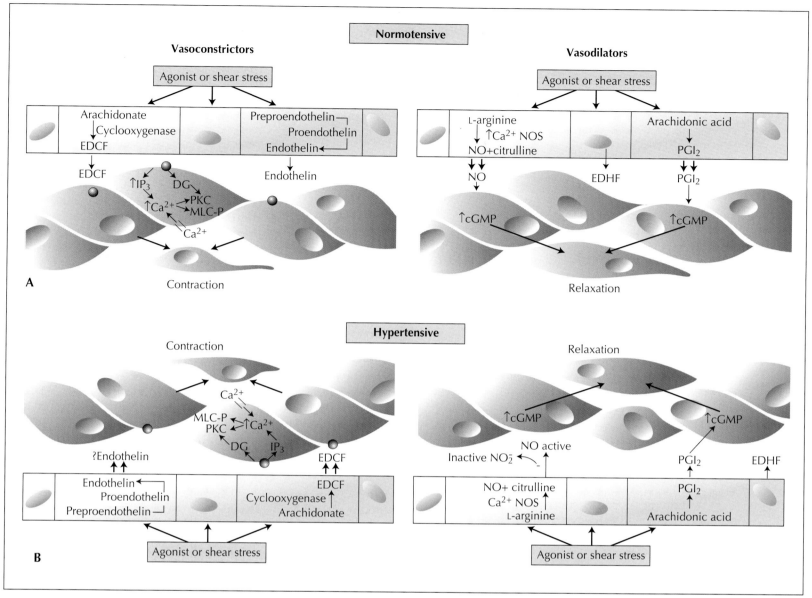

Figure 4-26. Endothelium-dependent vasodilator and vasoconstrictor mechanisms: modification in hypertension. Normal endothelial cells secrete both vasodilators—the most prominent of which are nitric oxide (NO), prostacyclin (PGI$_2$), and endothelium-derived hyperpolarizing factor (EDHF)—and vasoconstrictors, including endothelin and endothelium-derived contracting factor (EDCF) [31]. Vessel tone is dependent on the balance between these factors and on the ability of the smooth muscle cell to respond to them.

A, In normotensive vessels there is a predominance of vasodilator secretion. These substances may also contribute to the inhibition of smooth muscle cell growth or hypertrophy. The relative concentrations of the vasoconstricting/vasodilating agents are indicated by the relative sizes of the arrows and bold type in the illustration.

B, In hypertension, release of vasoconstrictor substances may predominate [4]. In addition, vasodilator release may be decreased or, alternatively, the vasodilator itself may be inactivated by superoxide anion. Under certain circumstances, endothelin also can

be growth-promoting, thereby contributing to smooth muscle cell hypertrophy or hyperplasia and intimal thickening. The biochemical pathways activated by endothelial agonists and by contracting and relaxing factors acting on smooth muscle can also be affected in hypertension. NO, produced by the conversion of L-arginine to citrulline, traverses the endothelial cell membrane, and activates the smooth muscle cell guanylate cyclase to generate intracellular cGMP. PGI$_2$ and EDCF are produced via cyclooxygenase action on arachidonic acid. PGI$_2$ relaxes vessels by increasing smooth muscle cell cAMP; the mechanism of action of EDCF is unknown. Endothelin is made and modified by endothelium. It then stimulates the phospholipase C pathway in smooth muscle to produce the second messengers inositol trisphosphate (IP$_3$) and diacylglycerol (DG), which in turn activate the Ca^{2+} and protein kinase C (PKC) signaling pathways. This leads to phosphorylation of the myosin light chain (MLC-P), causing contraction. Alterations of any of these signals could easily augment contraction or decrease the ability of the vessel to dilate.

FIGURE 4-27. Possible mechanisms responsible for defective endothelium-dependent vasodilatation in hypertension. As described earlier, nitric oxide is perhaps the most important of the endothelium-derived relaxing factors. Therefore, decreased production of nitric oxide or increased degradation by free radicals markedly impairs vasodilatation [32]. The smooth muscle itself may exhibit decreased responsiveness to ambient endothelium-derived vasodilators. Finally, an imbalance in the production of endothelium-derived relaxing and contracting factors to favor excess production of the latter may also contribute to defective vasodilatation.

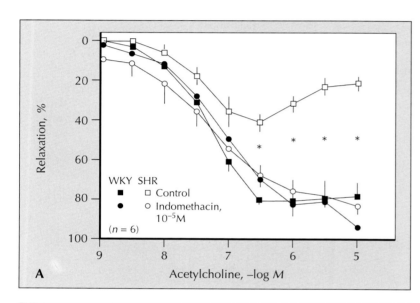

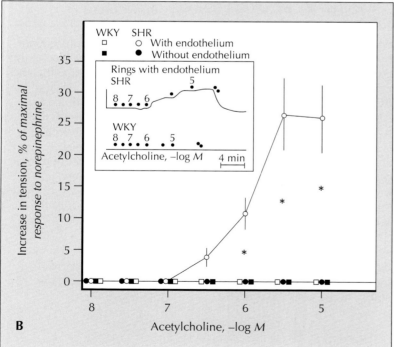

FIGURE 4-28. Enhanced endothelium-dependent constriction of rat aortic rings to acetylcholine in hypertensive animal models. In addition to nitric oxide, acetylcholine induces release of a cyclooxygenase-dependent product of arachidonic acid in the spontaneously hypertensive rat (SHR) that has been called endothelium-derived contracting factor (EDCF) [4].

A, The restoration of acetylcholine-induced relaxation by the cyclooxygenase inhibitor indomethacin in the SHR aorta. These results indicate that a cyclooxygenase-derived constricting factor is being stimulated in the hypertensive, but not the normotensive, rat strain. **B,** In the SHR the acetylcholine-stimulated contraction is dependent on the presence of the endothelium. Acetylcholine produced a contraction in the SHR aorta with endothelium but did not contract the SHR aorta without endothelium, nor did it contract the normotensive Wistar-Kyoto (WKY) rat aorta with or without endothelium. The *inset* shows an original isometric tracing from intact aortas from WKY and SHR. These results indicate that in the SHR model, acetylcholine releases an endothelium-dependent constrictor that overwhelms the dilator effect of acetylcholine-induced nitric oxide release. Whether similar endothelium-dependent vasoconstrictors play a role in the pathogenesis of any subset of human hypertension remains to be determined. *Asterisks* indicate $P < 0.05$; each data point is mean ± SEM. M—molar. (*Adapted from* Lüscher and Vanhoutte [4].)

AGENTS INVOLVED IN VASCULAR SMOOTH MUSCLE GROWTH AND EXTRACELLULAR MATRIX PRODUCTION

Angiotensin II
Endothelin
Vasopressin
Epidermal growth factor
Serotonin
Fibroblast growth factor
Epiregulin

Thrombin
Insulin-like growth factor-I
Platelet-derived growth factor
Transforming growth factor-β
Catecholamines
Reactive oxygen species

FIGURE 4-29. Agents involved in vascular smooth muscle growth. Vascular smooth muscle cells respond to a variety of classic growth factors and to vasoconstricting agents that can act as growth factors under certain circumstances. The agents listed in this table contribute to both hypertrophy (*eg*, angiotensin II) and hyperplasia (*eg*, platelet-derived growth factor). In addition, they increase extracellular matrix production, which may have a major role in vascular remodeling.

FACTORS INHIBITING VASCULAR SMOOTH MUSCLE CELL GROWTH

Heparinoids
Nitric oxide
Prostacyclin
Atrial natriuretic peptide

FIGURE 4-30. Factors that inhibit vascular smooth muscle cell growth. Vascular smooth muscle is also under the influence of many growth-inhibitory factors. Under normal conditions the organism maintains a balance between growth-promoting and growth-inhibiting factors such that there is no net arterial growth. However, diminished production of normal inhibitory agents, such as those listed here, can shift the balance toward abnormal growth of smooth muscle.

ABNORMALITIES IN MEMBRANE CHANNELS IN HYPERTENSION
[FOR ADDITIONAL DISCUSSION OF THIS SUBJECT SEE CHAPTERS 1 AND 3]

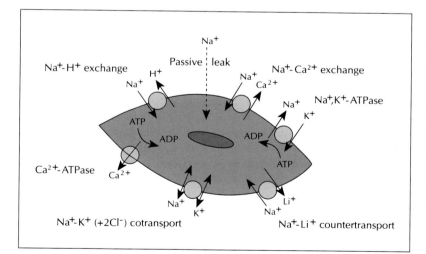

FIGURE 4-31. Ion transport mechanisms in vascular smooth muscle. Alterations in Ca^{2+} and Na^+ content and transport have been identified in hypertension. Many membrane channels and transporters participate in the regulation of these ions. The important molecules and their functional significance are indicated in this diagram. Na^+ enters the cell through Na^+-H^+ exchange, Na^+-Ca^{2+} exchange, Na^+-Li^+ countertransport, passive leak, and Na^+-K^+($+2Cl^-$) cotransport. Na^+ exits the cell mainly via the Na^+, K^+-ATPase. Ca^{2+} enters the cell via voltage-gated and receptor-operated Ca^{2+} channels (not shown) and is extruded by Na^+-Ca^{2+} exchange and the plasma membrane Ca^{2+}-ATPase. Perturbation of any one of these ion mechanisms can lead to abnormal Na^+ or Ca^{2+} regulation.

MEMBRANE ION TRANSPORT OR CONTENT ABNORMALITIES THAT HAVE BEEN REPORTED IN HUMAN ESSENTIAL HYPERTENSION

Increased Ca^{2+} concentration in platelets

Decreased Na^+-Ca^+ exchange

Decreased Ca^{2+}-ATPase activity

Decreased activity of the Na^+, K^+-ATPase leading to increased intracellular Na^+ concentration

Increased Na^+ content in red and white blood cells

Low Na^+, K^+/($^+$2Cl-) cotransport activity

Increased Na^+-Li^+ countertransport

Increased Na^+-H^+ exchange

FIGURE 4-32. Membrane ion transport or content abnormalities that have been reported in human essential hypertension. Studies of ion transport and content in cells from hypertensive patients are numerous. Virtually all of the transporters identified in Figure 4-31 have been examined in hypertension, and many have been found to be altered in platelets or erythrocytes of subsets of hypertensive patients. This table summarizes the abnormalities identified in various cell types in human essential hypertension. In the following figures, each will be considered separately.

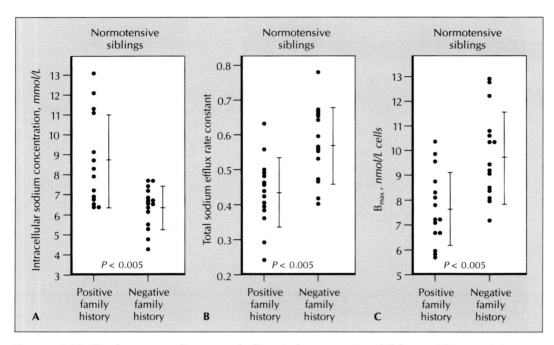

FIGURE 4-33. Erythrocyte sodium metabolism in hypertensive children with essential or secondary hypertension, with or without a family history of hypertension. The normotensive siblings of hypertensive patients had a higher intracellular sodium concentration

(**A**) and a lower sodium efflux rate (**B**) and number of Na^+, K^+-ATPase–dependent (ATPase, adenosine triphosphatase) pump sites (**C**). Hypertensive parents also had higher intracellular sodium and lower sodium efflux rates and number of Na^+, K^+-ATPase–dependent pump sites. These findings were not secondary to hypertension, because normotensive siblings with a positive family history of hypertension exhibited features of erythrocyte sodium metabolism that were similar to those of the hypertensive children. These data provide strong evidence for hereditary transmission of abnormalities of membrane sodium transport, in general, and of Na^+, K^+-ATPase, in particular, in families with a predisposition to developing hypertension. If these abnormalities are also expressed in vascular smooth muscle, they could contribute significantly to the functional abnormalities involved in the pathogenesis of hypertension. (*Adapted from* Deal *et al.* [33].)

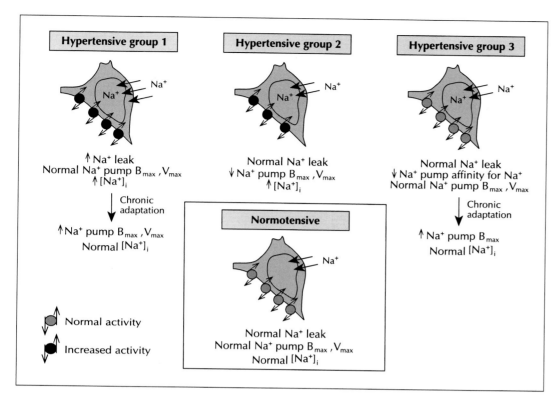

Figure 4-34. Alterations in Na$^+$ pump activity in different populations of hypertensive patients. The diversity of observations concerning alterations in Na$^+$, K$^+$-ATPase activity in blood-formed elements in hypertensive groups can be largely explained by considering the actual physiologic change observed. When this is taken into account, it appears that there are subpopulations of hypertensive patients who exhibit different defects in, and different abilities to compensate for, pump activity. In one group of patients (hypertensive group 1), the Na$^+$ leak is increased, but the B$_{max}$ and V$_{max}$ of the pump are normal, leading to increased intracellular Na$^+$. The increased intra-

cellular Na$^+$ stimulates pump activity, and some of these patients undergo chronic adaptation in which the number of Na$^+$ pumps is increased, returning intracellular Na$^+$ to normal.

In a second group (hypertensive group 2), the V$_{max}$ and number of Na$^+$ pumps are decreased in the face of a normal Na$^+$ leak, leading to increased intracellular Na$^+$. Pump "activity" of the diminished number of pumps is compensatorily increased, however. A third group of patients (hypertensive group 3) exhibits a normal Na$^+$ leak, normal Na$^+$ pump B$_{max}$ and V$_{max}$, but decreased affinity of the pump for Na$^+$. The resulting increased intracellular Na$^+$ sometimes leads to an increase in the number of Na$^+$ pumps, normalizing intracellular Na$^+$. The existence of three groups of patients with differing aspects of abnormalities in Na$^+$ handling helps to explain some of the contradictory information in the literature. Thus, although Na$^+$ may be important in essential hypertension, Na$^+$, K$^+$-ATPase abnormalities may not occur in all patients, and some groups of patients will be better able to compensate than others. The precise relationship between these abnormalities and the pathogenesis of essential hypertension remains to be determined. (*Adapted from* Aviv and Lasker [34].)

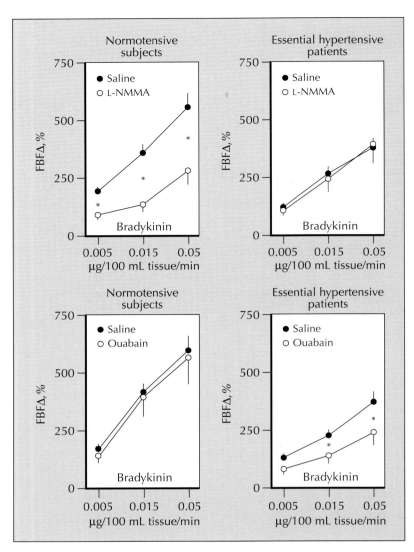

FIGURE 4-35. Evidence that vasodilation in response to bradykinin in essential hypertensive patients is mediated by an ouabain-sensitive pathway in compensation for deficient nitric oxide availability. In normotensive subjects, the increase in forearm blood flow induced by bradykinin was influenced strikingly by L-NMNA, an agent that interferes with nitric oxide production, and thus suggests that the effect of bradykinin on the normal forearm circulation reflects activation of nitric oxide synthesis and release. This response is unaffected by ouabain. In essential hypertensive patients, however, inhibition of nitric oxide production by the inhibitor L-NMMA has no effect on brady kinin-induced increases in blood flow, indicating that an ouabain-sensitive mechanism has developed that contributes to increased blood flow in patients with hypertension challenged with bradykinin. This mechanism could involve an endothelial-dependent hyperpolarizing factor. (*Adapted from* Taddei *et al.* [35].)

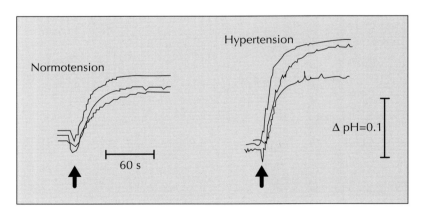

FIGURE 4-36. Increased Na^+/H^+ exchanger activity in platelets from normotensive and hypertensive subjects. Platelets were loaded with an indicator of intracellular pH (BCECF) and were stimulated with thrombin (*arrows*). Platelets from hypertensive patients showed a more rapid rise in pH (0.55 ± 0.1 dpH_i/min) than did those from normotensives (0.26 ± 0.01 dpH_i/min) and had a higher total increase in pH_i (0.15 ± 0.04 vs 0.08 ± 0.015). Basal pH_i values were not different. Increased activity of the Na^+/H^+ antiporter has been

observed in erythrocytes, leukocytes, and platelets from subsets of human hypertensive patients. Increased activity of the exchanger has also been observed in skeletal muscle using ^{31}P magnetic resonance imaging [36]. It is assumed that the alterations in antiporter activity observed in blood cells and in skeletal muscle reflect a generalized abnormality in all cell types. The increased activity does not appear to be affected by treatment of hypertension or by its duration or severity. Therefore, the alteration in antiporter activity may be a fundamental feature of the disease in the subsets of patients in whom it occurs [37]. However, the Na^+/H^+ antiporter does not appear to be a candidate gene for hypertension, since it does not segregate closely with the hypertensive phenotype or with other genes predisposing to hypertension [38]. Increased Na^+/H^+ exchanger activity appears to be one of several genetically controlled abnormalities of membrane ion transport that contribute to the development of the hypertensive phenotype. The lack of close linkage of gene expression with phenotypic expression illustrates the multifactorial (genetic and environmental) nature of the disease. A mechanistic link between increased antiporter activity and hypertension has not been established but may relate to increased agonist responsiveness or to enhanced cellular proliferation. (*Adapted from* Rosskopf *et al.* [39].)

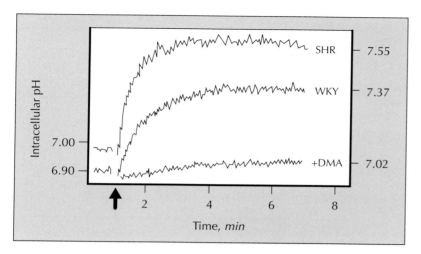

FIGURE 4-37. Evidence for enhanced Na^+/H^+ exchanger activity in cultured vascular smooth muscle cells of an animal model of hypertension as compared with cells from a normotensive control strain. Cells were loaded with a fluorescent indicator of intracellular pH and acidified with an ionophore in sodium-free medium. When sodium was added (*arrow*) the cells from spontaneously hypertensive rats (SHR) increased their pH (as reflected by the increase in the fluorescence signal) more rapidly than did those from Wistar-Kyoto (WKY) rats (*two upper tracings*). The sodium-dependent alkalinization was dependent on the Na^+/H^+ exchanger in both cell types, as indicated by blockade with the specific blocker dimethylamiloride (DMA). These data extend the observations in human blood cells and suggest that the enhanced antiporter activity is, in fact, expressed in vascular cells in this hypertensive model. (*Adapted from* Berk et al. [40].)

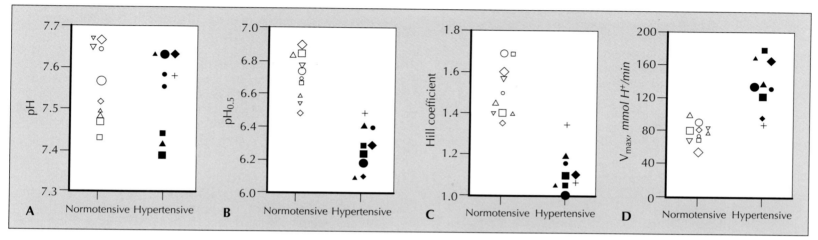

FIGURE 4-38. Persistence of the hypertensive Na^+/H^+ exchanger phenotype in Epstein-Barr virus immortalized immunoblasts from patients with essential hypertension. Peripheral lymphocytes from patients exhibiting the enhanced Na^+/H^+ exchanger phenotype were immortalized with Epstein-Barr virus and cultured. **A,** The enhanced antiporter activity phenotype persisted in culture. The resting pH was not different in cells from normotensive and hypertensive subjects (**B**). The $pH_{0.5}$ (the pH at which the antiporter is half-maximally activated) is lower in the hypertensive (6.32 ± 0.23) than the normotensive (6.72 ± 0.15) subject, indicating enhanced activity ($P < 0.002$; **C**). The Hill coefficient is lower in cells from hypertensives, whereas the V_{max} (maximum activity) is higher (**D**). Both of these measurements indicate increased activity of the Na^+/H^+ exchanger. The increase in V_{max} is not associated with increased expression of mRNA for the antiporter. The mechanism for the alteration in its kinetics and enhanced activity remains to be determined. These findings do provide compelling evidence for genetic factors (as opposed to features of the in vivo neural, humoral, or physical milieu) being important in determining abnormal functions of the Na^+/H^+ antiporter in certain groups of hypertensive patients [37]. Each symbol represents values from a single cell line. (*Adapted from* Rosskopf et al. [37].)

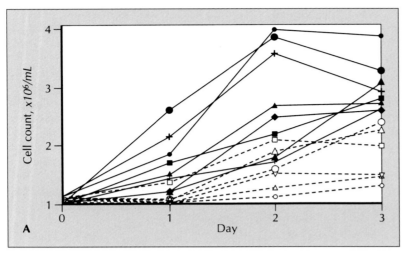

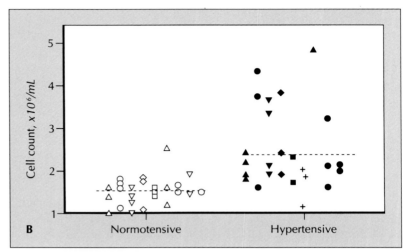

FIGURE 4-39. Growth pattern of immortalized lymphoblasts from normotensive and hypertensive patients who express abnormalities in Na^+/H^+ antiporter activity. **A,** Time course of lymphoblast proliferation of cells from normotensive (*open symbols; dashed lines*) and from hypertensive (*closed symbols; solid lines*) individuals. **B,** The reproducibility of the enhanced proliferation of immortalized lymphoblasts from hypertensive (*closed symbols*) and normotensive (*open symbols*) donors. Cells from each group were plated at the same initial density and then counted on day 2. Each symbol represents an individual cell line and the number of deter-

minations is represented by the number of symbols. The *dashed lines* represent the means of determinations in each category. These data confirm that cells from hypertensive subjects reproducibly grow faster than do those from normotensive subjects. Because growth of vascular smooth muscle cells (to compromise luminal diameter) is a characteristic of arterioles in hypertension, it may be that a generalized enhancement of the Na^+/H^+ exchanger may facilitate this growth. A direct causal role in enhanced growth is possible but cannot be inferred from the available data. (*Adapted from* Rosskopf *et al.* [37].)

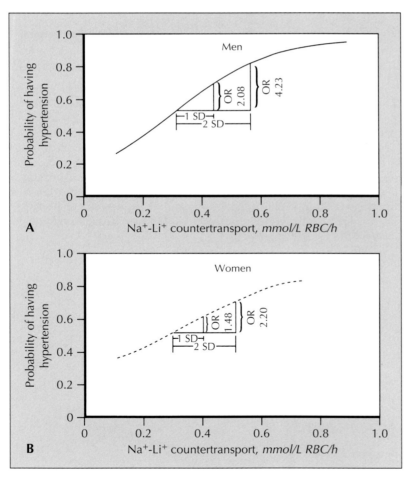

FIGURE 4-40. Predicted possibility of hypertension as a function of Na^+-Li^+ countertransport in erythrocytes from white men (**A**) and women (**B**) aged 47 to 89 years. The plots are based on the partial logistic regression coefficients for sodium-lithium countertransport in models encompassing other predictor traits, which include age, body weight, apolipoprotein CI, and apolipoprotein AI (in women). The odds ratio (OR) for the probability of having hypertension as a function of one or two SD increases in Na^+-Li^+ countertransport are depicted. These data provide evidence that increased activity of the Na^+-Li^+ countertransport is a risk factor for the development of hypertension. Although the mechanistic relationship between increased Na^+-Li^+ countertransporter activity and hypertension is unclear, even assuming that the defect is expressed in vascular smooth muscle cells, the data provide further evidence that defects in membrane ion transport mechanisms constitute an underlying risk for the development of hypertension that may interact with other genetic or environmental factors to produce the hypertensive phenotype. The contributions of increased Na^+-Li^+ transporter activity to the risk for developing hypertension is emphasized by the fact that the odds of having hypertension were increased 5.2-fold in men with the transporter genotype that is associated with elevated exchange [41]. RBC—red blood cell. (*Adapted from* Turner *et al.* [42].)

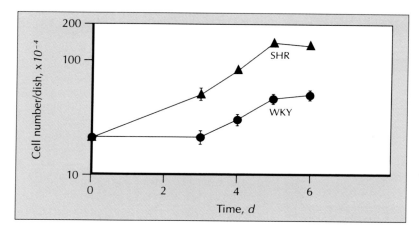

FIGURE 4-41. Proliferation of cultured early-passage vascular smooth muscle cells from spontaneously hypertensive rats (SHR) and Wistar-Kyoto (WKY) rats. The growth rate is increased in the cells from SHR as opposed to control WKY rats. The former exhibit enhanced Na^+/H^+ exchanger activity that may be related to the increase in growth rate. These data lend credence to the possibility that the increased proliferation rate of Epstein-Barr immortalized lymphoblasts depicted in Figure 4-39 may also have implications for vascular smooth muscle growth in human hypertension exhibiting the genotype associated with enhanced antiporter activity. (*Adapted from* Berk *et al.* [40].)

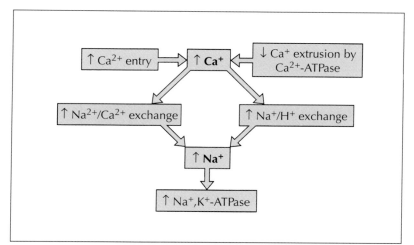

FIGURE 4-42. Role of calcium in hypertension. An alternative theory concerning the primary cellular defect in human hypertension centers on the calcium ion, rather than on sodium [34]. In this scenario, an increased level of intracellular Ca^{2+} ion due to either increased Ca^{2+} influx or decreased Ca^{2+} extrusion by the Ca^{2+}-ATPase is the initiating event in ion imbalance. Although the extrusion capacity of the Ca^{2+}-ATPase in platelets from essential hypertensive patients is higher than that of normotensive patients, the ability of this enzyme to respond to calmodulin stimulation is diminished in hypertension, resulting in an inability to maintain normal Ca^{2+} homeostasis [43]. The increase in intracellular Ca^{2+} stimulates Na^+-Ca^{2+} exchange and promotes Na^+-H^+ exchange leading to an increased intracellular Na^+ concentration and stimulation of Na^+, K^+-ATPase activity. Although the exact sequence of events remains unclear, the net effect would be an increase in intracellular Ca^{2+} and Na^+ levels, resulting in enhanced vasoconstriction.

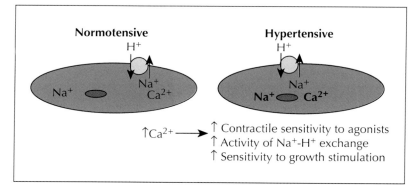

FIGURE 4-43. Unifying concept linking increased growth and contractility with ion abnormalities in vascular smooth muscle in hypertension. It has become apparent that human hypertension is associated with abnormalities of ion transport in vascular smooth muscle that result in an increase in intracellular Na^+ and Ca^{2+}. The increase in intracellular Ca^{2+}, by mechanisms discussed in Figure 4-42, could enhance contractile sensitivity to agonists and increase activity of the Na^+-H^+ exchanger. The resulting alkalinization, as well as the increased calcium, could lead to increased sensitivity to growth stimulation. Therefore, most of the important pathophysiologic features of the disease are potentially explainable in the context of abnormalities of ion transport.

CHARACTERISTICS OF HYPERTENSION

Interaction of environmental and genetic factors

Both structural and functional changes in arterioles leading to increased resistance

Structural changes resulting from growth or remodeling of the vessel due to the positive influence of growth factors or the removal of growth inhibitors

Functional abnormalities involving endothelial and vascular smooth muscle dysfunction

Abnormalities in membrane ionic control mechanisms likely underlying abnormalities in both contraction and growth

FIGURE 4-44. Characteristics of hypertension. Hypertension is caused by the interaction of environmental and genetic factors. It is characterized by both structural and functional changes in arterioles, leading to increased resistance. Structural changes result from growth or remodeling of the vessel due to the positive influence of growth factors or to the removal of growth inhibitors. Functional abnormalities involve endothelial and vascular smooth muscle dysfunction. Abnormalities in membrane ion control mechanisms probably underlie the abnormalities in both contraction and growth.

We wish to thank Lynda Prickett-Mathews for editorial assistance and Carolyn Morris for typing the manuscript.

REFERENCES

1. Berk BC, Alexander RW: Biology of the vascular wall in hypertension. In *The Kidney*. Edited by Brenner BM. Philadelphia: WB Saunders; 1995:2049–2070.

2. Reilly DF, Gordon D, Schwartz SM: Determination and comparison of the aortic polyploid smooth muscle content of human hypertensive subjects and normotensive controls. *Acta Physiol Scand* 1988, 571:181–188.

3. Folkow B, Hallback M, Lundgren Y, *et al.*: Background of increased flow resistance and vascular reactivity in spontaneously hypertensive rats. *Acta Physiol Scand* 1970, 80:93–106.

4. Lüscher TF, Vanhoutte PM: Endothelium-dependent contraction to acetylcholine in the aorta of the spontaneously hypertensive rat. *Hypertension* 1986, 8:344–348.

5. Moncada S, Palmer RM, Higgs EA: Nitric oxide: physiology, pathophysiology and pharmacology. *Pharmacol Rev* 1991, 43:109–142.

6. Hüttner I, Gabbiani G: Vascular endothelium in hypertension. In *Hypertension*. Edited by Genest J, Kuchel O, Hamet P, Cantin M. New York: McGraw-Hill; 1983.

7. Treasure CB, Klein JL, Vita JA, *et al.*: Hypertension and left ventricular hypertrophy are associated with impaired endothelium-mediated relaxation in human coronary resistance vessels. *Circulation* 1993, 87:86–93.

8. Harrison DG: Endothelial function and oxidant stress [review]. *Clin Cardiol* 1997, 20 (11 Suppl 2):II-11-7.

9. Hagashi Y, Sasaki S, Nakagawa K, *et al.*: Endothelial function and oxidative stress in renovascular hypertension. *N Engl J Med* 2002, 346:1954–1962.

10. Linder L, Kiowski W, Buhler FR, *et al.*: Indirect evidence for release of endothelium-derived relaxing factor in human forearm circulation in vivo: blunted response in essential hypertension. *Circulation* 1990, 81:1762–1767.

11. Owens GK, Schwartz SM: Vascular smooth muscle cell hypertrophy and hyperploidy in the Goldblatt hypertensive rat. *Circ Res* 1983, 53:491–501.

12. Halpern W, Warshaw DM, Mulvany MJ: Mechanical and morphological properties of arterial resistance vessels in young and old spontaneously hypertensive rats. *Circ Res* 1979, 45:250–259.

13. Harper RN, Moore MA, Marr MC, *et al.*: Arteriolar rarefaction in the conjunctiva of human essential hypertensives. *Microvasc Res* 1978, 16:369–372.

14. Fagrell B, Gundersen J: Capillary blood flow in the nail fold in relation to the digital systolic blood pressure. *Vasa* 1975, 4:250–257.

15. Wolf S, Arend O, Schulte K, *et al.*: Quantification of retinal capillary density and flow velocity in patients with essential hypertension. *Hypertension* 1994, 23:464–467.

16. Doyle AE, Fraser JRE: Vascular reactivity in hypertension. *Circ Res* 1961, 9:755–761.

17. Ushio-Fukai M, Zafari AM, Fukui T, *et al.*: p22phox is a critical component of the superoxide-generating NADH/NADPH oxidase system and regulates angiotensin II-induced hypertrophy in vascular smooth muscle cells. *J Biol Chem* 1996, 271:23317–23321.

18. Rajagopalan S, Kurz S, Münzel T, *et al.*: Angiotensin II mediated hypertension in the rat increases vascular superoxide production via membrane NADH/NADPH oxidase activation: contribution to alterations of vasomotor tone. *J Clin Invest* 1996, 97:1916–1923.

19. Bech-Laursen J, Rajagopalan S, Tarpey M, *et al.*: A role of superoxide in angiotensin II- but not catecholamine-induced hypertension. *Circulation* 1997, 95:588–593.

20. Nakazono K, Watanabe N, Matsuno K, *et al.*: Does superoxide underlie the pathogenesis of hypertension? *Proc Natl Acad Sci U S A* 1991, 88:10045–10048.

21. Fukui T, Ishizaka N, Rajagopalan S, *et al.*: p22phox mRNA expression and NADPH oxidase activity are increased in aortas from hypertensive rats. *Circ Res* 1997, 80:45–51.

22. Russo C, Olivieri O, Girelli D, *et al.*: Anti-oxidant status and lipid peroxidation in patients with essential hypertension. *J Hypertens* 1998, 16:1267–1271.

23. Landmesser U, Cai H, Dikalov S, *et al.*: Role of p47^{phox} in vascular oxidative stress and caused by angiotensin II. *Hypertension* 2002, 40:511–515.

24. Somers MJ, Mavromatis K, Galis ZS, Harrison DG: Vascular superoxide production and vasomotor function in hypertension induced by deoxycorticosterone acetate-salt. *Circulation* 2000, 101(14):1722–1728.

25. Laursen JB, Somers M, Kurz S, *et al.*: Endothelial regulation of vasomotion in apoE-deficient mice: implications for interactions between peroxynitrite and tetrahydrobiopterin. *Circulation* 2001, 103(9):1282–1288.

26. Hong HJ, Hsiao G, Cheng TH, Yen MH: Supplemention with tetrahydrobiopterin suppresses the development of hypertension in spontaneously hypertensive rats. *Hypertension* 2001, 38(5):1044–1048.

27. Fukai T, Siegfried MR, Ushio-Fukai M, *et al.*: Modulation of extra-cellular superoxide dismutase expression by angiotensin II and hypertension. *Circ Res* 1999, 85:23–28.

28. Imig JD, Falck JR, Wei S, *et al.*: Epoxygenase metabolites contribute to nitric oxide-independent afferent arteriolar vasodilation in response to bradykinin. *J Vasc Res* 2001, 38:247–255.

29. Fleming I: Cytochrome p450 and vascular homeostasis. *Circ Res* 2001, 89:753–762.

30. Fisslthaler B, Popp R, Kiss L, *et al.*: Cytochrome P450 2C is an EDHF synthase in coronary arteries. *Nature* 1999, 401:493–497.

31. Griendling KK, Alexander RW: Cellular biology of blood vessels. In *Hurst's The Heart*. Edited by Schlant RC, Alexander RW, O'Rourke R, *et al.* New York: McGraw-Hill; 1994:31–45.

32. Harrison D: The endothelial cell. *Heart Dis Stroke* 1992, 1:95–99.

33. Deal JE, Shah V, Goodenough V, *et al.*: Red cell membrane sodium transport: possible genetic role and use in identifying patients at risk of essential hypertension. *Arch Dis Child* 1990, 65:1154–1157.

34. Aviv A, Lasker N: Proposed defects in membrane transport and intracellular ions as pathogenetic factors in essential hypertension. In *Hypertension: Pathophysiology, Diagnosis, and Management*. Edited by Laragh JH, Brenner BM: New York: Raven Press; 1990:923–937.

35. Taddei S, Ghiadoni L, Virdis A, *et al.*: Vasodilation to bradykinin is mediated by an ouabain-sensitive pathway as a compensatory mechanism for impaired nitric oxide availability in essential hypertensive patients. *Circulation* 1999, 100:1400–1405.

36. Dudley CRK, Taylor DJ, Ng LL, *et al.*: Evidence for abnormal Na^+/H^+ antiport activity detected by phosphorus nuclear magnetic resonance spectroscopy in exercising skeletal muscle of patients with essential hypertension. *Clin Sci* 1990, 79:791–797.

37. Rosskopf D, Fromter E, Siffert W: Hypertensive sodium-proton exchanger phenotype persists in immortalized lymphoblasts from essential hypertensive patients. *J Clin Invest* 1993, 92:2553–2559.

38. Lifton RP, Hunt SC, Williams RR, *et al.*: Exclusion of the Na^+/H^+ antiporter as a candidate gene in human essential hypertension. *Hypertension* 1991, 17:8–14.

39. Rosskopf D, Dusing R, Siffert W: Membrane sodium-proton exchange and primary hypertension. *Hypertension* 1993, 21:607–617.

40. Berk BC, Vallega G, Muslin AJ, *et al.*: Spontaneously hypertensive rat vascular smooth muscle cells in culture exhibit increased growth and Na^+/H^+ exchange. *J Clin Invest* 1989, 83:822–829.

41. Rebbeck TR, Turner ST, Michels V, *et al.*: Genetic and environmental explanations for the distribution of sodium-lithium countertransport in pedigrees from Rochester, MN. *Am J Hum Genet* 1991, 48:1092–1104.

42. Turner ST, Rebbeck TR, Sing CF: Sodium-lithium countertransport and probability of hypertension in caucasians 47 to 89 years old. *Hypertension* 1992, 20:841–850.

43. Resink TJ, Tkachuk VA, Erne P, *et al.*: Platelet membrane Ca^{2+}-ATPase: blunted calmodulin-stimulation in essential hypertension. *J Hypertens* 1985, 3:S37–S40.

Cardiovascular Risk Assessment in Hypertension

William B. Kannel

Hypertension, along with the dyslipidemia and glucose intolerance that often accompanies it, plays a major role in the development of coronary disease, stroke, peripheral artery disease, and heart failure. The accelerated atherogenesis it promotes is a complex process involving coexistent risk factors, all of which impair endothelial function. The prevalence of hypertension and these major cardiovascular disease (CVD) risk factors is still unacceptably high. Hypertensive persons have significantly increased total and low-density lipoprotein (LDL) cholesterol, elevated triglycerides, and impaired glucose tolerance that augment the hazard of elevated blood pressure.

Hypertension increases CVD incidence two- to threefold. The risk ratio imposed is greatest for heart failure, but coronary disease is the most common hazard, equaling in incidence all the other hypertensive sequelae combined. Unrecognized myocardial infarctions are particularly common, necessitating periodic electrocardiogram (ECG) surveillance to detect them. CVD risk increases incrementally with the blood pressure even within the high-normal range. Because moderate blood pressure elevation is much more prevalent than severe elevations, a large fraction of CVD attributable to hypertension derives from seemingly innocuous levels of hypertension. Systolic blood pressure is now accepted as a greater adverse influence than diastolic pressure, particularly in the elderly, and isolated systolic hypertension is shown to confer substantial CVD risk. Furthermore, the CVD hazard of systolic hypertension appears to increase the greater the accompanying pulse pressure.

Other risk factors should be routinely sought and measured in all patients with hypertension because of the tendency for dyslipidemia and impaired glucose tolerance to cluster with elevated blood pressure. Hypertension occurs in isolation in only about 20% of patients. The size of the cluster of accompanying risk factors mirrors weight gain and loss. The burden of coexistent risk factors promoted by visceral adiposity and insulin resistance profoundly affects the CVD hazard of hypertension. High-risk hypertension is that accompanied by one or more of the following: a high total/high-density lipoprotein (HDL)-cholesterol ratio, impaired glucose tolerance, left ventricular hypertrophy, tachycardia, cardiomegaly, proteinuria, and cigarette smoking. The urgency and choice of treatment should take into account these associated risk factors, as well as the character of the blood pressure elevation.

Global multivariable risk assessment of hypertension as a component of a CVD risk profile is readily accomplished for any of its CVD hazards using risk assessment algorithms based on Framingham Study data. Hypertensive persons are more optimally targeted for treatment after consideration of coexistent risk factors, and therapy should have as its goal improvement of the global risk. By quantifying the hazard, it is possible to avoid needlessly alarming mildly hypertensive persons with no other risk factors, or falsely reassuring those with multiple marginal risk factor levels.

Measures are available to improve all of the major risk factors that accompany hypertension using medication and changes in lifestyle. A lifestyle that promotes hypertensive CVD or elevated blood pressure itself includes lack of exercise, faulty diet, unrestrained weight gain, and cigarette smoking. Antihypertensive therapy for isolated systolic hypertension, the predominant variety in the elderly, is of proven effectiveness in preventing stroke and coronary disease and seems likely to also benefit the middle-aged. The efficacy of correcting abdominal obesity and insulin resistance is unproven, but these are known to promote the atherogenic dyslipidemia and impaired glucose tolerance that accompanies hypertension.

Despite the proven efficacy of vigorous control of blood pressure elevation of any variety, at any age, in both sexes, Joint National Committee (JNC) VI–recommended goals for hypertension treatment are not being achieved. This is particularly the case for systolic hypertension.

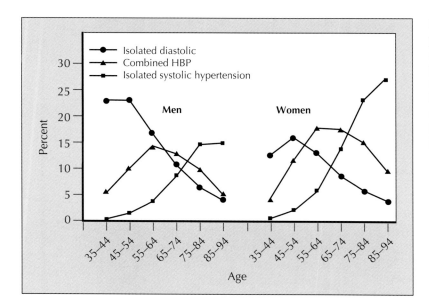

FIGURE 5-1. Prevalence of isolated systolic and diastolic blood pressure by age in each gender. The prevalence of isolated diastolic blood pressure declines sharply with age after age 55 years, whereas the prevalence of isolated systolic hypertension rises steeply from age 35 on. The prevalence of isolated systolic hypertension in women exceeds that in men at all ages beyond age 55. Isolated systolic hypertension is the dominant variety, accounting for about 60% of hypertension in the elderly. HBP—high blood pressure. (*Adapted from* Kannel [1].)

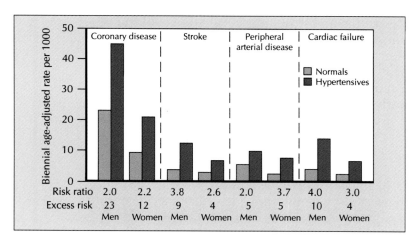

FIGURE 5-2. Risk of cardiovascular disease (CVD) events by hypertensive status in Framingham Study subjects ages 35 to 64 years. Hypertension contributes to atherosclerotic CVD sequelae of elevated blood pressure. Although risk ratios are higher for heart failure and stroke, coronary disease is the most common outcome of uncontrolled hypertension. Its incidence equals all the other CVD sequelae combined. (*Adapted from* Kannel [2].)

CLINICAL MANIFESTATIONS OF CORONARY HEART DISEASE BY HYPERTENSIVE STATUS

	\multicolumn{8}{c}{AGE-ADJUSTED RATE PER 1000}							
	ANGINA PECTORIS[†]		MYOCARDIAL INFARCTION[†]		SUDDEN DEATH[†]		TOTAL CHD[†]	
HYPERTENSIVE STATUS*	MEN	WOMEN	MEN	WOMEN	MEN	WOMEN	MEN	WOMEN
Normal	7.6	5.8	8.4	3.0	7.2	1.3	17.4	9.6
Mild	14.7	10.1	16.8	5.8	7.5	2.3	32.2	17.5
Definite	16.1	12.4	12.1	8.0	9.4	2.7	43.5	23.4

*Normal, < 140/90 mm Hg; mild, 140–159/90–94 mm Hg; definite, ≥ 160/95 mm Hg.
[†]All trends significant at $P < 0.001$; subjects 35–94 years of age.

FIGURE 5-3. Clinical manifestations of coronary heart disease (CHD) by hypertensive status: 30-year follow-up data from the Framingham Study. Hypertension predisposes to all clinical manifestations of coronary disease, including angina pectoris, myocardial infarction, and sudden death. This imposed risk is independent of other related risk factors including glucose intolerance, dyslipidemia, cigarette smoking, and left ventricular hypertrophy. (*Adapted from* Wilson and Kannel [3].)

MYOCARDIAL INFARCTIONS UNRECOGNIZED ACCORDING TO HYPERTENSIVE STATUS

	\multicolumn{6}{c}{UNRECOGNIZED MYOCARDIAL INFARCTIONS, %}					
	EXCLUDING DIABETICS*		EXCLUDING ANTI-HBP THERAPY*		EXCLUDING , LVH*	
HYPERTENSIVE STATUS	MEN	WOMEN	MEN	WOMEN	MEN	WOMEN
Normal	18.5	30.7	17.8	26.6	19.6	29.0
Mild	28.3	36.1	30.2	35.5	31.1	35.3
Definite	33.2	48.1	34.8	48.5	32.7	50.5

*Also excludes persons with CHD at examination immediately before MI.

FIGURE 5-4. Proportion of myocardial infarctions (MIs) that go unrecognized by hypertensive status. Hypertension is a powerful risk factor for MI that is often silent or unrecognized. Among hypertensive women who sustain an MI, approximately half are unrecognized; among men the fraction is one third. This is almost double the fraction in normotensive persons. This propensity for unrecognized MIs persists after exclusion of possible confounders such as diabetes, anti-hypertensive therapy, and electro-cardiogram-left ventricular hypertrophy (ECG-LVH). This is serious because unrecognized MIs carry the same prognosis as symptomatic MI patients who survive hospitalization. CHD—coronary heart disease; HBP—high blood pressure. (*Adapted from* Kannel *et al.* [4].)

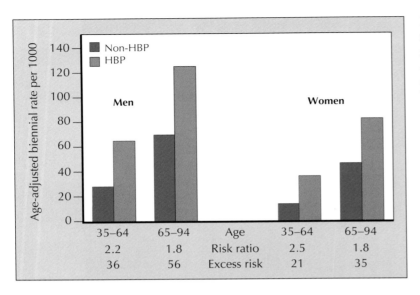

FIGURE 5-5. Risk of cardiovascular disease (including coronary disease, stroke, heart failure, and intermittent claudication) imposed by hypertension (> 60/90 mm Hg). Data are displayed by age for men and women. Hypertension remains relevant in the elderly. The risk ratio diminishes with age; however, this is offset by a higher absolute and excess risk in the elderly. Women appear to have lower absolute and excess risk than men at all ages; however, their relative risk compared with normotensive persons of the same sex is just as much as that for men. HBP—high blood pressure. (*Adapted from* Kannel [5].)

POPULATION ATTRIBUTABLE RISK OF CARDIOVASCULAR DISEASE BY JNC-VI BLOOD PRESSURE CATEGORY

FRAMINGHAM STUDY SUBJECTS AGES 65–94 Y

CVD ATTRIBUTABLE TO ELEVATED BLOOD PRESSURE, %		AMONG HYPERTENSIVE PERSONS ATTRIBUTABLE TO STAGES OF HYPERTENSION, %[*]				
		HIGH NORMAL, %	STAGE 1	STAGE 2	STAGE 3	ON MEDICATION
Men	31.6	6.6	25.1	22.5	12.9	32.9
Women	26.5	2.3	18.1	4.9	10.6	64.1

[*]High normal (130–139/85–89); stage 1 (140–159/90–99); stage 3 (> 180/110).

FIGURE 5-6. Population attributable risk for cardiovascular disease (CVD) by blood pressure category in elderly Framingham Study subjects. A substantial proportion of CVD in the elderly is attributable to hypertension, coming mostly from those with moderate blood pressure elevation. Odds ratios increase steeply with the blood pressure level, but because milder degrees of hypertension are much more common than severe hypertension, most of the CVD events arise from those who have seemingly innocuous blood pressure elevation. JNC—Joint National Committee. (*Adapted from* Kannel [6].)

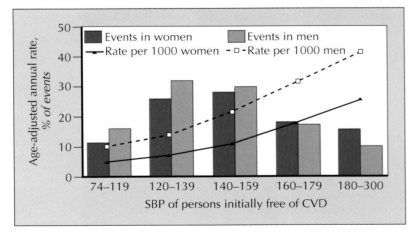

FIGURE 5-7. Annual rate and proportion of cardiovascular disease (CVD) events by level of systolic blood pressure (SBP). As demonstrated by 38-year follow-up data from the Framingham Study, in subjects ages 35 to 64 years, blood pressure exerts a continuous graded influence on CVD occurrence, but most events occur at pressures in the high-normal and mild-hypertensive range. Each 10-mm Hg increment in SBP increases risk 20% to 25% at ages 35 to 64 and by 13% to 14% at ages 65 to 94 years.

RELATION OF NONHYPERTENSIVE BLOOD PRESSURE CATEGORIES TO THE DEVELOPMENT OF CARDIOVASCULAR DISEASE

FRAMINGHAM STUDY SUBJECTS AGES 35–90 Y

10-Y CUMULATIVE INCIDENCE

BLOOD PRESSURE CATEGORY (MM HG)	WOMEN		MEN	
	AGE-ADJUSTED RATE, %	HAZARD RATIO	AGE-ADJUSTED RATE, %	HAZARD RATIO
Optimal (< 120/80)	1.9	1.0	5.8	1.0
Normal (120–129/80–84)	2.8	1.5	7.6	1.6
High-normal (130–139/85–89)	4.4	2.5	10.1	2.0

P value for trend across categories < 0.001 < 0.001.
Stratified by examination and adjusted for age, BMI, total cholesterol, diabetes, smoking.

FIGURE 5-8. Relation of nonhypertensive blood pressure to development of cardiovascular disease (CVD). In Framingham Study subjects ages 35 to 90 years, high-normal blood pressure (130–139/85–89 mm Hg) compared with optimal blood pressure (120/80) is associated with a risk factor–adjusted hazard ratio for CVD of 2.5 in women and 2.0 in men. There is a significant trend in CVD risk from optimal, to normal, to high-normal systolic blood pressure. BMI—body mass index. (*Adapted from* Vasan *et al.* [7].)

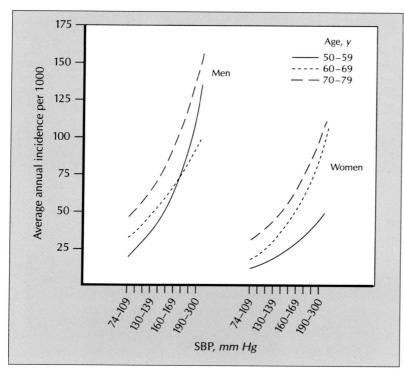

FIGURE 5-9. Risk of cardiovascular disease (CVD) by systolic blood pressure (SBP) in persons with normal diastolic blood pressure. No evidence exists to support the contention that the CVD sequelae of hypertension derive chiefly from the diastolic component of blood pressure. Risk of CVD in Framingham Study subjects increases in relation to systolic blood pressure even in persons whose diastolic blood pressure has not exceeded 95 mm Hg during 20 years of follow-up. The risk increases with systolic pressure at all ages in both men and women. (*Adapted from* Kannel [2].)

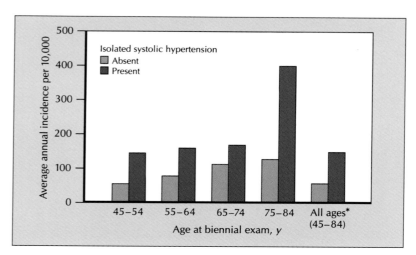

FIGURE 5-10. Risk of myocardial infarction with isolated hypertension (> 160/< 90 mm Hg) in men ages 35 to 84 years over 24 years of follow-up in the Framingham Study. Contrary to the prevailing belief, the impact of systolic blood pressure on CVD risk is greater than that of diastolic blood pressure, particularly in the elderly. In the elderly, isolated systolic hypertension is the most common type of hypertension and exerts a greater influence than isolated diastolic hypertension for CVD in general, and for myocardial infarction in particular (*P* < 0.001). (*Adapted from* Kannel [6]).

RISK OF CARDIOVASCULAR EVENTS BY PULSE PRESSURE: 30-YEAR FOLLOW-UP

FRAMINGHAM STUDY AGE-ADJUSTED RATE PER 1000

PULSE PRESSURE, *MM HG*	35–64 Y		65–94 Y	
	MEN	WOMEN	MEN	WOMEN
2–39	9	4	2	17
40–49	13	6	16	19
50–59	16	7	32	22
60–69	22	10	39	25
70–182	33	16	58	32
Regression coefficient				
Age-adjusted	0.024	0.025	0.024	0.014
Risk-factor adjusted	0.018	0.019	0.021	0.010
All trends significant *P* < 0.001.				

FIGURE 5-11. Risk of cardiovascular events by pulse pressure: Framingham Study (30-year follow-up). Isolated systolic hypertension signifies an elevated pulse pressure, and risk of cardiovascular disease (CVD) increases incrementally with the pulse pressure above and below age 65 in both sexes. The rela-tionship persists on adjustment for age and other associated CVD risk factors. There is a gradual shift from diastolic to systolic and pulse pressure as dominant predictors of coronary disease with increasing age. (*Adapted from* Kannel [1].)

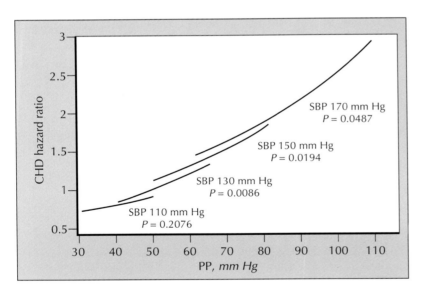

FIGURE 5-12. Impact of pulse pressure (PP) at specified levels of systolic blood pressure (SBP). Investigation of 1924 Framingham Study subjects ages 50 to 79 years without coronary heart disease (CHD) and not on antihypertensive therapy indicated that CHD risk increased at any SBP the lower the accompanying diastolic pressure suggesting that PP is an important determinant of the CHD hazard of blood pressure. Risk of CHD increases with PP at all levels of systolic blood pressure. Neither SBP nor diastolic blood pressure appears superior to PP as a predictor of CHD. (*Adapted from* Franklin *et al.* [8].)

INCREMENTAL INFLUENCE OF ANTECEDENT ELEVATED BLOOD PRESSURE ON CURRENT BLOOD PRESSURE RISK OF STROKE: THE FRAMINGHAM STUDY

INCREMENTAL INFLUENCE ON 10-Y RISK

RELATIVE RISK PER STANDARD DEVIATION INCREMENT*

WOMEN (AGE, Y)	SYSTOLIC BP	DIASTOLIC BP	PULSE PRESSURE
60	1.68 (1.25–2.25)	1.78 (1.33–2.38)	1.80 (1.14–2.58)
70	1.66 (1.28–2.14)	1.44 (1.11–1.88)	1.72 (1.31–2.27)
MEN (AGE, Y)			
60	1.92 (1.39–2.66)	1.73 (1.26–2.38)	1.82 (1.14–2.58)
70	1.30 (0.97–1.75)	1.14 (0.84–1.54)	1.37 (0.99–1.90)

*Relative risk is adjusted for diabetes and smoking status.

FIGURE 5-13. Incremental stroke risk imposed on current blood pressure (BP) by antecedent BP. The 10-year risk of 491 initial ischemic strokes was determined as a function of their 1- to 9-year average antecedent blood pressure adjusted for smoking, diabetes, and baseline BP. All components of antecedent BP further contribute to stroke risk in both hypertensive and nonhypertensive persons. Optimal prevention of late-life stroke requires rigorous control of mid-life BP. (*Adapted from* Seshadri *et al.* [9].)

RISK FACTOR CLUSTERING WITH ELEVATED BLOOD PRESSURE

FRAMINGHAM OFFSPRING AGES 19–74 Y

NUMBER OF RISK FACTORS	AFFLICTED WITH OTHER RISK FACTORS, %	
	MEN	WOMEN
None	19	17
One	26	27
Two	25	24
Three	22	20
Four or more	8	12

FIGURE 5-14. Risk factor clustering with hypertension in Framingham Study offspring ages 18 to 74 years. Hypertension seldom occurs in isolation of other risk factors. More than 80% of patients have one or more coexistent risk factors, and more than 30% have three or more risk factors in the top quintile of their distribution. Because the extent of clustering greatly influences the impact of elevated blood pressure, all hypertensive patients should be tested for the presence of other risk factors. Risk factors in the upper quintile include total cholesterol, body mass index, triglycerides, and glucose; for the bottom quintile, high-density lipoprotein cholesterol. (*Adapted from* Kannel *et al.* [10].)

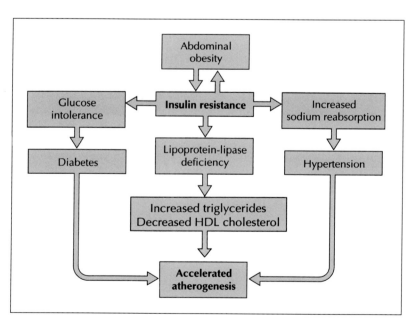

FIGURE 5-15. Risk factors cluster with hypertension because there appears to be a metabolic linkage binding them together. Factor analysis of Framingham Study data suggest that more than one factor underlies the clustering. Glucose intolerance and hypertension appear to be linked to the central syndrome through shared correlations with insulin levels and obesity. Insulin resistance alone does not appear to underlie all features of the "insulin resistance syndrome." However, insulin resistance promoted by abdominal obesity is thought to be responsible for at least some of the clustering of other risk factors with hypertension. Obesity is consistently incriminated as a major determinant of hypertension in population-based epidemiologic research. In the Framingham Study, it is estimated that 70% of hypertension evolving in the population is directly attributable to obesity. HDL—high-density lipoprotein. (*Adapted from* Kannel [6] and Meigs *et al.* [11].)

EXTENT OF RISK FACTOR CLUSTERING IN PERSONS WITH ELEVATED BLOOD PRESSURE BY BODY MASS INDEX

FRAMINGHAM STUDY PARTICIPANTS AGES 18 TO 74 Y

MEN		WOMEN	
BMI	AVERAGE NUMBER OF RISK FACTORS	BMI	AVERAGE NUMBER OF RISK FACTORS
< 23.7	1.68	< 20.8	1.80
23.7–25.5	1.85	20.8–22.3	2.00
25.6–27.2	2.06	22.4–23.9	2.22
27.3–29.5	2.28	24.0–26.8	2.20
> 29.5	2.35	> 26.8	2.66

FIGURE 5-16. Extent of risk factor clustering by body mass index (BMI). The average number of risk factors associated with elevated blood pressure in Framingham Study offspring ages 18 to 74 years increased stepwise with each increment in BMI with no discernible critical value. Risk factors clustering with weight and weight gain in persons with elevated blood pressure included reduced high-density lipoprotein cholesterol and elevated total cholesterol, triglycerides, and blood glucose. (*Adapted from* Kannel *et al.* [10].)

16-Y CORONARY HEART DISEASE INCIDENCE BY NUMBER OF CONCOMITANT RISK FACTORS

FRAMINGHAM STUDY OFFSPRING AGES 30–65 Y WITH ELEVATED BLOOD PRESSURE

NO OTHER RISK FACTORS	RELATIVE RISK	PREVALENCE, %	CHD, %	PAR
MEN				
None	1.0 (ref.)	22	14	—
One	1.33	29	24	0.09
Two or more	2.28	49	63	0.39
WOMEN				
None	1.0 (ref.)	18	5	—
One	2.05	28	18	0.23
Two or more	4.93	54	78	0.68

FIGURE 5-17. Incidence of coronary heart disease (CHD) by number of associated risk factors. In the Framingham Study hypertensive offspring ages 30 to 65 years, the 16-year incidence of CHD increased sharply with the number of associated risk factors. Two or more coexistent risk factors were present in 49% of the men and 54% of the women with hypertension. Of all the CHD events that occurred in hypertensive subjects, 63% in men and 78% in women occurred in those with two or more additional risk factors. Only 14% of the events in men and 5% in women occurred in hypertension unaccompanied by other risk factors. Top quintile risk factors were elevated total cholesterol, triglycerides, body mass index, and diabetes; bottom quintile risk factor: reduced high-density lipoprotein cholesterol. PAR—population attributable risk. (*Adapted from* Kannel *et al.* [10].)

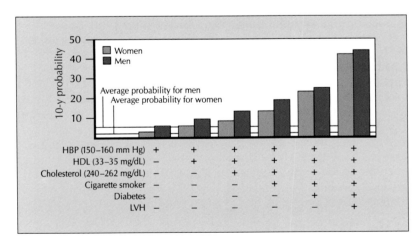

FIGURE 5-18. Risk of coronary disease in hypertension by increasing number of associated risk factors in Framingham Study subjects ages 42 to 43 years. The cluster of metabolically linked risk factors that usually accompany hypertension greatly influences the cardiovascular disease (CVD) hazard of the elevated blood pressure. Risk of coronary heart disease varies widely and is concentrated in those hypertensives who have one or more of the following additional risk factors: dyslipidemia, diabetes, left ventricular hypertrophy (LVH), or cigarette smoking. Coexistent risk factors exert a greater influence on the CVD outlook than the character (*ie,* systolic, diastolic) of the hypertension. It is essential to measure the other risk factors when evaluating patients with hypertension for treatment. HBP—high blood pressure; HDL—high-density lipoprotein. (*Adapted from* Kannel [5].)

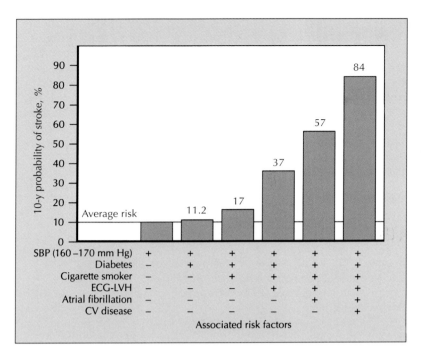

FIGURE 5-19. Probability of a stroke in mildly hypertensive Framingham Study men aged 63 to 65 years according to associated risk factors. As for coronary disease, hypertensive candidates for a stroke are those who have accompanying diabetes, left ventricular hypertrophy (LVH), or the cigarette habit—particularly if they have already developed coronary disease, heart failure, or atrial fibrillation. Risk varies widely depending on the burden of these associated risk factors. CV—cardiovascular; ECG—electrocardiogram; SBP—systolic blood pressure. (*Adapted from* Kannel [2].)

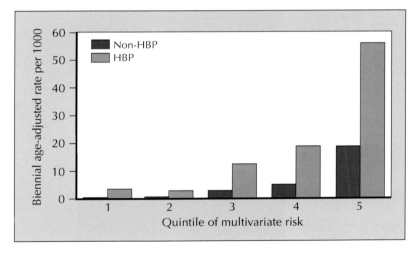

FIGURE 5-20. Risk of heart failure in hypertension by quintile of multivariable risk. In Framingham Study men ages 35 to 94 years, cardiac failure tended to occur in hypertensive persons who have one or more indications of impaired cardiac function such as left ventricular hypertrophy, radiographic cardiomegaly, a rapid resting heart rate, heart murmur, or reduced vital capacity. Risk of heart failure increases in proportion to the number of these impairments and with the presence of coronary disease or diabetes. HBP—high blood pressure. (*Adapted from* Kannel *et al.* [12].)

BENEFIT OF QUITTING SMOKING IN HYPERTENSIVE PATIENTS

	DECREASE IN CORONARY ATTACK IN 2 YEARS, %	
CIGARETTES PER DAY	MEN	WOMEN
10 (1/2 pack)	19	24
20 (1 pack)	34	40
40 (2 packs)	57	64

FIGURE 5-21. Benefit of quitting smoking in hypertensive patients. Based on 20-year follow-up data from the Framingham Study, it is estimated that persons who quit smoking can reduce their risk of coronary attacks by 20% to 60%. The benefit of quitting increases the more the patient smokes and can be achieved regardless of how long the patient has previously smoked. Upon quitting, risk of cardiovascular disease is reduced promptly to half that of those who continue to smoke. Risk decreases to the nonsmoker's level within 2 years if smoking abatement is sustained. Counseling against cigarette smoking should have a high priority in the preventive management of hypertension.

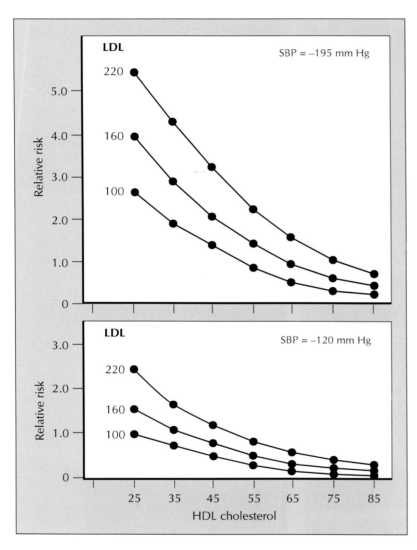

FIGURE 5-22. Relative risk of coronary disease according to high-density lipoprotein cholesterol (HDL-C), low-density lipoprotein cholesterol (LDL-C), and systolic blood pressure (SBP) in men aged 50 to 70 years who participated in the Framingham Study. Dyslipidemia, which often accompanies hypertension, greatly increases its cardiovascular disease hazard. Among hypertensive persons, the greater the total/HDL or LDL/HDL cholesterol ratio, the greater its coronary heart disease (CHD) potential. This ratio, which reflects the net effect of the two-way traffic of cholesterol entering and leaving the arterial intima, constitutes the most efficient lipoprotein profile for predicting CHD. At any LDL-C level, CHD risk is greater the lower the accompanying HDL-C, and at any HDL-C level, risk increases in accordance with the LDL-C level. Control of blood lipids is an important feature of optimal preventive management of hypertension (*Adapted from* Kannel [13].)

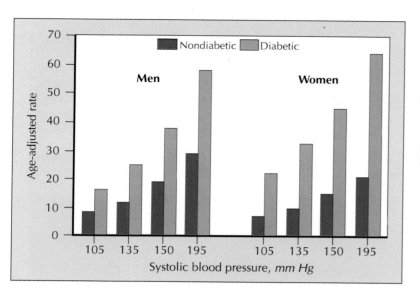

FIGURE 5-23. Risk of peripheral artery disease by systolic blood pressure and diabetic status in Framingham Study patients aged 65 years over 26-year follow-up. This risk was estimated in patients who did not smoke, had cholesterol levels of 185 mg/dL, and had no left ventricular hypertrophy. Even in these otherwise low-risk patients, diabetes almost doubles the risk. Even lesser degrees of glucose intolerance greatly augment the risk for cardiovascular disease (CVD) sequelae of hypertension. Diabetes eliminates the CVD advantage hypertensive women have over men. (*Adapted from* Kannel and McGee [14].)

RISK REDUCTION WITH CALCIUM CHANNEL BLOCKERS IN DIABETICS AND NONDIABETIC HYPERTENSIVES

	SYST-EUR STUDY	
	RISK REDUCTION, %	
	DIABETICS	NONDIABETICS
Outcomes		
Overall mortality	55*	6
CVD mortality	76*	13
CVD events	69	26
Stroke	NS	38
Cardiac events	NS	21

Adjusted relative hazards: *P <0.05.

FIGURE 5-24. Risk reduction with calcium channel blockers in diabetic versus nondiabetic hypertensives in the Syst-Eur Study. The benefit of blood pressure control is especially great in the diabetic hypertensive patient for all outcomes including overall and cardiovascular disease (CVD) mortality, CVD events, stroke, and cardiac events. This was also found in the Systolic Hypertension in the Elderly (SHEP) trial using diuretic-based therapy. NS—not significant (*Adapted from* Tuomilehto *et al.* [15].)

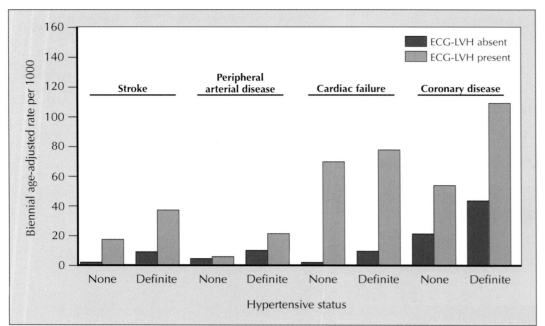

FIGURE 5-25. Risk of cardiovascular events by hypertensive and electrocardiogram–left ventricular hypertrophy (ECG-LVH) status. Based on 32 years of follow-up in the Framingham Study, in men aged 35 to 64 years, it is evident that ECG-LVH is an ominous harbinger of cardiovascular disease in persons with hypertension. Hypertension, obesity, and diabetes are major determinants of LVH in the general population. When it occurs, it greatly escalates risk of all the major sequelae of hypertension including coronary disease, heart failure, stroke, and even peripheral artery disease.

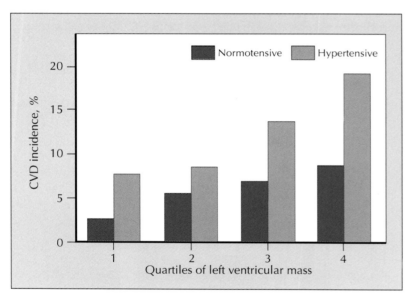

FIGURE 5-26. Four-year cardiovascular disease (CVD) rates in women participating in the Framingham Study according to echo–left ventricular hypertrophy (Echo-LVH) and hypertensive status. Echocardiographic examination provides a more sensitive and specific indication of the extent of LVH in terms of wall thickness and left ventricular mass than does the ECG or chest film. There is a continuous graded relationship of left ventricular mass to the rate of development of CVD in hypertensive persons. There is no discernable critical degree of left ventricular mass that separates presumed compensatory from pathologic hypertrophy in either normotensive or hypertensive persons. (*Adapted from* Levy *et al.* [16].)

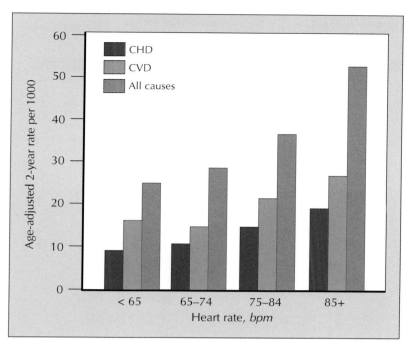

FIGURE 5-27. Association of heart rate with mortality in hypertensive men in the Framingham Study. Hypertensive persons tend to have more rapid heart rates than do those who are normotensive. The hazard of deaths from major cardiovascular disease (CVD) sequelae of hypertension tends to increase the higher the heart rate accompanying their hypertension. Occurrence of fatal CVD events is more strongly influenced by the heart rate than are nonfatal sequelae. bpm—beats per minute; CHD—coronary heart disease. (*Adapted from* Gillman *et al.* [17].)

CARDIOVASCULAR DISEASE PREVALENCE IN HYPERTENSION (≥ 160/95 MM HG)

| | PERCENT WITH CV CONDITION | | | |
| | AGE 35–64 | | AGE 65–89 | |
PERSON-EXAMINATIONS	MEN	WOMEN	MEN	WOMEN
Person-examinations, *n*	650	443	237	438
Angina	4.0%	4.5%	12.2%	16.0%
MI	4.8%	1.8%	11.9%	4.6%
CHF	0.6%	1.0%	3.0%	4.9%
Stroke	1.0%	0.7%	9.5%	4.9%
IC	2.0%	2.6%	9.0%	6.2%
CVD (≥ 1)	—	8.5%	31.4%	26.9%

FIGURE 5-28. Prevalence of cardiovascular disease (CVD) by hypertension status in Framingham Study men and women ages 35 to 64 and 65 to 89 years. Many hypertensive persons already have overt CVD when first encountered. They should be queried and examined carefully for its presence. Among those older than 65, 27% to 31% will have one or more CVD conditions. These associated conditions markedly influence the subsequent risk of CVD events and the choice of therapy for the hypertension. CHF—congestive heart failure; IC—intermittent claudication; MI—myocardial infarction. (*Adapted from* Kannel [5].)

A. ESTIMATION OF 10-Y RISK OF CORONARY DISEASE FOR MEN

FRAMINGHAM STUDY MULTIVARIABLE POINT SCORES

AGE	POINTS	TOTAL CHOLESTEROL	POINTS	HDL-C	POINTS
35–39	0	< 160 mg/dL	–3	< 35 mg/dL	2
40–44	1	160–199 mg/dL	0	35–44 mg/dL	1
45–49	2	200–239 mg/dL	1	45–49 mg/dL	0
50–54	3	240—279 mg/dL	2	50–59 mg/dL	0
55–59	4	> 280 mg/dL	–2	> 60 mg/dL	–2

SYSTOLIC BP	DIASTOLIC BP					DIABETES	POINTS	SMOKER	POINTS
	< 80	80–84	85–89	90–99	> 100				
< 120						No	0	No	0
120–129	0	0	0	2	3	Yes	2	Yes	2
130–139	0	0	1	2	3				
140–159	2	2	2	2	3				
> 160	3	3	3	3	3				

COMPARATIVE CHD RISK

AGE	AVERAGE 10-Y RISK, %
35–39	5
40–44	7
45–49	11
50–54	14
55–59	16
60–64	21
65–69	25
70–74	30

CORONARY DISEASE RISK

TOTAL POINTS	10-Y RISK, %	TOTAL POINTS	10-Y RISK, %
1	3	8	16
2	4	9	20
3	5	10	25
4	7	11	31
5	8	12	37
6	10	13	45
7	13	> 14	> 53

FIGURE 5-29. A and **B**, Estimation of 10-year coronary heart disease (CHD) risk using Framingham Multivariable Scores. Because hypertension is usually accompanied by additional risk factors, the urgency for treatment should be based on a global risk assessment. Gender-specific prediction equations have been formulated to estimate CHD risk according to age, diabetes, smoking, Joint National Committee-V blood pressure, and National Cholesterol Education Program total cholesterol categories.

Continued on next page

FRAMINGHAM STUDY MULTIVARIABLE POINT SCORES

AGE	POINTS	TOTAL CHOLESTEROL	POINTS	HDL-C	POINTS
35–39	–4	< 160 mg/dL	–2	< 35 mg/dL	5
40–44	0	160–199 mg/dL	0	35–44 mg/dL	2
45–49	3	200–239 mg/dL	1	45–49 mg/dL	1
50–54	6	240—279 mg/dL	1	50–59 mg/dL	0
55–59	7	> 280 mg/dL	–2	> 60 mg/dL	–3

SYSTOLIC BP	DIASTOLIC BP					DIABETES	POINTS	SMOKER	POINTS
	< 80	80–84	85–89	90–99	> 100	No	0	No	0
< 120						Yes	4	Yes	2
120–129	-3	0	0	2	3				
130–139	0	0	0	2	3				
140–159	2	2	2	2	3				
> 160	3	3	3	3	3				

CORONARY DISEASE RISK

POINTS	10-Y RISK, %	POINTS	10-Y RISK, %
1	2	8	7
2	3	9	8
3	3	10	11
4	4	11	11
5	4	12	15
6	5	13	17
7	6	14	18
8	7	15	20
9	8	16	24
10	10	> 17	> 27

COMPARATIVE CHD RISK

AGE	AVERAGE 10-Y RISK, %
35–39	< 1
40–44	2
45–49	5
50–54	8
55–59	12
60–64	12
65–69	13
70–74	14

FIGURE 5-29. (Continued) The accuracy of this categorical approach is comparable with CHD prediction when continuous risk factor variables are used. Using the Framingham point scores, it is possible to pull together all the relevant information to make a quantitative estimate of the absolute and relative risk of a coronary event by simply adding designated points for each risk factor. BP—blood pressure; HDL-C—high-density lipoprotein cholesterol. (*Adapted from* Wilson *et al.* [18].)

CONTROL OF SYSTOLIC VERSUS DIASTOLIC BLOOD PRESSURE

FRAMINGHAM STUDY PARTICIPANTS 1990 TO 1995

	ALL HYPERTENSIVE SUBJECTS, %	ON TREATMENT, %
Control of		
Systolic BP (< 140 mm Hg)	32.7	49.0
Diastolic BP (< 90 mm Hg)	82.9	89.7
Both (< 140/90 mm Hg)	29.0	47.8

FIGURE 5-30. Control of systolic versus diastolic blood pressure (BP) in Framingham Study hypertensive participants, 1990 to 1995. Consistent with data from elsewhere, control of systolic pressure in the Framingham Study is particularly poor (49%) compared with diastolic BP in persons on treatment for hypertension. Poor systolic BP control in the Framingham Study was associated with older age, obesity, and left ventricular hypertrophy. (*Adapted from* Lloyd-Jones *et al.* [19].)

FAILURE TO REACH JNC-VI BLOOD PRESSURE GOALS IN SPECIFIED HYPERTENSION SUBGROUPS

		NOT A GOAL, %	
PATIENT SUBGROUP	GOAL	SYSTOLIC	DIASTOLIC
Uncomplicated	< 140/90	64	26
Black	< 140/90	62	37
Elderly	< 140/90	78	9
Diabetics	<130/85	81	24

FIGURE 5-31. Failure to reach Joint National Committee (JNC)-VI blood pressure goals in specified subgroups of hypertensive persons. Many patients are failing to achieve JNC-VI recommended blood pressure goals. The JNC-VI blood pressure goals for hypertensive patients are less than 140/90 mm Hg for uncomplicated patients to less than 130/85 mm Hg for diabetes or impaired renal function. Blood pressure is poorly controlled in 26% of persons with hypertension. This is predominantly due to failure to reach goals for systolic pressure in all subgroups including blacks, the elderly, people with diabetes, and those with uncomplicated hypertension. Among people with diabetes, 81% are not at their recommended systolic blood pressure goal. Of those with uncomplicated hypertension, 64% are not achieving the JNC systolic blood pressure recommended goal. Failure to control pressure in the elderly and in people with diabetes is particularly unfortunate, because the benefits of blood pressure control are greatest in these hypertensive patients. (*Adapted from* JNC-VI and National Health and Nutrition Examination Survey III [20,21].)

REFERENCES

1. Kannel WB: Elevated systolic blood pressure as a cardiovascular risk factor. *Am J Cardiol* 2000, 85:251–255.

2. Kannel WB: Epidemiology of essential hypertension: the Framingham experience. *Proc Royal Coll Phys Edinb* 1991, 21:273–287.

3. Wilson PWF, Kannel WB: Hypertension, other risk factors and the risk of cardiovascular disease. In *Hypertension: Pathophysiology, Diagnosis and Management,* vol 1, edn 2. Edited by Laragh JH, Brenner BM. New York: Raven Press; 1995:99–114.

4. Kannel WB, Dannenberg AL, Abbott RD: Unrecognized myocardial infarction and hypertension: the Framingham Study. *Am Heart J* 1985, 109:581–585.

5. Kannel WB: Potency of vascular risk factors as the basis for antihypertensive therapy. *Eur Heart J* 1992, 13:(suppl G)34–42.

6. Kannel WB: Prospects for prevention of cardiovascular disease in the elderly. *Prev Cardiol* 1998, 1:32–39.

7. Vasan RS, Larson MG, Leip EP, *et al.*: Impact of high-normal blood pressure on the risk of cardiovascular disease. *N Engl J Med* 2001, 345:1291–1297.

8. Franklin SS, Kahn SA, Wong NA, *et al.*: Is pulse pressure useful in predicting risk for coronary heart disease? The Framingham Study. *Circulation* 1999, 100:354–360.

9. Seshadri S, Wolf PA, Beiser A, *et al.* Elevated midlife blood pressure increases stroke risk in elderly persons: the Framingham Study. *Arch Intern Med* 2001, 161:2343–2350.

10. Kannel WB, Wilson PWF, Silbershatz H, D'Agostino RB: Epidemiology of risk factor clustering in elevated blood pressure. In *Multiple Risk Factors in Cardiovascular Disease.* Edited by Goto AM Jr *et al.* Netherlands: Kluwer Academic Publishers, 1998.

11. Meigs JB, D'Agostino RB, Wilson PWF, *et al.*: Risk variable clustering in the insulin resistance syndrome: the Framingham Offspring Study. *Diabetes* 1997, 46:1594–1600.

12. Kannel WB, D'Agostino RB, Silbershatz H, *et al.*: Profile for estimating risk of heart failure. *Arch Intern Med* 1999, 159:1197–1204.

13. Kannel WB: High-density lipoproteins: epidemiologic profile and risks of coronary artery disease. *Am J Cardiol* 1993, 52:9–13B.

14. Kannel WB, McGee DL: Update on epidemiologic features of intermittent claudication: the Framingham Study. *J Am Geriatr Soc* 1985, 33:13–18.

15. Tuomilehto J, Rastenyte D, Berkenhager WH, *et al.*: Effect of calcium channel blockade in older patients with diabetes and systolic hypertension. *N Engl J Med* 1999, 340:677–684.

16. Levy D, Garrison MS, Savage DD, *et al.*: Left ventricular mass and incidence of CHD in an elderly cohort: the Framingham Study. *Ann Intern Med* 1989, 110:101–107.

17. Gillman MW, Kannel WB, Belanger AJ, D'Agostino RB: Influence of heart rate on mortality among persons with hypertension: the Framingham Study. *Am Heart J* 1993, 125:1148–1154.

18. Wilson PWF, D'Agostino RB, Levy D, *et al.* : Prediction of coronary heart disease using risk factor categories. *Circulation* 1998, 97:1837–1847.

19. Lloyd-Jones DM, Evans JC, Larson MG, *et al.* : Differential control of systolic and diastolic blood pressure: factors associated with lack of blood pressure control in the community. *Hypertension* 2000, 36:504–509.

20. The Sixth Report of the Joint National Committee on Prevention: Evaluation and treatment of high blood pressure. *Arch Intern Med* 1997, 157:2413–2446.

21. *Third National Health and Nutrition Examination Survey (Phase 2)* [CD-ROM]. Hyattesville, MD: National Center for Health Statistics; 1991–1994.

Secondary Hypertension: Adrenal and Nervous Systems

Emmanuel L. Bravo

In most cases of hypertension, the cause is not clear. Such cases are usually termed *essential hypertension*. In the remainder, a specific cause can be identified. The percentage of individuals with so-called *secondary hypertension* ranges from more than 5% of all hypertensive patients presenting in a community clinical practice to more than 30% in referral centers. It is especially important to identify patients with secondary hypertension because correction of the cause will often cure—not merely palliate—the disorder. Of equal importance is the fact that detailed study of patients with secondary hypertension may offer important clues regarding the cause and management of essential hypertension.

This chapter discusses the abnormalities of the adrenal glands (*ie*, cortex and medulla) and nervous system that are responsible for a large fraction of secondary hypertension cases.

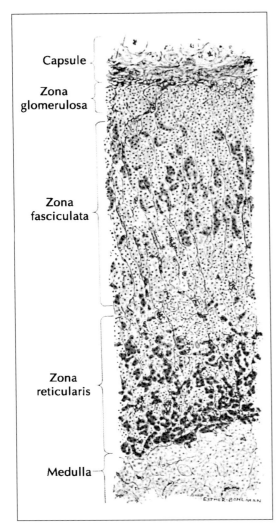

FIGURE 6-1. Adrenal histology in cross-section. The adrenal cortex can cause hypertension through overproduction of deoxycorticosterone (DOC), aldosterone, and cortisol. DOC and aldosterone are mineralocorticoids that produce hypertension through salt and water retention. Cortisol is a glucocorticoid but causes hypertension, in part, by exerting a mineralocorticoid effect because of incomplete metabolism at target tissues. The best-defined circumstances in which DOC plays a significant role in hypertension are DOC-producing tumors and in syndromes characterized by a deficiency of 11β- or 17α-hydroxylation of steroids [1,2]. The latter are usually congenital but may be induced by excessive production of estrogen [3] or androgen [4] from either a benign or malignant tumor.

The adrenal cortex consists of three anatomic zones: zona glomerulosa (ZG), zona fasciculata (ZF), and zona reticularis (ZR). The ZG forms an ill-defined zone around the periphery of the cortex; it is present locally and is never prominent in the normal gland. The cells have relatively small amounts of cytoplasm in which few lipids are seen. The ZF comprises most of the cortex and consists of cells with abundant amounts of cholesterol and its esters in the cytoplasm, causing the cells to appear vacuolated in paraffin-embedded sections. These cells are called clear cells and form columns that extend from either the capsule or the ZG to the ZF. The ZR is the innermost zone of the adrenal cortex adjacent to the adrenal medulla, and consists of networks of interconnecting cells that differ greatly in size, shape, and density. There are much smaller numbers of lipid droplets in these cells. ZR mitochondria are remarkably similar to those of the ZF cells but contain flattened cristae.

Whereas the ZG produces aldosterone, there is some evidence that the ZF and ZR represent different morphologic appearances of a single unit, with both cell types capable of producing cortisol, androgen, and estrogen. Adrenocorticotropic hormone, however, increases cortisol secretion by the clear cells of the ZF but not by the compact cells of the ZR. Mallory azan stain. (*Adapted from* Forsham [5].)

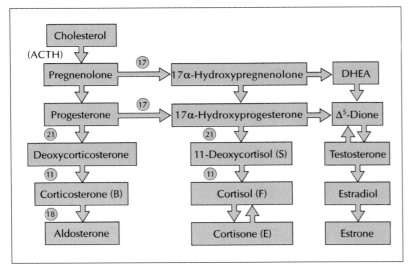

FIGURE 6-2. Pathways of adrenal steroidogenesis. The principal adrenocortical products are aldosterone, cortisol (F), and dehydroepiandrosterone (DHEA) sulfate. The enzymes that transform cholesterol, the main precursor, to the active principal reside in different subcellular particles. The system or systems that transform cholesterol to pregnenolone together with 11β-hydroxylase are found in all mitochondria, while the 18-oxidase system necessary for aldosterone formation resides only in the mitochondria of zona glomerulosa (ZG) cells. The remaining enzymes are located in the endoplasmic reticulum.

The structure, growth, and secretory activity of the ZG are regulated largely by angiotensin II and changes in the concentrations of sodium and potassium in plasma, whereas the zona reticularis (ZR) and zona fasciculata (ZF) are regulated entirely by adrenocorticotropic hormone (ACTH). Only cortisol inhibits ACTH release when present in higher-than-physiologic levels in blood. A decline in cortisol results in ACTH release, thereby raising the level of cortisol that in turn inhibits ACTH release. This continuous feedback inhibition of ACTH by cortisol may be interrupted at any time by an overriding mechanism, such as any stressful situation, an ACTH-producing tumor, or a cortisol-producing tumor of the adrenal cortex. *Letters in parentheses* are designations for steroids. *Circled numbers* represent the following hydroxylases: 11—11β-hydroxylase; 17—17α-hydroxylase; 18—18-hydroxylase; 21—21α-hydroxylase.

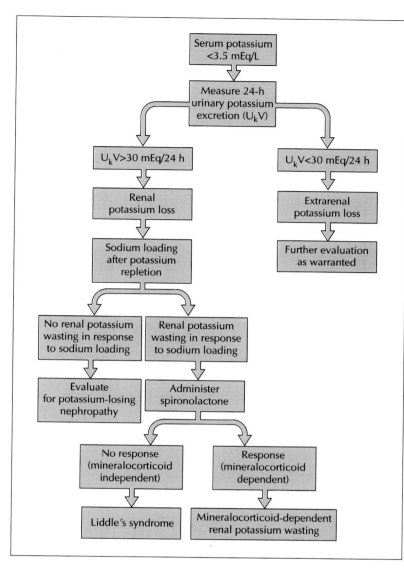

FIGURE 6-3. Algorithmic approach to suspected mineralocorticoid-induced hypertension, which is usually associated with spontaneous hypokalemia [6]. Although hypokalemia is often simply a side effect of diuretics, evaluation is recommended under the following circumstances: diuretic therapy results in serum potassium less than 3.0 mEq/L even if levels normalize when diuretics are withdrawn; oral potassium supplementation and potassium-sparing agents fail to maintain serum potassium values greater than 3.5 mEq/L in a patient on diuretics; or serum potassium levels fail to normalize after 4 weeks of diuretic abstinence.

The initial assessment and subsequent studies should be designed to answer three questions: Is potassium loss renal or extrarenal? If renal, is it steroid- or nonsteroid-dependent? If steroid-dependent, what is its cause? A 24-hour urinary potassium excretion greater than 30 mEq/24 h when the serum potassium is equal to or less than 3.4 mEq/L usually reflects renal potassium wasting, whereas lower excretion rates suggest extrarenal loss caused by diarrhea, vomiting, or laxative abuse. Renal wasting should be investigated further after adequate repletion of total body potassium with oral chloride potassium supplementation. Salt-loading (oral sodium of 250 mEq/24 h for 5 to 7 days) that results in hypokalemia with renal potassium wasting suggests an exaggerated exchange mechanism of sodium for potassium at distal tubular sites mediated by inappropriate secretion of electrolyte-active steroids. An exception to this rule is Liddle's syndrome, a familial, nonsteroid-dependent renal potassium wasting disorder associated with hypokalemia and hypertension (*see* below). Response to spironolactone (50 mg four times daily for 3 to 5 days) can demonstrate conclusively whether renal potassium wasting is truly mineralocorticoid-dependent. If spironolactone produces an elevation in the serum potassium level with concomitant reduction in urinary excretion, potassium wasting is probably mediated by electrolyte-active steroids.

The demonstration of true mineralocorticoid-dependent renal potassium wasting warrants further diagnostic studies to determine the most effective treatment. The determination of dexamethasone responsiveness is the final step in the evaluation, to be undertaken if the physician suspects familial primary aldosteronism. This glucocorticoid-responsive aldosteronism should be suspected in patients with a family history of aldosteronism when imaging techniques fail to reveal anatomic abnormalities in the adrenal glands. Administration of dexamethasone, in doses of 0.5 mg four times daily, usually results in remission of hypertension and hypokalemia in 10 to 14 days.

Liddle's syndrome is an autosomal dominant disorder that mimics the signs and symptoms of mineralocorticoid excess [7]. The fault appears to lie with continuously avid sodium channels in the distal nephron, resulting in excessive salt absorption and potassium wasting (despite negligible aldosterone production) and severe hypertension [8]. A prominent feature is premature death due to stroke or heart failure. The clinical manifestations can be corrected by triamterene and amiloride, but not by spironolactone. Triamterene and amiloride directly block the sodium channel, whereas spironolactone inhibits sodium absorption by binding the aldosterone receptor. (*Adapted from* Bravo [6].)

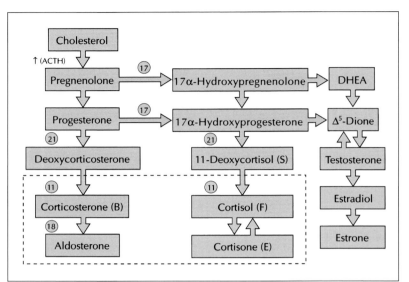

FIGURE 6-4. Abnormalities of steroid production in patients with 11β-hydroxylase deficiency syndrome. Deficiency of 11β-hydroxylase results in reduced production of cortisol, corticosterone, and aldosterone. Subsequent overproduction of adrenocorticotropic hormone (ACTH) drives the pathway in the zona fasciculata leading to increased production of deoxycorticosterone (DOC), which produces a type of mineralocorticoid hypertension. There is also increased formation of dehydroepiandrosterone (DHEA) and androstenedione, which produces hypergonadism. Excess DOC may also contribute to the hypertension associated with ectopic ACTH excess syndrome and in DOC-producing adrenocortical adenomas. Deficiency of 11β-hydroxylase is confirmed by demonstrating increased levels of plasma 11-deoxycortisol (S) and urinary tetrahydro-S and 17-ketosteroids. The *dashed area* encloses the steroids reduced in 11β-hydroxylase deficiency. *Letters in parentheses* are designations for steroids. *Circled numbers* represent the following hydroxylases: 11—11β-hydroxylase; 17—17α-hydroxylase; 18—18-hydroxylase; 21—21α-hydroxylase.

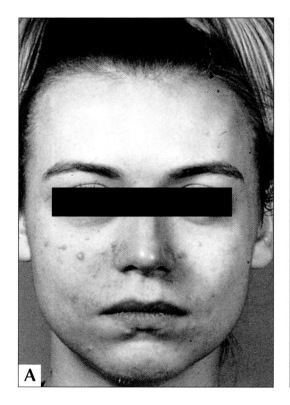

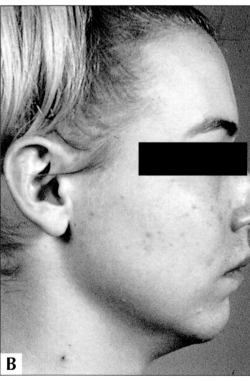

FIGURE 6-5. Findings on physical examination provide the most important clues to the presence of enzymatic deficiency. Virilization in females or precocious puberty with advanced masculinization in males (caused by increased androgen production) are prominent features of 11β-hydroxylase deficiency. **A** and **B,** The physical characteristics of a patient with 11β-hydroxylase deficiency syndrome. These features are the result of excess androgen production. There is prominent recession of the hairline characteristic of male baldness, and the patient also has dark hair on the upper lip and acne.

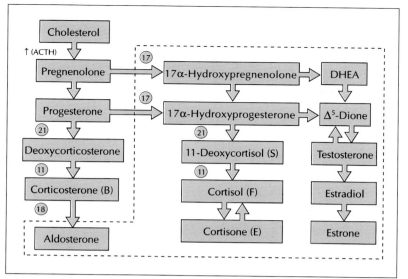

FIGURE 6-6. Abnormalities in steroid production in the 17α-hydroxylase deficiency syndrome. This syndrome results in reduced production of 17α-OH progesterone and the distal steroids in the 17-hydroxy pathway, deoxycortisol, and cortisol. Resultant overproduction of adrenocorticotropic hormone (ACTH) stimulates the uninvolved 17-deoxy pathway to increase the levels of progesterone, deoxycorticosterone (DOC), corticosterone (B), 18-OH DOC, and 18-hydroxycorticosterone. Because DOC causes salt and water retention, total suppression of renin synthesis and subsequent suppression of aldosterone result.

Deficiency of 17α-hydroxylase also causes reduced production of all adrenal and gonadal androgens, including testosterone, dehydroepiandrosterone (DHEA), and androstenedione, which results in a form of hypergonadotropic hypogonadism and abnormalities of sexual development (*dashed area*). Increased production of DOC and corticosterone as well as decreased androgen secretion establish the diagnosis of 17α-hydroxylase deficiency. In both 11β- and 17α-hydroxylase deficiency disorders, dexamethasone, by inhibiting ACTH release, decreases DOC production, thereby resulting in normalization of arterial blood pressure and serum potassium concentration. *Letters in parentheses* are steroid designations. *Circled numbers* represent the following hydroxylases: 11—11β-hydroxylase; 17—17α-hydroxylase; 18—18-hydroxylase; 21—21α-hydroxylase.

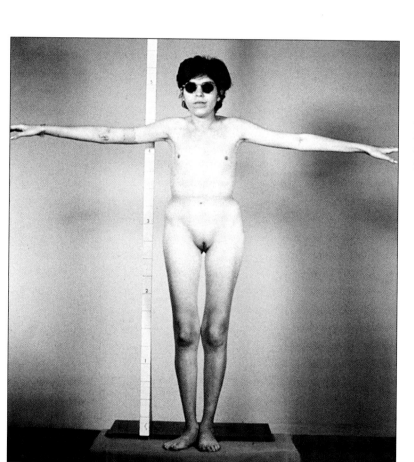

FIGURE 6-7. Physical characteristics of a patient with 17α-hydroxylase deficiency syndrome. The hypogonadal consequences of the enzyme deficiency account for most of the clinical features of the disorder. Women with primary amenorrhea have disproportionately long limbs relative to the trunk, absent axillary and pubic hair, infantile breast and genitalia development, an absent uterus, and an incomplete vagina. In men, the testes do not produce testosterone, causing decreased masculinization; male patients also have reduced axillary and pubic hair and ambiguous genitalia.

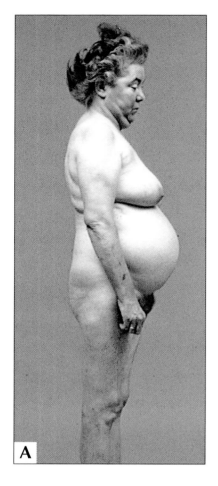

A

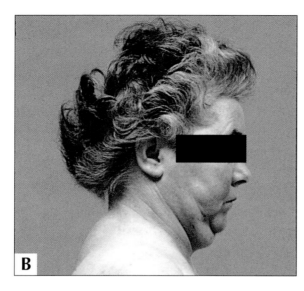

B

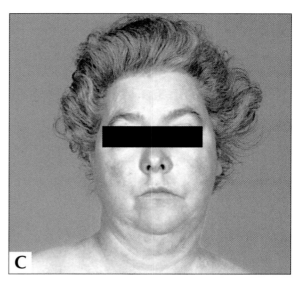

C

FIGURE 6-8. Physical features of Cushing's syndrome. The recognizable causes of Cushing's syndrome include Cushing's disease (72%), ectopic adrenocorticotropic hormone (ACTH) excess (12%), adrenal adenoma (8%), carcinoma (6%), and hyperplasia (4%). The typical clinical presentation of Cushing's syndrome includes truncal obesity, moon facies, hypertension, plethora, muscle weakness and fatigue, hirsutism, emotional disturbances, and typical purple skin striae. Carbohydrate intolerance or diabetes, amenorrhea, loss of libido, easy bruising, and spontaneous fracture of ribs and vertebrae may also be encountered. Patients with ectopic ACTH excess may not have the typical manifestations of cortisol excess but may present with hyperpigmentation of the skin, severe hypertension, and marked hypokalemic alkalosis.

A, There is centripetal distribution of fat associated with significant atrophy of the thigh muscles. B, Side view of the patient revealing a buffalo hump. C, Facial features show the characteristic moon facies with a malar flush. Also obvious are the full supraclavicular fat pads.

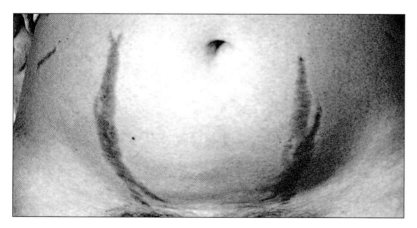

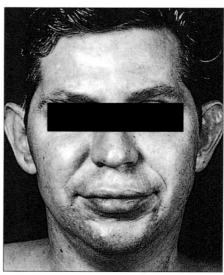

FIGURE 6-9. Abdominal striae caused by excess cortisol production. The striae can also be found along the inner aspects of the upper arms and thighs as well as along the lateral aspects of the breasts. The striae that result from excess cortisol production are purple and can thus be distinguished from the stretch marks produced by obesity or pregnancy, which are whitish or pale.

FIGURE 6-10. Facial features of patients with ectopic adrenocorticotropic hormone excess. The face has a bronzelike tint caused by hyperpigmentation from overproduction of melano-cyte-stimulating hormone. The characteristic moon facies is absent. (*From* Bravo [6]; with permission.)

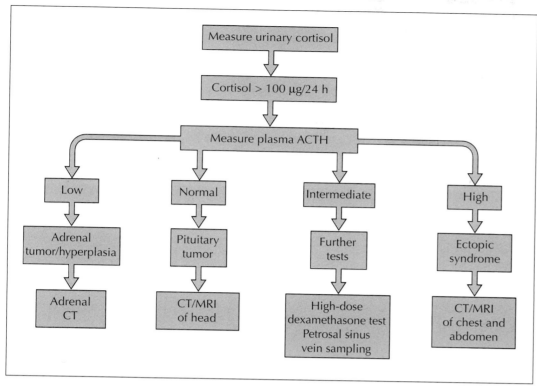

FIGURE 6-11. Differential diagnosis of Cushing's syndrome. Although it is cumbersome to perform, the determination of 24-hour urinary free cortisol is the best available test for documenting endogenous hypercortisolism. A level above 100 µg/24 h suggests excessive cortisol production. There are virtually no false-negative results. False-positive results may, however, be obtained in non-Cushing's hypercortisolemic states (*eg*, stress, chronic strenuous exercise, psychiatric states, glucocorticoid resistance, and malnutrition). If differentiation between pituitary and ectopic sources cannot be made based on plasma levels alone, pharmacologic manipulation of adrenocorticotropic hormone (ACTH) secretion should be performed (*ie*, high-dose dexamethasone suppression test or inferior petrosal sinus sampling for ACTH after corticotropin-releasing hormone administration).

The overnight dexamethasone suppression test requires only a blood collection for serum cortisol the morning after the patient has taken a 1.0-mg dose of dexamethasone at 11 PM the previous evening. In normal subjects, cortisol levels at 8 AM will be suppressed to 5.0 µg/dL or less. When the presence of the syndrome has been verified by appropriate biochemical testing, the cause must be identified. Radioimmunoassay of plasma ACTH is the procedure of choice for pinpointing the basis of hypercortisolism. In patients with ACTH-independent Cushing's syndrome, ACTH levels have usually been suppressed to less than 5 pg/mL. In contrast, patients with the ACTH-dependent form tend to have either normal or elevated levels, usually greater than 10 pg/mL. In patients with Cushing's disease, ACTH release can be inhibited only at much higher doses of dexamethasone

(2 mg every 6 hours for 2 days). The established criterion for the test is that suppression of the 24-hour urine and plasma steroids to less than 50% of baseline indicates pituitary Cushing's syndrome. Failure to suppress to less than 50% of baseline is considered consistent with an ectopic source of ACTH or ACTH-independent Cushing's syndrome.

Surgical resection of a pituitary or ectopic source of ACTH or of a cortisol-producing adrenocortical tumor is the treatment of choice for Cushing's syndrome. For pituitary Cushing's syndrome, transsphenoidal pituitary adenomectomy is the treatment of choice but total hypophysectomy may be required in patients with diffuse hyperplasia or large pituitary tumors. Bilateral adrenalectomy for Cushing's disease is universally successful in alleviating the hypercortisolemic state; however, 10% to 38% of individuals may later develop pituitary tumors and hyperpigmentation (Nelson's syndrome). Radiotherapy (*ie*, external pituitary irradiation, seeding the pituitary bed with yttrium or gold) has also been used with occasionally good results. The long-acting analogue SMS 201-995 (octreotide or sandostatin) has been used with varied success to treat ectopic ACTH syndromes; some benefit has been reported in Cushing's disease and Nelson's syndrome. Cyproheptadine has had limited success in the treatment of Cushing's disease. Ketoconazole, an inhibitor of several steroid biosynthetic pathways, has been used for rapid correction of hyper-cortisolism awaiting definitive intervention. Mitotane (o,p'-DDD), an insecticide derivative, induces destruction of the zonae reticularis and fasciculata with relative sparing of the zona glomerulosa. Mitotane has been used to treat Cushing's syndrome associated with adrenal carcinoma or to suppress cortisol secretion in Cushing's disease.

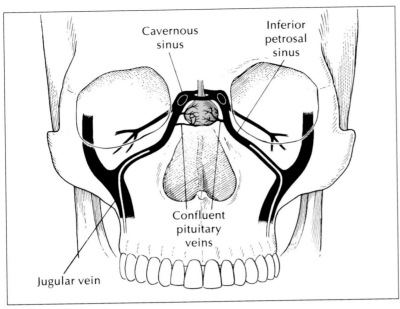

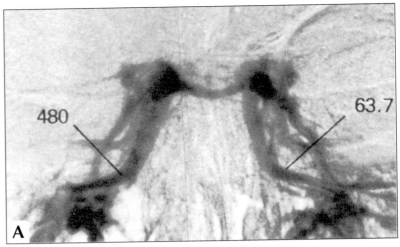

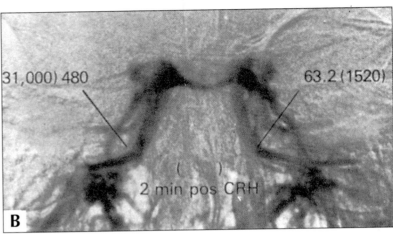

FIGURE 6-12. Catheter sampling for a bilateral simultaneous sample of the inferior petrosal sinus. Inferior petrosal sinus sampling for adrenocorticotropic hormone (ACTH) after corticotropin-releasing hormone (CRH) administration has an accuracy of nearly 100% in distinguishing pituitary from nonpituitary sources of ACTH. The criterion currently used after CRH administration is that the ACTH gradient between the inferior petrosal sinus and the peripheral site will be greater than 2 if the patient has pituitary Cushing's syndrome. Once biochemical evidence gives an indication of the tumor location, either CT or MRI can be performed for confirmation.

A major problem in the differential diagnosis of ACTH-dependent Cushing's syndrome is separating pituitary Cushing's syndrome from the ectopic ACTH syndrome. Both entities may present with similar clinical and laboratory features. In addition, even the most sophisticated radiographic technique may fail to visualize pituitary microadenomas and ectopic ACTH-secreting tumors. Bilateral inferior petrosal venous sinus and peripheral venous catheterization with simultaneous collection of samples for measurement of ACTH is the most accurate method for localizing the source of ACTH production.

During the procedure, venous blood from the anterior pituitary drains into the cavernous sinus and subsequently into the superior and inferior petrosal sinuses. Catheters are led into each inferior petrosal sinus via the ipsilateral femoral vein. The location of the catheters is confirmed radiographically by injection of radiopaque solution. Samples for measuring plasma ACTH are collected from each inferior petrosal sinus and a peripheral vein at 0, 3, 5, and 10 minutes after injection of 1 µg/kg CRH. (*Adapted from* Oldfield *et al.* [9].)

FIGURE 6-13. Inferior petrosal sinuses before (**A**) and after (**B**) ovine corticotropin-releasing hormone (oCRH) was administered. The *numbers in A* indicate plasma immunoreactive–adrenocorticotropic hormone (ACTH) concentrations before oCRH was administered. In *B*, the *numbers in parentheses* indicate plasma immunoreactive–ACTH concentrations 2 minutes after administration of 1 µg/kg oCRH. Patients with the ectopic ACTH syndrome have no ACTH concentration gradient between the inferior petrosal sinus and the peripheral sample. An increased gradient (≥ 2.0) of plasma ACTH between any or both of the inferior petrosal sinuses is highly suggestive of pituitary Cushing's syndrome. (*From* Kamilaris and Chrousos [10]; with permission.)

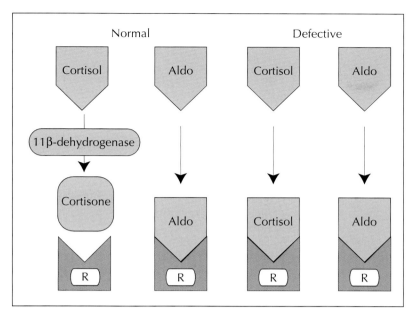

FIGURE 6-14. Activation of mineralocorticoid receptors by cortisone. 11β-hydroxysteroid dehydrogenase (OHSD) deficiency syndromes caused by this enzyme deficiency result in excessive activation of mineralocorticoid receptors (R) by a steroid dependent on adrenocorticotropic hormone (ACTH), rather than by the conventional mineralocorticoid agonist [11]. This steroid appears to be cortisol. It has been shown that mineralocorticoid receptors in the distal nephron have equal affinity for their two ligands—aldosterone (Aldo) and cortisol—but are protected from cortisol by the presence of 11β-dehydrogenase, which inactivates cortisol to cortisone [12]. The 11,18-hemiacetal structure of aldosterone protects it from the action of 11β-dehydrogenase so that aldosterone gains specific access to the receptors. When this mechanism is defective either because of congenital 11β-dehydrogenase deficiency or enzyme inhibition (by either licorice or carbenoxolone), then intrarenal levels of cortisol increase, and cortisol causes inappropriate activation of mineralocorticoid receptors [13–15]. The resulting antinatriuresis and kaliuresis cause hypertension and hypokalemia. Biochemically, there are elevations in urinary-free cortisol excretion and the ratio of the urinary metabolites of cortisol to those of cortisone and prolongation of the half-life of tritiated cortisol. Plasma cortisol concentrations usually are not elevated. The signs and symptoms are reversed by spironolactone or dexamethasone and are exacerbated by administration of physiologic doses of cortisol. (*Adapted from* Walker and Edwards [16].)

HYPERTENSIVE SYNDROMES SECONDARY TO HYPERSECRETION OF ALDOSTERONE

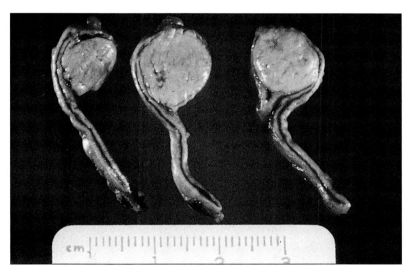

FIGURE 6-15. Pathologic characteristics of an aldosterone-producing tumor. Primary aldosteronism is an uncommon cause of hypertension, but is nevertheless an important disorder to recognize in hypertensive patients. First, the associated hypertension can be severe, and cardiovascular and renal complications tend to occur. Second, removal of the tumor often results in cure of hypertension or at the very least renders

it more responsive to medical therapy. Third, knowledge of the presence of the disorder allows the physician to formulate a rational and specific therapeutic regimen, resulting in better compliance and better blood pressure control.

In the classic form of primary aldosteronism (Conn's syndrome), excessive aldosterone production results from a unilateral adrenocortical adenoma. In approximately one third of all patients, the adrenal glands may show hyperplasia of the zona glomerulosa, with or without micronodular changes (idiopathic hyperaldosteronism). Rarely, the syndrome can result from either an adrenal or ovarian carcinoma. In certain patients, the hypertension and biochemical abnormalities can be corrected by administration of dexamethasone. This form of aldosteronism in which aldosterone secretion is regulated by adrenocorticotropic hormone is hereditary and can be remedied by glucocorticoids. Recent studies demonstrate that this disorder is caused by a mutation in the zona fasciculata 11β-hydroxylase, which confers methyl oxidase activity. Such mutations result in ectopic expression of aldosterone synthase in adrenal fasciculata.

Aldosterone-producing tumors arise from the zona glomerulosa cells of the adrenal cortex. Such tumors characteristically measure from 1 to 3 cm in diameter and are golden yellow on cross-section. The tumors are homogenous, and may or may not be encapsulated; atrophy of the adjacent adrenal cortical tissue may be seen.

FIGURE 6-16. Clinical clues to the presence of primary aldosteronism. Primary aldosteronism can occur at all ages, although in most reported series, most patients were in their 30s, 40s, and 50s. Aldosterone-producing adenomas occur more commonly in women than in men. In contrast, idiopathic hyperaldosteronism is sometimes more common in men. Whites seem to be more prone to the disease than are blacks. The symptoms are usually related to hypokalemia or to the complications of hypertension. Many patients are, however, completely asymptomatic, and the disorder is detected either at routine examination for serum electrolyte values or during assessment of diuretic-induced hypokalemia or refractory hypertension. The blood pressure can range from normal (rare) to

mildly elevated or very high. Some patients have been reported to enter the malignant phase of hypertension. Vascular complications, such as stroke and coronary attacks, occur in approximately one fourth of all patients.

Primary aldosteronism should be considered in all patients with spontaneous hypokalemia, moderately severe hypokalemia induced by conventional doses of potassium-wasting diuretics, or refractory hypertension. Hypokalemia, whether spontaneous or provoked, provides an important clue to the presence of the disorder. Plasma renin activity measurements are of limited use in screening patients for the presence of primary aldosteronism because of the large number of false-positive and false-negative results. The plasma aldosterone–plasma renin activity ratio has been used to define the appropriateness of plasma renin activity for the circulating concentrations of aldosterone. One serious drawback of this test is the inherent variability of plasma levels of aldosterone even in the presence of a tumor. Another is that the drugs used during the test can result in either marked suppression or prolonged stimulation of renin long after their discontinuance.

The measurement of the 24-hour urinary aldosterone excretion rate provides greater sensitivity and specificity than does the measurement of plasma aldosterone concentration. Spontaneous hypokalemia of less than 3.0 mEq/L, an anomalous postural decrease in plasma aldosterone concentration, and plasma 18-hydroxycorticosterone values 100 ng/dL or greater distinguish an adenoma from hyperplasia. For localization of an adenoma, adrenal CT can accurately locate tumors 1.5 cm in diameter or larger. If CT is inconclusive, adrenal venous sampling for aldosterone and cortisol levels should be done.

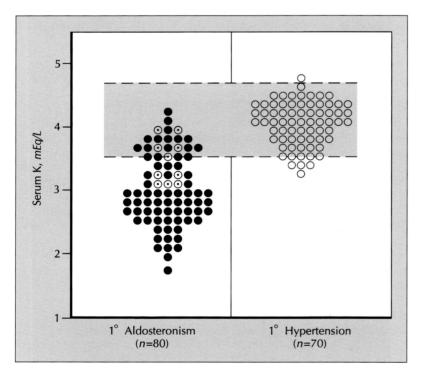

FIGURE 6-17. Serum potassium concentrations in cases of primary aldosteronism and essential hypertension. Patients were age- and sex-matched. No medication had been given for at least 2 weeks, and the patients were on an isocaloric diet containing 110 mEq of sodium and 80 mEq of potassium per day for 5 days. Blood was drawn between 8 AM and 9 AM after an overnight fast and at least 30 minutes of supine rest. Each point represents the mean of at least three determinations. For patients with primary aldosteronism, *solid circles* represent adenomas (*n* = 70) and *open circles with dotted centers* represent hyperplasia (*n* = 10). The *shaded area* represents 95% CI (3.5 to 4.6 mEq/L) of values obtained from 60 healthy subjects.

Twenty-two patients (27.5%) with primary aldosteronism (17 with tumors and five with hyperplasia) had fasting serum potassium values of 3.5 mEq/L or greater, whereas four patients (5.7%) with essential hypertension had values below 3.5 mEq/L. Serum potassium values below 3.0 mEq/L were usually associated with the presence of a tumor. Ten patients (six of 17 with tumors and four of five with hyperplasia) remained persistently normokalemic, despite intake of high dietary sodium for 3 days. (*Adapted from* Bravo *et al.* [17].)

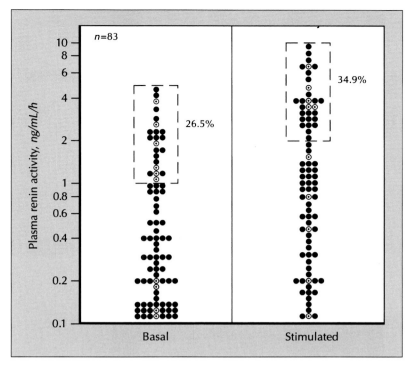

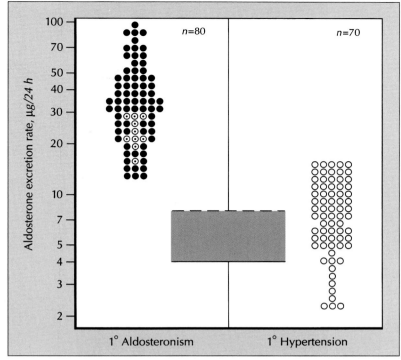

FIGURE 6-18. Stimulated plasma renin activity in primary aldosteronism. Clinical conditions and patient identification are the same as in Figure 6-17. Plasma renin activity was estimated by radioimmunoassay of generated angiotensin I. Blood for the measurement of plasma renin activity was drawn after 4 days of sodium deprivation. On the morning after 3 to 5 days of normal dietary sodium, basal activity was measured after an overnight fast followed by 30 minutes of supine rest. Stimulated activity was measured under similar conditions after 4 days of sodium deprivation. *Solid circles* represent patients with adenoma (*n* = 73) and *open circles with dotted centers* represent those with hyperplasia (*n* = 10). Approximately 26% of patients had normal-to-high plasma renin activity in the basal state, and approximately 35% had values of at least 2.0 ng/mL after sodium deprivation (*boxed areas*). Based on the stimulated activity, 42% of patients had false-negative results. Using a value of 2.0 ng/mL or less after 4 days of sodium deprivation as the reference value, the sensitivity and specificity of the test were 64% and 83%, respectively. (*Adapted from* Bravo [18].)

FIGURE 6-19. Aldosterone excretion rate after 3 days of high dietary sodium intake. Clinical conditions and patient identification are the same as in Figure 6-16. Urine was collected on the third day of high sodium intake. The level of aldosterone in the urine was measured by a radioimmunoassay technique as the pH 1.0 conjugate 18-glucuronide metabolite. The *shaded area* represents the mean (4.0 µg/24 h) and +2 SD (8.0 µg/24 h) of values obtained from 47 healthy subjects. No patient with primary aldosteronism had a value within the 95% normal range. Ten patients (14%) with primary hypertension had values that fell within the range obtained in patients with primary aldosteronism. Using a reference value of greater than 14 µg/24 h after a high sodium intake for 3 days, the sensitivity and specificity of the test were 96% and 93%, respectively. (*Adapted from* Bravo *et al.* [17].)

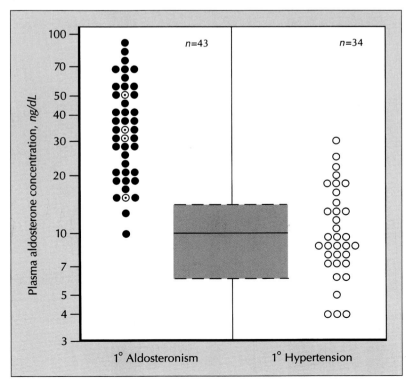

FIGURE 6-20. Plasma aldosterone concentration after 3 days of high dietary sodium intake. Clinical conditions and patient identification are the same as in Figure 6-17. Aldosterone in plasma was measured by a radioimmunoassay technique. The *shaded area* represents the 95% CIs of values (5.3 to 13.7 ng/dL) obtained from 47 healthy subjects. Seventeen patients (39%) with primary aldosteronism had values that fell within the range obtained in patients with primary hypertension. This gave a false-negative rate of 39.5%. Using a reference value of greater than 22 ng/dL after high sodium intake for 3 days, the sensitivity and specificity of the test were 72% and 91%, respectively. (*Adapted from* Bravo *et al.* [17].)

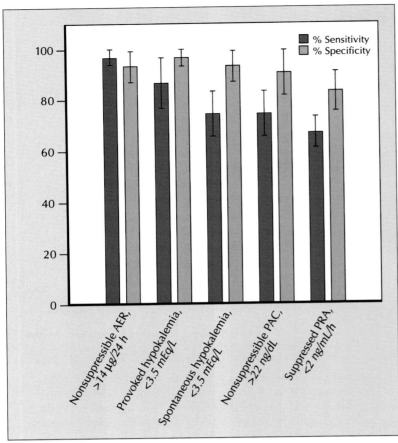

FIGURE 6-21. Sensitivity and specificity of screening tests for primary aldosteronism. The single best test that identifies patients with primary aldosteronism is measurement of aldosterone excretion rate (AER) after salt loading. Measurement of plasma aldosterone concentration (PAC) is much less sensitive. Suppressed plasma renin activity (PRA) is the least sensitive test, perhaps because of the large number of essential hypertensive patients with suppressed PRA. In untreated patients, demonstration of significant hypokalemia (serum potassium ≤ 3.0 mEq/L) with renal wasting (24-hour urinary potassium > 30 mEq/L), PRA less than 1.0 ng/mL, and elevated plasma (> 22 ng/dL) and urinary aldosterone (> 14 μg/24 h) values makes the diagnosis unequivocal. (*Adapted from* Bravo [19].)

FIGURE 6-22. Biochemical confirmation of adenoma versus hyperplasia as a cause of primary aldosteronism. A patient with the clinical features of primary aldosteronism is more likely to have an adenoma in the presence of moderately severe hypokalemia, an anomalous postural decrease in plasma aldosterone concentration during ambulation, and an overnight recumbent plasma 18-hydroxycorticosterone (18-OHB) greater than 100 ng/dL. Plasma 18-OHB of less than 100 ng/dL or plasma aldosterone that increases with ambulation does not, however, completely rule out the presence of a tumor.

Although it is rare for patients with hyperplasia to have 18-OHB values greater than 100 ng/dL, approximately 30% (false-negative rate) of patients with adenomas will have values less than 100 ng/dL. Similarly, it is very rare for the level of aldosterone in the plasma of patients with hyperplasia to decline with ambulation; however, approximately 40% (false-negative rate) of patients will have increased rather than decreased levels of plasma aldosterone with ambulation. Urinary values of 18-hydroxycortisol have been shown to be elevated in patients with adenoma but normal in patients with hyperplasia.

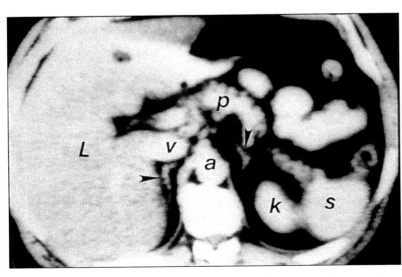

FIGURE 6-23. Computed tomography scan of the normal adrenal glands (*arrowheads*). The right adrenal gland is the sliver of tissue behind the inferior vena cava (v). The left adrenal gland is the inverted y-shaped tissue that is bordered by the aorta (a), the tail of the pancreas (p), and the top of the kidney (k). L—liver; S—spleen.

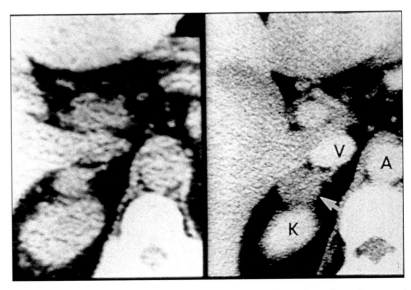

FIGURE 6-24. Computed tomography scan of a right adrenal tumor (*arrow*) before (*left*) and after (*right*) contrast injection. The tumor is located between the vena cava (v) and the upper pole of the kidney (k). A—aorta.

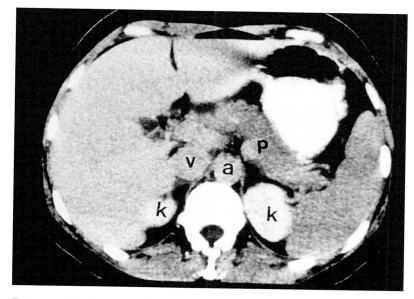

FIGURE 6-25. Computed tomography scan of a left adrenal tumor. The tumor is the low attenuation mass bordered by the aorta (a), pancreas (p), and kidney (k). v—vena cava. (*From* Bravo [19]; with permission.)

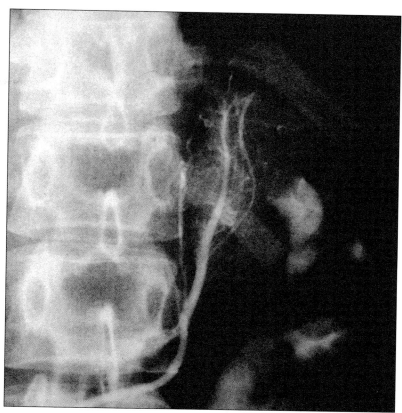

FIGURE 6-26. Venography of a left adrenal tumor. Because of their small size, nonvascular nature, and tendency to displace veins, aldosterone-producing tumors are more clearly visualized by adrenal venography than by arteriography.

DIAGNOSTIC ACCURACY OF IMAGING TECHNIQUES IN ADRENOCORTICAL DISORDERS

		TRUE POSITIVES, %	
DISORDER	PATIENTS, *n*	NP-59	CT
Cushing's syndrome	28	93	90
Primary aldosteronism	58	88	91
Nonfunctional tumors	13	100	89

FIGURE 6-27. Diagnostic accuracy of iodocholesterol NP-59 scanning and CT in adrenocortical disorders. As demonstrated, NP-59 has a greater percentage of true-positive results in the diagnosis of Cushing's syndrome and nonfunctional tumors; CT is a better diagnostic imaging method for primary aldosteronism. (*Adapted from* Guerin *et al.* [20].)

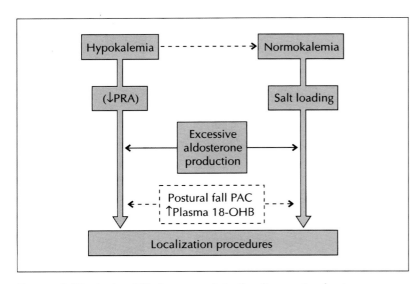

FIGURE 6-28. A simplified approach to the diagnosis of primary aldosteronism. Priority of evaluation should be given to patients with a history of spontaneous hypokalemia, marked sensitivity to potassium-wasting diuretics, or refractory hypertension in whom other causes of secondary hypertension (*ie*, renal parenchymal disease, renovascular disease, pheochromocytoma) have been

eliminated. Patients with significant hypokalemia, suppressed plasma renin activity (PRA) (< 2 ng/mL), or an increased aldosterone excretion rate (> 14 μg/24 h) have unequivocal evidence of primary aldosteronism. Patients with equivocal findings will require salt loading. This evaluation can be accomplished on an outpatient basis by adding 10 to 12 g sodium chloride to the patient's daily diet in addition to determining the values of serum potassium concentration and 24-hour urinary excretion of sodium, potassium, and aldosterone after 7 days of high salt intake. A 24-hour urinary sodium value of at least 250 mEq gives some assurance that the patient has ingested the amount of salt prescribed.

Under these conditions, an aldosterone excretion rate greater than 14 μg/24 h suggests inappropriate aldosterone production. The development of hypokalemia or suppressed PRA are corroborative data, but their absence does not rule out a diagnosis of inappropriate aldosterone production. Demonstration of a postural decrease in plasma aldosterone concentration (PAC) and overnight recumbent plasma 18-hydroxycorticosterone (OHB) greater than 100 ng/dL indicate the presence of an adenoma. For localization, adrenal CT should be performed first and considered diagnostic if an adrenal mass is clearly identified. When the results of CT are inclusive, adrenal venous sampling for aldosterone levels may be performed. (*Adapted from* Bravo [18].)

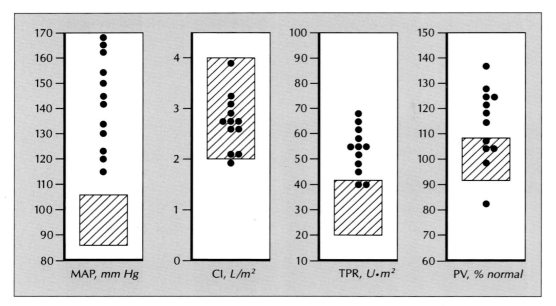

FIGURE 6-29. Hemodynamic features of primary aldosteronism. The mean arterial pressure (MAP) is maintained by increased total peripheral resistance (TPR). Plasma volume (PV) is either increased or (inappropriately) normal despite the increased MAP. Cardiac index (CI) remains essentially within normal limits. Understanding the hemodynamic profile helps design the appropriate medical regimen for patients with primary aldosteronism. Thus, administration of a diuretic or a vasodilator appears to be the most rational option for the medical management of such patients. The *cross-hatched areas* indicate 95% CIs.

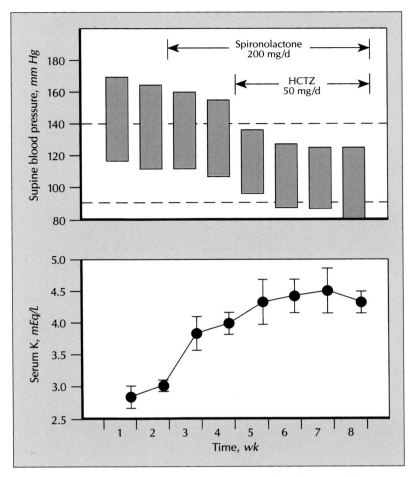

FIGURE 6-30. Diuretic therapy in patients with primary aldosteronism. An average of 10 blood pressure readings were taken at home by each patient for this assessment. Serum potassium values were measured at the end of each week of observation. Administration of 200 mg/d (50 mg four times daily) of spironolactone increased serum potassium with little or no effect on arterial pressure. The addition of hydrochlorothiazide (HCTZ), 50 mg/d (25 mg twice daily), immediately reduced blood pressure while serum potassium concentration remained normal. (*Adapted from* Bravo *et al.* [21].)

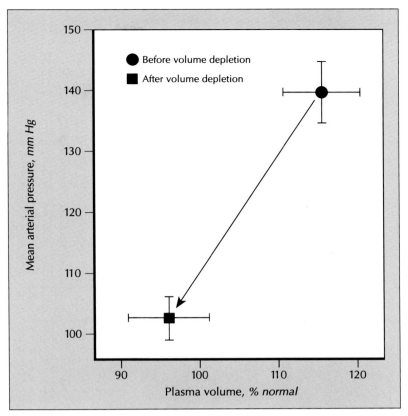

FIGURE 6-31. Relationship between the decrease in plasma volume and reduction of arterial blood pressure (*n* = 28). Before treatment, mean arterial pressure averaged 138 mm Hg while plasma volume averaged 116% of normal. As plasma volume was reduced by diuretic therapy, mean arterial pressure was concomitantly decreased. These findings reemphasize the importance of plasma volume in the maintenance of hypertension.

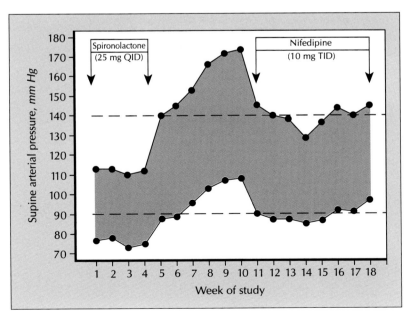

FIGURE 6-32. Calcium antagonists have been proposed as alternative agents to diuretics in the treatment of primary aldosteronism. This concept emerged from the demonstration that in vitro calcium antagonists inhibit aldosterone biosynthesis. This illustration compares diuretics and calcium antagonists in the treatment of primary aldosteronism. It shows that spironolactone, a diuretic, is a better antihypertensive than is nifedipine, a calcium antagonist. In addition, contrary to in vitro studies, nifedipine has little or no effect on aldosterone biosynthesis in vivo and, as a result, the metabolic abnormalities of hyperaldosteronism remain uncorrected. Systolic and diastolic blood pressures are weekly averages of blood pressures taken at home twice daily. The *broken lines* define the normal limits of systolic and diastolic blood pressures. (*Adapted from* Bravo [22].)

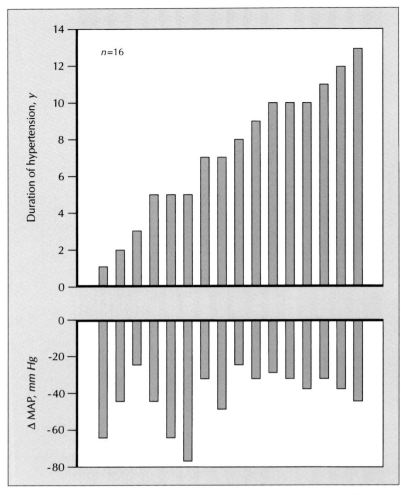

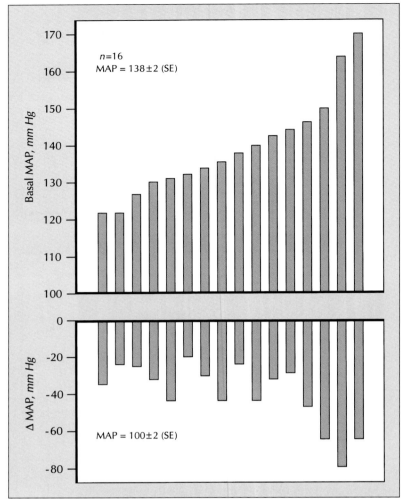

FIGURE 6-33. The influence of duration of hypertension on blood pressure response after surgery. Surgery is indicated in patients with solitary adenomas, especially if the tumor is larger than 5.0 cm in diameter or is secreting other steroids, in patients with poor blood pressure control, and in patients with intolerable side effects of drug therapy. In most cases, surgical excision of aldosterone-producing adenomas leads to normotension as well as reversal of biochemical abnormalities. In patients with residual hypertension, surgery renders arterial pressure easier to control with medications. The duration of hypertension is arranged in increasing length. The change in blood pressure is that observed at least 1 year after surgical removal of an adenoma. There was no relationship between the duration of hypertension and the blood pressure response after surgery. MAP—mean arterial pressure. (*Adapted from* Bravo [23].)

FIGURE 6-34. The influence of the severity of hypertension on blood pressure response after surgery. The basal blood pressure (before surgery) is arranged in order of increasing severity. The corresponding change in blood pressure is that observed at least 1 year after surgical removal of an adenoma. There was no relationship between the severity of hypertension before surgery and the blood pressure response after surgery. MAP—mean arterial pressure. (*Adapted from* Bravo [23].)

EFFICACY OF LONG-TERM MEDICAL MANAGEMENT OF ALDOSTERONE-PRODUCING ADENOMAS

PATIENT	AGE y	SEX	FOLLOW-UP y	BLOOD PRESSURE AT PRESENTATION* mm Hg	MOST RECENT BLOOD PRESSURE* mm Hg	ELECTROLYTE LEVELS AT DIAGNOSIS† SODIUM	POTASSIUM	CHLORIDE	CARBON DIOXIDE	ELECTROLYTE LEVELS AT LAST FOLLOW-UP† SODIUM	POTASSIUM	CHLORIDE	CARBON DIOXIDE
1	65	M	5	170/94	120/80	145	3.1	105	30	140	5.2	110	28
2	69	M	12	164/65	157/86	141	3.2	98	35	141	3.9	104	30
3	63	M	11	178/96	130/95	141	2.9	100	28	144	4.0	107	26
4	43	F	8	180/104	124/82	140	3.0	98	31	137	4.1	105	25
5	39	F	5	184/132	128/80	141	3.9	102	29	140	3.7	106	28
6	76	M	9	174/100	116/74	143	2.9	104	29	139	4.7	103	23
7	68	M	6	180/105	195/76	140	3.1	98	32	142	4.2	109	28
8	69	M	5	190/95	130/70	144	2.9	103	29	140	4.1	104	21
9	59	M	7	180/116	145/99	144	2.4	102	35	139	4.3	104	30
10	55	M	8	180/110	140/74	145	3.0	102	30	142	4.6	104	30
11	59	M	6	165/102	112/68	142	3.0	106	30	142	4.8	108	30
12	50	M	6	177/117	115/80	144	3.1	102	31	143	4.5	104	27
13	44	M	6	160/110	130/82	141	3.0	106	29	140	4.3	103	29
14	54	F	8	160/98	142/60	144	3.4	106	29	142	4.7	108	25
15	52	F	13	150/104	104/76	142	3.3	105	24	137	4.4	106	25
16	52	F	5	168/102	128/91	143	2.7	102	32	141	3.6	106	32
17	54	F	17	180/110	101/71	143	3.0	105	33	139	4.4	101	30
18	59	M	8	176/116	158/78	142	2.6	106	29	138	4.6	101	27
19	44	F	9	190/122	122/78	142	2.6	98	32	137	3.6	98	26
20	61	F	14	160/110	144/72	145	2.9	103	35	140	3.7	113	29
21	68	F	5	166/108	111/78	143	2.6	103	30	146	4.5	108	26
22	66	M	11	178/108	150/92	141	3.0	101	31	142	3.8	102	26
23	73	M	10	178/100	107/66	143	3.8	99	31	143	4.8	105	24
24	56	M	15	200/125	128/85	141	3.2	102	32	139	4.6	102	26

*Blood pressure values are the average of at least three measurements.
†Levels are measured in millimoles per liter.

FIGURE 6-35. Efficacy of long-term medical management of aldosterone-producing adenomas (APAs). The study included 24 patients (15 men) with documented APA who received medical therapy for at least 5 years (range 5 to 17 years). Patients were followed two to three times yearly. Blood pressure was measured in the seated and standing positions at each ambulatory visit. The average of three measurements of each position was calculated. Blood for the measurements of serum electrolytes, creatinine, blood urea nitrogen, plasma renin activity, and plasma aldosterone were measured at each visit after an overnight fast and 30 minutes of supine rest. The blood pressure levels and serum electrolyte values at diagnosis and last follow-up are shown. From the time of diagnosis to the last follow-up, systolic blood pressure decreased from 175 mm Hg to 129 mm Hg (95% CI for difference, 37.1–53.8 mm Hg). Diastolic blood pressure decreased from 106 mm Hg to 79 mm Hg (95% CI for difference, 20.8–33.9 mm Hg). Serum potassium increased from 3.0 mmol/L to 4.3 mmol/L (95% CI for difference, 1.1–1.5 mmol/L). At the time of the most recent follow-up, four patients were receiving a single potassium-sparing diuretic—either amiloride, 20 to 40 mg/d, or spironolactone, 50 to 200 mg/d. Twenty were receiving a potassium-sparing diuretic and other antihypertensive agent(s); one other in 13, two others in six, and three others in one. During follow-up, no patient had stroke, myocardial infarction, or developed cardiac failure or renal dysfunction. None had evidence of malignant transformation of the APA. Only five had a noticeable increase (≥ 0.5 cm) in size of the adrenal tumor as measured by CT. This study shows that medical management is a viable option for controlling blood pressure and normalizing serum potassium concentration in patients with APA. (Adapted from Ghose et al. [24].)

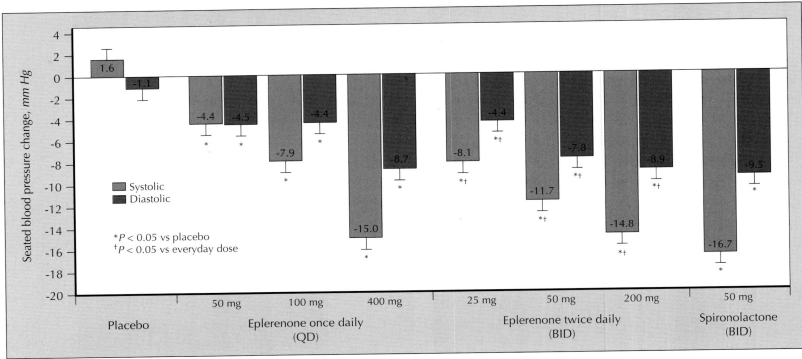

FIGURE 6-36. Comparison of eplerenone once daily, twice daily, and spironolactone on (seated) systolic and diastolic blood pressure. Spironolactone has traditionally been used to treat primary aldosteronism and as a potassium-sparing diuretic in the treatment of hypertension and congestive heart failure. However, its use has been limited by progestational and antiandrogenic side effects, including gynecomastia, impotence, and menstrual irregularities. In the near future, a more selective aldosterone antagonist, eplerenone, will be available, providing benefits equal to but with fewer side effects than spironolactone. *Weinberger et al.* [25] demonstrated that eplerenone is efficacious in the treatment of mild-to-moderate hypertension. Eplerenone in daily doses of 50 ($n = 54$), 100 ($n = 49$), and 400 mg ($n = 56$) for 5 weeks significantly reduced blood pressure compared with placebo ($n = 53$). Eplerenone lowered blood pressure in a dose-dependent manner with minimal effect on heart rate. Reductions in systolic blood pressure were greater than those in diastolic blood pressure. In general, adjusted mean changes from baseline to final visit in systolic and diastolic blood pressure for twice-daily 50 mg and daily 100 mg of eplerenone dosing were approximately 50% and 75% of those observed with the twice-daily 50 mg of spironolactone. Adjusted means are from the analysis of covariance model with treatment and center as factors and baseline as covariate.

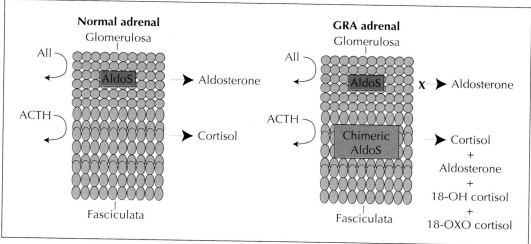

FIGURE 6-37. Glucocorticoid-remediable aldosteronism (GRA). GRA is an inherited autosomal-dominant disorder that mimics an aldosterone-producing adenoma [26]. GRA is caused by a genetic mutation that results in a hybrid or chimeric gene product fusing nucleotide sequences of the 11β-hydroxylase and aldosterone synthase genes [27,28]. Characterization of this chimeric gene indicates that it arose from unequal crossing between 11β-hydroxylase and aldosterone synthase genes [29]. These two genes are located in close proximity to human chromosome 8, are 95% homologous in nucleotide sequence, and have identical intron-exon structure. The structure of the duplicated gene contains 5′ regulatory sequences conferring adreno-corticotropic hormone (ACTH) responsiveness of 11β-hydroxylase fused to more distal coding sequences of the aldosterone synthase gene. Therefore, this hybrid gene is expected to be regulated by ACTH and, in addition, to have aldosterone synthase activity. This hybrid gene allows ectopic expression of aldosterone synthase activity in the ACTH-regulated zona fasciculata, which normally produces cortisol. This enzyme thereby oxidizes the C-18 carbon of a steroid precursor, such as corticosterone or cortisol, leading to the production of aldosterone and the hybrid steroids 18-hydroxy and 18-oxycortisol. This abnormal gene duplication can readily be detected by the Southern blotting test, allowing for direct genetic screening for this disorder with a small blood sample.

An important clinical clue is the age of onset of hypertension. Patients with GRA typically are diagnosed with high blood pressure as children; conversely, patients with other mineralocorticoid excess disorders, such as aldosterone-producing adenomas and idiopathic hyperplasia, usually are diagnosed in their thirties to sixties. The strong family history of hypertension that is often associated with the early death of affected family members resulting from cerebrovascular accidents characteristically is seen in some families with GRA.

No controlled studies have been done on the treatment of patients with GRA. Theoretically, the suppression of ACTH with exogenous glucocorticoid should correct all GRA abnormalities; however, this therapy may be limited by untoward complications resulting from excess glucocorticoids [30]. Another theoretical concern with glucocorticoid treatment is that patients may undergo a brief period of mineralocorticoid insufficiency when therapy is initiated before the renin-angiotensin axis recovers fully. Additional treatment modalities are aimed at mineralocorticoid receptor blockade with spironolactone or inhibition of the mineralocorticoid-sensitive distal tubule sodium channel with amiloride. (*Adapted from* Lifton *et al.* [28].)

PHEOCHROMOCYTOMA

IMPORTANT FACTS ABOUT PHEOCHROMOCYTOMAS

About 30% of pheochromocytomas reported in the literature are found either at autopsy or at surgery for an unrelated problem

35% to 76% of pheochromocytomas discovered at autopsy are clinically unsuspected during life

The average age of diagnosis in those whose disease was discovered before death was 48.5 y, while the average in those diagnosed at autopsy was 65.8 y

Death was usually attributed to cardiovascular complications

FIGURE 6-38. Important facts about pheochromocytomas. Pheochromocytoma is a tumor of neuroectodermal origin that produces excessive quantities of catecholamines, thereby causing hypertension with a constellation of signs and symptoms that can mimic several other acute medical and surgical disorders. Early recognition, accurate localization, and appropriate management of benign pheochromocytomas nearly always result in complete cure. If unrecognized, these tumors cause lethal disease that can lead to significant cardiovascular morbidity and mortality and particularly to sudden death during surgical and obstetric procedures.

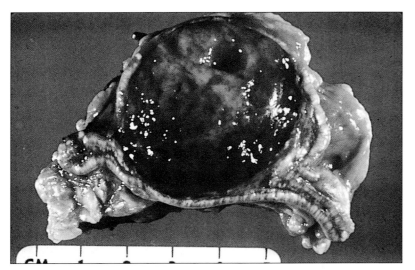

FIGURE 6-39. Typical gross pathologic features of an adrenal pheochromocytoma. The specimen is ovoid and encapsulated, surrounded by a rim of yellow tissue grossly resembling adrenal cortex. The lesion is rubbery to moderately firm and is pale gray to dusky brown. Pheochromocytomas have a strong affinity for chromium salts. Immersion in chromium salt fixative (Zenker's or potassium dichromate solution) changes the tumor from the usual pale gray appearance to a dark black color as cytoplasmic catecholamines are oxidized.

CLINICAL CONDITIONS LIKELY TO BE CONFUSED WITH PHEOCHROMOCYTOMA

β-Adrenergic hyperresponsiveness
Acute state of anxiety
Angina pectoris
Acute infections
Autonomic epilepsy
Hyperthyroidism
Idiopathic orthostatic hypotension
Cerebellopontine angle tumors
Acute hypoglycemia
Acute drug withdrawal
  Clonidine
  β-Adrenergic blockade
  α-Methyldopa
  Alcohol
Vasodilator therapy
  Hydralazine
  Minoxidil
Factitious administration of sympathomimetic agents
Tyramine ingestion in patients on monoamine oxidase inhibitors
Menopausal syndrome with migraine headaches

FIGURE 6-40. Differential diagnosis of pheochromocytoma. Among these are the most common disorders that are confused with pheochromocytoma. (*Adapted from* Bravo [31].)

PRIORITIES FOR DETECTION OF PHEOCHROMOCYTOMA

Patients with the triad of episodic headaches, tachycardia, and diaphoresis (with or without associated hypertension)

Family history of pheochromocytoma

"Incidental" suprarenal masses

Patients with a multiple endocrine adenomatosis syndrome, neurofibromatosis, or von Hippel-Lindau disease

Adverse cardiovascular responses to anesthesia, to any surgical procedure, or to certain drugs (*eg*, guanethidine, tricyclics, thyrotropin-releasing hormone, naloxone, or antidopaminergic agents)

FIGURE 6-41. Priorities for detection of pheochromocytoma. The detection of pheochromocytoma requires a high degree of clinical alertness. Pheochromocytoma usually occurs as a sporadic event. These tumors have, however, been associated with other clinical syndromes, such as von Recklinghausen's disease, von Hippel-Lindau disease, Werner's syndrome (multiple endocrine neoplasia [MEN] type I), Sipple's syndrome (MEN type IIA), mucocutaneous neuroma (MEN type IIB), acromegaly, and Cushing's syndrome. Most patients present with labile hypertension, diaphoresis, headaches, and tachycardia with or without palpitations; however, as many as 30% of all reported cases were unsuspected during life and the tumors were found either at autopsy or during surgery for an unrelated condition.

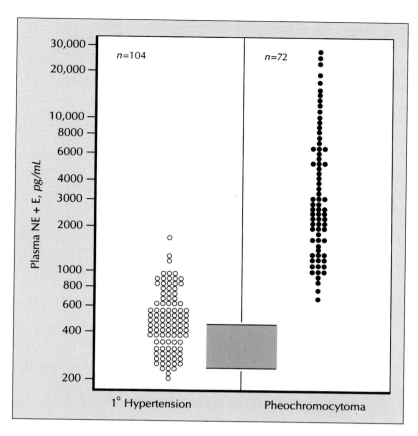

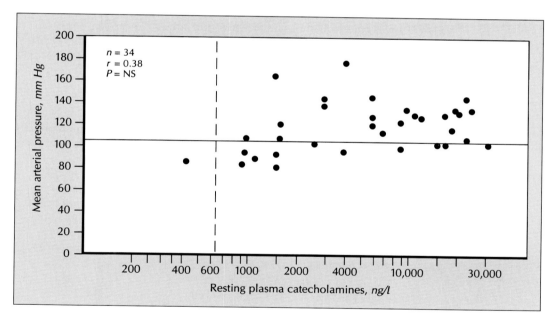

FIGURE 6-42. Supine resting plasma catecholamines in patients with essential hypertension or proven pheochromocytoma. The definitive diagnosis of pheochromocytoma rests primarily on laboratory test results. Most patients with proven pheochromocytoma have elevated plasma catecholamine levels ($\geq$ 2000 pg/mL) that are markedly higher than those seen in other conditions. For the patients shown in this figure, blood being measured for plasma catecholamines was drawn between 8 AM and 9 AM after an overnight fast and 30 minutes of supine rest. Caffeine and nicotine were not allowed for at least 3 hours before blood was drawn.

The *shaded area* represents the mean (260 pg/mL) + 2 SD (500 pg/mL) of values in 47 sex- and age-matched normotensive healthy adults. For patients with essential hypertension, the mean and + 2 SD are 516 and 950 pg/mL, respectively. Four of 72 patients (5.5%) with proven pheochromocytoma had values that fell within the upper 95% confidence limits for essential hypertensive patients; however, 22 patients had values that overlapped with the highest values obtained in essential hypertensive patients. These individuals required either a clonidine suppression test or a glucagon stimulation test for definitive diagnosis. NE + E——norepinephrine plus epinephrine. (*Adapted from* Bravo and Gifford [32].)

FIGURE 6-43. Relationship between blood pressure and plasma catecholamines in pheochromocytoma. The *broken line* indicates the mean + 3 SD for plasma catecholamines; the *solid line* indicates the upper limits of mean arterial pressure. No relationship between the height of blood pressure and circulating catecholamines was noted. This finding suggests that patients may be normotensive or asymptomatic even in the presence of pathologically elevated circulating catecholamines. (*Adapted from* Bravo *et al.* [33].)

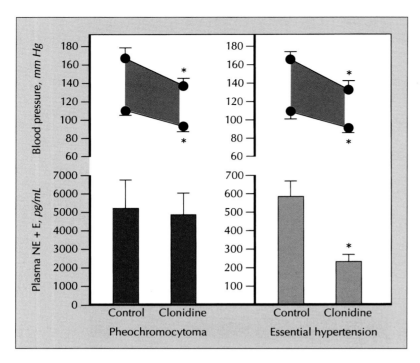

FIGURE 6-44. Blood pressure and plasma catecholamine responses to oral clonidine (3 hours after a single oral dose) in patients with pheochromocytoma (*n* = 35) and essential hypertension (*n* = 117). Despite differing levels of plasma catecholamines, clonidine decreases blood pressure to the same degree in patients with essential hypertension as in those with pheochromocytoma. These results suggest that the sympathetic nervous system is intact in patients with pheochromocytoma and indicate that high concentrations of catecholamines at sites of synaptic release appear to have a greater influence on vasoconstriction than do circulating levels. All values are mean ± SE. *Asterisks* indicate *P* < 0.01. NE+E—norepinephrine plus epinephrine. (*Adapted from* Bravo and Gifford [34].)

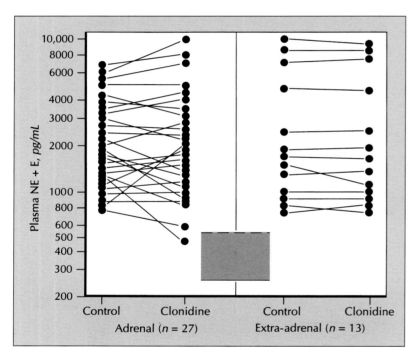

FIGURE 6-45. Clonidine suppression test in pheochromocytoma. The test is based on the principle that normal increases in plasma catecholamines are mediated through activation of the sympathetic nervous system. In patients with pheochromocytoma, the increases result from diffusion of excess catecholamines from the tumor into the circulation, bypassing the normal storage and release mechanisms. Thus, clonidine should not suppress catecholamine release in patients with pheochromocytoma but will suppress catecholamine release in patients in whom release is neurogenically mediated.

The *shaded area* represents the mean (260 pg/mL) and the 95% upper confidence limits (500 pg/mL) of values obtained from 47 normal subjects. Values shown for clonidine represent the lowest values reached (at either 2 or 3 hours) after oral administration of 0.3 mg. A normal response is reduction of plasma catecholamines of at least 50% from baseline and below 500 pg/mL. Blood pressure and heart rate should be recorded every 30 minutes during the test. The results were compared with those of sex- and age-matched subjects with essential hypertension. Plasma catecholamine values fell below 500 pg/mL in all but one patient with essential hypertension. Only one patient with pheochromocytoma had a plasma catecholamine value below 500 pg/mL. NE + E—norepinephrine plus epinephrine. (*Adapted from* Bravo [35].)

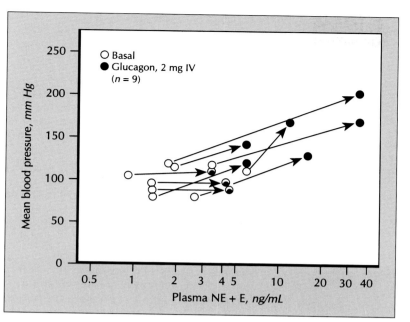

FIGURE 6-46. Glucagon stimulation test for pheochromocytoma. The glucagon stimulation test is used when clinical findings strongly suggest a pheochromocytoma but catecholamine production is equivocal or nearly normal. In practice, a plasma catecholamine level of 1000 pg/mL or less requires a stimulation test. Glucagon is given as a intravenous bolus dose of 2.0 mg. Blood pressure is taken every 30 seconds. A positive test requires an increase of at least threefold or over 2000 pg/mL in plasma catecholamines 1 to 3 minutes after drug administration. A simultaneous increase in blood pressure of at least 20/15 mm Hg is desirable but not essential. In the subjects for this figure, three had unaltered blood pressure despite marked increases in simultaneously measured plasma catecholamines (*half-filled circles*). NE+E—norepinephrine plus epinephrine. (*Adapted from* Bravo and Gifford [32].)

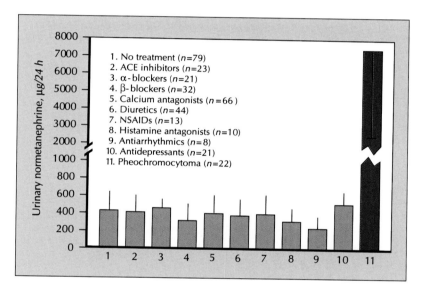

FIGURE 6-47. Urinary normetanephrine values in hypertensive patients on various types of drugs. Normetanephrine in urine was measured by high-pressure liquid chromatography. None of the commonly used antihypertensive agents interfered with the measurement of normetanephrine in urine. Values represent mean ± SD. ACE—angiotensin-converting enzyme; NSAID—nonsteroidal anti-inflammatory drug.

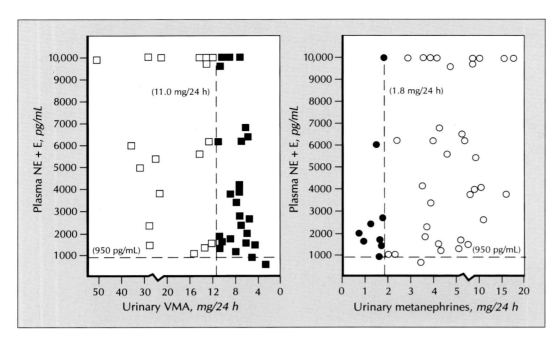

FIGURE 6-48. Comparison of simultaneously measured indexes of catecholamine production in 43 patients with surgically confirmed pheochromocytoma. *Closed symbols* indicate values within the limits of those obtained in essential hypertensives. *Open symbols* represent values outside the limits of those obtained in essential hypertension. Twenty-five of the 43 patients (58%) had false-negative rates for urinary vanillylmandelic acid (VMA). For total urinary metanephrines plus normetanephrines, nine patients (21%) had false-negative results. In one patient, all three biochemical determinations were within the hypertensive range; in another patient, an elevated level of urinary metanephrines plus normetanephrines was the only biochemical abnormality; and in three other patients, the only abnormal result was an elevated level of plasma catecholamines. Therefore, the false-negative rate for plasma catecholamines was 4.6%. The *vertical broken lines* represent the 95% upper confidence limits for urinary VMA and total urinary metanephrines in 30 subjects with essential hypertension. The *horizontal broken lines* indicate the 95% upper confidence limit for essential hypertensive patients. NE + E—norepinephrine plus epinephrine. (*Adapted from* Bravo and Gifford [32].)

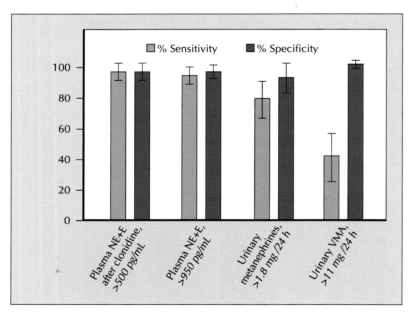

FIGURE 6-49. Sensitivity and specificity of various tests for pheochromocytoma. Measurement of plasma catecholamines appears to be the most sensitive test, and measurement of urinary vanillylmandelic acid (VMA) seems to be the least sensitive. When levels of catecholamines are elevated, all three tests provide excellent specificity. A combination test of plasma catecholamines and 24-hour urinary metanephrines provides nearly 100% accuracy (sensitivity and selectivity) in the diagnosis of pheochromocytoma. NE + E—norepinephrine plus epinephrine. All values are mean ± 2 SE.

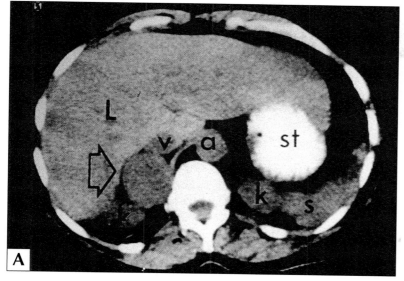

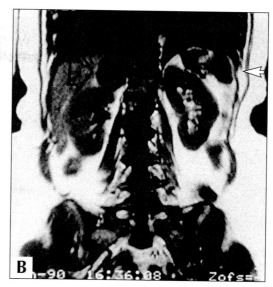

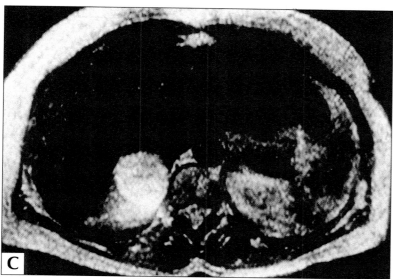

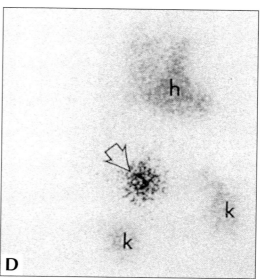

FIGURE 6-50. Three modalities used to localize pheochromocytomas. CT can accurately detect tumors larger than 1.0 cm and has a localization precision of approximately 98%, although it is only 70% specific. CT is the most widely applied and accepted modality for the anatomic localization of pheochromocytomas. MRI is equally sensitive to CT and lends itself to in vivo tissue characterization, which is not possible with CT. MRI is nearly 100% sensitive but is only 67% specific. Scintigraphic localization with radioiodinated ^{131}I-meta-iodobenzylguanidine (MIBG) provides both anatomic and functional characterization. Although this modality is less sensitive than CT and MRI, it has a specificity of 100%. Ninety-seven percent of pheochromocytomas are found in the abdominal region, with most found in the adrenal glands. Less likely sites are the thorax (2% to 3%) and the neck (1%). Multiple tumors may arise in 10% of adults. Familial pheochromocytomas are frequently bilateral or arise from multiple sites. Pheochromocytomas occurring in children are more commonly bilateral and more frequently lie outside the adrenal glands than they do in adults. Tumor localization not only serves to confirm the diagnosis of pheochromocytoma but also assists the surgeon in planning the surgical strategy. Advances in noninvasive imaging techniques now provide safe and reliable means of localizing pheochromocytomas, regardless of their location.

A, CT of the adrenal glands (*arrow*). **B,** Coronal (*arrow*) and **C,** sagittal MRI sections of the abdomen, respectively. Pheochromocytomas demonstrate high signal intensity on a T_2-weighted image, unlike a benign tumor, which has a low signal intensity. **D,** Scintigraphic localization of a pheochromocytoma (*arrow*) with radioiodinated ^{131}I-MIBG. This modality provides both anatomic and functional characterization of a tumor. Because ^{131}I-MIBG is actively concentrated in sympathomedullary tissue through the catecholamine pump, the administration of drugs that block the reuptake mechanism (*eg*, tricyclic antidepressants, guanethidine, labetalol) may result in false-negative results. a—aorta; h—heart; k—kidney; L—liver; s—spleen; st—stomach; v—vena cava. (**A,C,D,** *from* Bravo *et al.* [36]; with permission; **B** *from* Bravo [37]; with permission.)

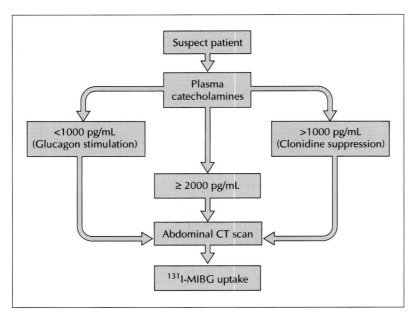

FIGURE 6-51. Diagnostic strategies in pheochromocytoma. Priority of evaluation is given to patients with the signs and symptoms detailed in Figure 6-40. Concentrations of plasma norepinephrine and epinephrine are measured after the patient has rested in a supine position for at least 30 minutes. Caffeine and nicotine are prohibited for at least 3 hours before testing. Values of 2000 pg/mL or greater are considered pathognomonic for pheochromocytoma. Values between 1000 and 2000 pg/mL require a clonidine suppression test. Abdominal CT or MRI is then performed in patients with clinical and biochemical features suggestive of pheochromocytoma. Approximately 5% of patients may have plasma catecholamines of 1000 pg/mL or less. If the clinical presentation strongly suggests pheochromocytoma in these patients, further evaluation should be performed. Such evaluation may include measurement of urinary catecholamine metabolites or a glucagon stimulation test. For patients with arterial pressure greater than 160/100 mg Hg or if coexistent medical problems make sudden increases in blood pressure risky, pretreatment with 10 mg of oral nifedipine, 30 minutes before testing, will attenuate any increases in blood pressure without interfering with catecholamine release. MIBG—meta-iodobenzylguanidine.

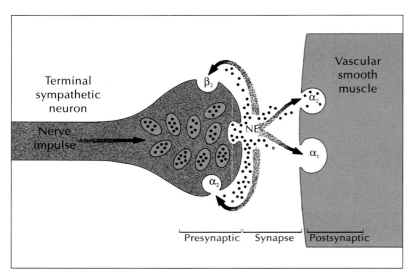

FIGURE 6-52. Pharmacologic effect of norepinephrine. The medical management of pheochromocytoma has been dominated by attempts to prevent hypertensive crises mediated by catecholamine-induced stimulation of α-adrenergic receptors. For control of blood pressure, use of α-blocking agents has been the longstanding treatment of choice. Phenoxybenzamine hydrochloride (10 to 20 mg three or four times daily) has been used most commonly. Theoretic advantages of phenoxybenzamine relate to its ability to permit vascular volume repletion and to block α receptors noncompetitively. As a result, it is difficult for released catecholamines to overcome the blocking effect; however, phenoxybenzamine produces significant orthostatic hypotension. It also blocks presynaptic α2 receptors, thereby enhancing norepinephrine release and leading to reflex tachycardia. Phenoxybenzamine may also prolong and contribute to blood pressure reduction that follows removal of the tumor or masks the presence of residual pheochromocytoma. Despite adequate blockage of α receptors, total elimination of cardiovascular disturbances is seldom achieved and significant elevations of blood pressure often occur during surgical manipulations of the tumor. (*Adapted from* Taylor [38].)

PERIOPERATIVE HEMODYNAMIC VARIABLES

	OPEN, n=20	LAPAROSCOPIC, n=14	P VALUE
Mean preoperative blood pressure*, *mm Hg*	140±18/78±10	144±13/74±14	0.50
Highest blood pressure*, *mm Hg*	191±33/98±25	194±19/106±19	0.50
Hypertension[†]	0.5 (0–5)	1.0 (0–3)	0.41
SBP ≥ 200 mm Hg[†]	0 (0–4)	0 (0–2)	0.70
Lowest blood pressure*, *mm Hg*	88±14/50±13	98±19/57±8	0.05
Hypotension[†]	2.0 (0–6)	0 (0–2)	0.005
Highest heart rate, *bpm*	104±15	101±24	0.78
Heart rate ≥ 110 bpm[†]	0 (0–3)	0 (0–3)	0.36
Lowest heart rate, *bpm*	61±11	60±9	0.81
Heart rate ≥ 50 bpm[†]	0 (0–1)	0 (0–5)	0.81
Patients requiring treatment for hypertension[‡], *n*	17.0	13.0	0.63
Patients requiring treatment for hypotension[§], *n*	9.0	1.0	0.02

*Systolic and diastolic blood pressure presented as the standard deviation; *P* value based on the test.

[†]Median number of episodes for one patient, with the range in parentheses; *P* value based on the Jackson-Whitney U test.

[‡]Includes patients who intraoperatively received at least one of the following treatments: nitroglycerin, sodium nitroprusside, β-blocker, α/β-blocker, or a calcium channel antagonist.

[§]Includes patients who intraoperatively received at least one of the following treatments: phenylephrine, dopamine, or epinephrine.

FIGURE 6-53. Perioperative hemodynamic variables. Until recently, pheochromocytoma was removed only through an open approach. With technologic advances and experience in minimally invasive techniques, the tumor can now be removed safely and successfully with laparoscopic surgery. In this study, 14 pheochromocytoma patients who underwent laparoscopic surgery were compared with 20 patients who underwent the traditional open approach. The intraoperative hemodynamic values during laparoscopic surgery (adrenalectomy) were comparable with those of open surgery. However, in patients undergoing laparoscopy, intraoperative hypotension was less severe (mean lowest blood pressure, 98/57 mm Hg vs 80/50 mm Hg; P=0.05) and hypotensive episodes were less frequent (median 0 vs two episodes; P=0.005). The median estimated blood loss was 100 mL (range, 100 to 200 mL) in the laparoscopy group and 400 mL (range, 150 to 1500 mL) in the open group (P=0.0001). Surgery time was no different between the two groups (196± 69 for open vs 177± 59 minutes for laparoscopy). Patients who underwent laparoscopy had a faster postoperative course. Time to ambulation was sooner (1.5 vs 4 days; P=0.002), oral food intake resumed sooner (median 1 vs 3.5 days; P=0.001), and duration of hospitalization was much shorter (median 3 vs 7.5 days; P=0.001). (*Adapted from* Sprung *et al.* [39].)

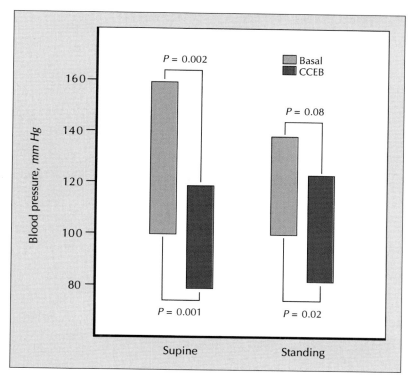

FIGURE 6-54. Blood pressure response to calcium antagonists in pheochromocytoma. *Bars* represent the mean systolic and diastolic blood pressures from 10 patients with surgically diagnosed pheochromocytoma. Patients received either verapamil-SR (120 to 240 mg daily; *n* = 5) or nifedipine-XL (30 to 90 mg daily; *n* = 5) for 6 to 8 weeks. The blood pressure values reported here were obtained immediately before drug administration and before the surgical procedure. Calcium antagonists maintained blood pressure at normal levels, and patients were symptom-free throughout the period of study. Before drug treatment, patients had reductions in systolic blood pressure with standing. This was completely eliminated during treatment. Surgical extirpation of the tumor is the only definitive method of treatment and should be advised for all patients unless the risks are unacceptable.

Even in cases where the tumor has already metastasized, debulking of large primary tumors is sometimes indicated to control hypertension and other symptoms. Appropriate antihypertensive drugs are used to manage hypertension for control of symptoms and to prepare patients for surgery. The α-adrenergic blocking agents, namely phenoxybenzamine hydrochloride (10 to 20 mg three or four times daily) and prazosin hydrochloride (1 to 10 mg twice daily), are most commonly used. Experience with the newer α_1-adrenergic blocking agents, terazosin and doxazosin, is limited and unpublished. Calcium channel blockers have been used successfully to control blood pressure in patients with pheochromocytoma. Because they do not produce *overshoot hypotension* or orthostatic hypotension, calcium channel blockers may be used safely in normotensive patients who have occasional episodes of paroxysmal hypertension. These agents may also prevent catecholamine-induced coronary vasospasm and myocarditis. In addition, they have none of the complications associated with chronic use of α-adrenergic blockers. CCEB—calcium channel entry blockers. (*Adapted from* Canale and Bravo [40].)

1. Rodriguez-Portales JA, Arteaga E, Lopez-Morena JR, *et al.*: Zona glomerulosa function after lifelong suppression in two siblings with the hypertensive virilizing form of congential adrenal hyperplasia. *J Clin Endocrinol Metab* 1988, 66:349–354.

2. Biglieri EG, Herron MA, Brust N: 17-Hydroxylation deficiency in man. *J Clin Invest* 1966, 45:1946–1954.

3. Saadi HF, Bravo EL, Aron DC: Feminizing adrenocortical tumor: steroid hormone response to ketoconazole. *J Clin Endocrinol Metab* 1990, 70:540–543.

4. Azziz R, Boots LR, Parker CR, *et al.*: 11β-Hydroxylase deficiency in hyperandrogenism. *Fertil Steril* 1991, 55:733–741.

5. Forsham PH: The adrenal cortex. In *Textbook of Endocrinology*, edn 4. Edited by Williams RH. Philadelphia: WB Saunders; 1968:287–379.

6. Bravo EL: What to do when potassium is low or high. *Diagnosis* 1988, 10:1–6.

7. Liddle GW, Bledsoe T, Coppage WS: A familial renal disorder stimulating primary aldosteronism but with negligible aldosterone secretion. *Trans Assoc Am Physicians* 1963, 76:19.

8. Botero-Velez M, Curtis JJ, Warnock DG: Liddle's syndrome revisited: a disorder of sodium reabsorption in the distal tubule. *N Engl J Med* 1994, 300:178–181.

9. Oldfield EH, Chrousos GP, Schulte HM, *et al.*: Preoperative localization of ACTH-secreting pituitary microadenomas by bilateral and simultaneous inferior petrosal venous sinus sampling. *N Engl J Med* 1985, 312:100–103.

10. Kamilaris TC, Chrousos GP: Adrenal diseases. In *Diagnostic Endocrinology*. Edited by Moore WT, Eastman RC. Philadelphia: BC Decker; 1990:79–199.

11. Arriza JL, Weinberger C, Cerelli G: Cloning of human mineralo-corticoid receptor complementary DNA: structural and functional kinship with the glucocorticoid receptor. *Science* 1987, 237:268–275.

12. Edwards CRW, Stewart PM, Burt D, *et al.*: Localization of 11β-hydroxysteroid dehydrogenase: tissue specific protector of the mineralocorticoid receptor. *Lancet* 1988, 2:986–989.

13. Funder JW, Pearce PT, Smith R, *et al.*: Mineralocorticoid action: target tissue specificity is enzyme, not receptor, mediated. *Science* 1988, 242:583–585.

14. Brem AS, Matheson KL, Conca T, *et al.*: Effect of carbenoxolone on glucocorticoid metabolism and Na transport in toad bladder. *Am J Physiol* 1989, 257 (4 Pt 2):F700–F704.

15. Farese RV, Biglieri EG, Shackleton CHL, *et al.*: Licorice-induced hypermineralocorticoidism. *N Engl J Med* 1991, 325:1223–1227.

16. Walker BR, Edwards ERW: Licorice-induced hypertension and syndromes of apparent mineralocorticoid excess. *Endocrinol Metab Clin North Am* 1994, 23:359–377.

17. Bravo EL, Tarazi RC, Dustan HP, *et al.*: The changing clinical spectrum of primary aldosteronism. *Am J Med* 1983, 74:641–651.

18. Bravo EL: Primary aldosteronism. *Urol Clin North Am* 1989, 16:481–486.

19. Bravo EL: Primary aldosteronism. *Cardiol Clin* 1988, 6:509–515.

20. Guerin CK, Wahner HW, Gorman CA, *et al.*: Computed tomographic scanning versus radioisotope imaging in adreno-cortical diagnosis. *Am J Med* 1983, 75:653–657.

21. Bravo EL, Dustan HP, Tarazi RC: Spironolactone as a non-specific treatment for primary aldosteronism. *Circulation* 1973, 48:491–498.

22. Bravo EL: Calcium channel blockage with nifedipine in primary aldosteronism. *Hypertension* 1986, 8(suppl I):I-191–I-194.

23. Bravo EL: Pheochromocytoma and mineralocorticoid hypertension. In *Current Therapy in Nephrology and Hypertension*, edn 3. Edited by Glassock RJ. Philadelphia: BC Decker; 1992:386–391.

24. Ghose RP, Hall PM, Bravo EL: Medical management of aldosterone-producing adenomas. *Ann Intern Med* 1999, 131:105–108.

25. Weinberger MH, Roniker B, Krause AL, *et al.*: Eplerenone, a selective aldosterone blocker in mild-to-moderate hypertension. *Am J Hypertens* 2002, 15:709–716.

26. Sutherland DJ, Ruse JL, Laidlaw JC: Hypertension, increased aldosterone secretion, and low plasma renin activity relieved by dexamethasone. *Can Med Assoc J* 1966, 95:1109–1119.

27. Lifton RP, Dluhy RG, Powers M, *et al.*: A chimeric 11-hydroxylase/aldosterone synthase gene causes glucocorticoid-remediable aldosteronism and human hypertension. *Nature* 1992, 355:262–265.

28. Lifton RP, Dluhy RG, Powers M, *et al.*: Hereditary hypertension caused by chimeric gene duplications and ectopic expression of aldosterone synthase. *Nat Genet* 1992, 2:66–74.

29. Pascoe L, Curnow KM, Slutsker L, *et al.*: Glucocorticoid-suppressible hyperaldosteronism results from hybrid genes created by unequal crossovers between CYP11B1 and CYP11B2. *Proc Natl Acad Sci U S A* 1992, 89:8327–8331.

30. Woodland E, Tunny TJ, Hamlet SM, *et al.*: Hypertension corrected and aldosterone responsiveness to renin-angiotensin restored by long-term dexamethasone in glucocorticoid-suppressible hyperal-dosteronism. *Clin Exp Pharmacol Physiol* 1985, 12:245–248.

31. Bravo EL: The syndrome of primary aldosteronism and pheochro-mocytoma. In *Diseases of the Kidney*. Edited by Shrier RW, Gosschalk CV. Boston: Little, Brown & Co; 1993:1475–1503.

32. Bravo EL, Gifford RW: Pheochromocytoma: diagnosis, localization and management. *N Engl J Med* 1984, 311:1298–1303.

33. Bravo EL, Tarazi RC, Gifford RW, Jr, Stewart BH: Circulating plasma and urinary catecholamines in pheochromocytoma: diagnostic and pathophysiologic implications. *N Engl J Med* 1979, 301:682–686.

34. Bravo EL, Gifford RW: Pheochromocytoma. In *Endocrinology and Metabolism Clinics of North America*. Edited by Ober KP. Philadelphia: WB Saunders; 1993:329–341.

35. Bravo EL: Adrenal medullary function. In *Diagnostic Endocrinology*. Edited by Moore WT, Eastman RC. Philadelphia: BC Decker; 1990:217–226.

36. Bravo EL, Gifford RW, Manger WM: Adrenal medullary tumors: pheochromocytoma. In *Endocrine Tumors*. Edited by Mazzaferri EL, Samaan NA. Boston: Blackwell Scientific Publications; 1993:426–447.

37. Bravo EL: Evolving concepts in the pathophysiology, diagnosis, and treatment of pheochromocytoma. *Endocr Rev* 1994, 15:356–368.

38. Taylor SH: Pharmacotherapeutic stature of doxazosin and its role in coronary risk reduction. *Am Heart J* 1988, 16:1735–1747.

39. Sprung J, O'Hara JF, Jr, Gill IS, *et al.*: Anesthetic aspects of laparoscopic and open adrenalectomy for pheochromocytoma. *Urology* 2000, 55:339–343.

40. Canale MP, Bravo EL: Calcium channel entry blockers are effective and safe in the preoperative management of pheochromocytoma [abstract]. *Hypertension* 1993, 21:560.

CHAPTER 7

ANTIHYPERTENSIVE AGENTS: MECHANISMS OF DRUG ACTION

Bernard Waeber and Hans R. Brunner

Hypertension is a major risk factor for the development of cardiovascular diseases. There is a direct relationship between blood pressure and the incidence of stroke and coronary events [1]. Even modest elevations in blood pressure (both systolic and diastolic) are associated with an increased health risk. Hypertension also predisposes to left ventricular hypertrophy and chronic renal failure [2,3].

Antihypertensive treatment clearly has beneficial effects on cardiovascular morbidity and mortality, as shown in a meta-analysis of 14 randomized primary prevention trials involving nearly 37,000 patients [4]. This analysis demonstrated that a reduction in diastolic blood pressure of 5 to 6 mm Hg reduces cardiovascular mortality by 21%, fatal and nonfatal stroke by 42%, and fatal and nonfatal coronary heart disease by 14%. It now appears that elderly patients also benefit from drug-induced blood pressure reduction. Treating elderly hypertensive patients (even those with isolated systolic hypertension) significantly reduces the occurrence of fatal and nonfatal cardiovascular complications [5].

Official guidelines propose that patients with diastolic blood pressure of 90 mm Hg or higher or systolic blood pressure of 140 mm Hg or higher on several visits be considered hypertensive [6,7]. Conservative management (decreased sodium and alcohol consumption, weight reduction in obese patients, increased physical activity, and cessation of smoking) should be the first step in treating patients with slightly elevated blood pressures; antihypertensive drugs should be added if further control of blood pressure is necessary. The goal of intervention is to reduce blood pressure below 130 mm Hg systolic and 85 mm Hg diastolic by means of an individualized well-tolerated treatment regimen.

Currently available antihypertensive drugs, administered alone or in combination, normalize blood pressure in nearly all hypertensive patients, regardless of the underlying pathogenetic mechanisms responsible for blood pressure elevation. Modern pharmacology offers a broad choice of compounds that lower blood pressure by interfering with different pressor systems. This greatly facilitates the therapeutic approach, making it possible to find the most suitable treatment, in terms of both efficacy and tolerability, for each patient.

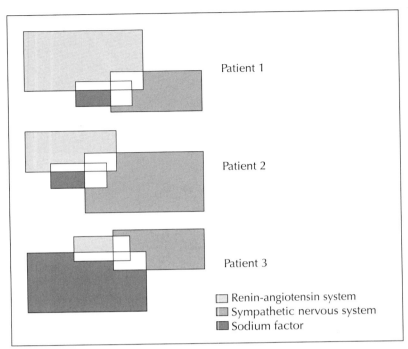

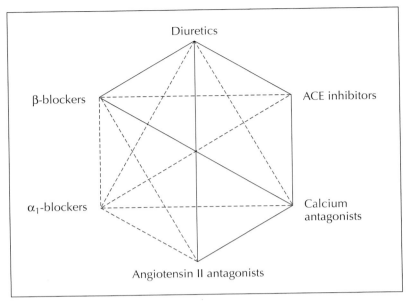

FIGURE 7-1. Heterogeneity of hypertension. Essential hypertension is a heterogeneous disease. Various pressor mechanisms might be responsible for the blood pressure elevation, including stimulation of the renin-angiotensin system, overactivity of the sympathetic nervous system, or an increase in total body sodium [8–10]. In everyday practice, the exact contribution of these different factors to the pathogenesis of hypertension cannot be predicted in individual patients. This illustration represents three hypertensive patients exhibiting similar blood pressures. In one patient, the abnormal blood pressure results primarily from an exaggerated renin secretion. In the second, an enhanced sympathetic tone plays the preponderant role. In the third, the sodium factor is predominant.

FIGURE 7-2. First-line antihypertensive drugs. Different classes of antihypertensive agents are proposed as first-line treatment for hypertension, *ie*, diuretics, β- (and α-) adrenergic blockers, angiotensin-converting enzyme (ACE) inhibitors, angiotensin II antagonists, and calcium antagonists [6,7]. These agents reduce blood pressure by various mechanisms. They are therefore more or less effective, depending on the prevailing pathogenic factors in a given hypertensive patient. There is no reliable way to predict a positive response (*ie*, normalized blood pressure) to a specific therapeutic approach. A patient may respond favorably to one class of drugs exclusively or to several types of antihypertensive agents. Some patients may remain hypertensive regardless of the drug used as monotherapy. When necessary, different types of antihypertensive agents can be combined. Some drug associations are particularly effective, as indicated by the *thick lines* [11].

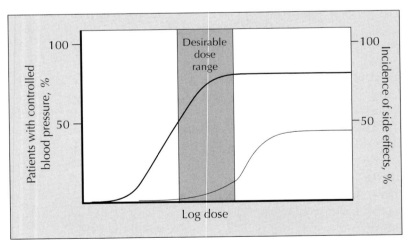

FIGURE 7-3. Dose response to antihypertensive drugs. The ability of antihypertensive agents to lower blood pressure is dose-dependent, but the dose response is generally quite flat [12]. This illustration demonstrates such a relationship. Increasing the dose of a given medication allows control of blood pressure in a larger percentage of patients. The favorable results, however, are often associated with a progressive rise in the incidence of side effects. Fortunately, with many drugs, side effects occur at somewhat higher doses. The desirable dose range should be chosen not only to normalize blood pressure in the largest fraction of hypertensive patients but also to be well tolerated. Selecting good responders to small doses of antihypertensive agents minimizes the risk of causing adverse effects.

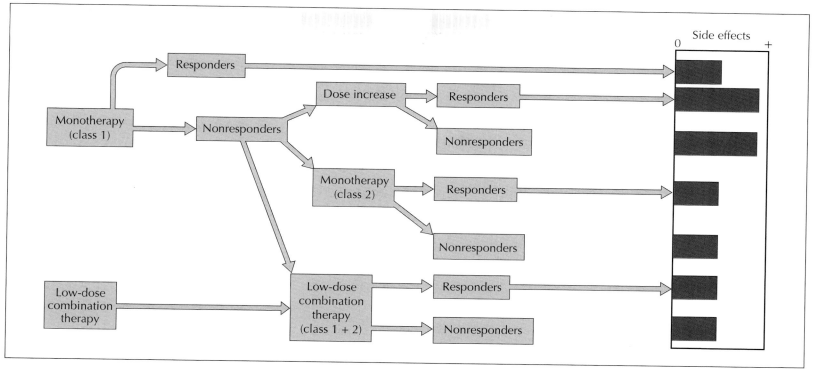

FIGURE 7-4. Sequential monotherapy and low-dose combination therapy. A rational approach to treatment of hypertensive patients is sequential monotherapy [12]. According to this concept, attempts are made to normalize blood pressure as often as possible with antihypertensive drugs given as monotherapy and to treat patients sequentially with two or more types of antihypertensive agents.

Several weeks are usually needed to assess whether a drug is both effective and well tolerated. When necessary, drugs belonging to different classes can be associated. In such cases, low-dose combinations should be used to minimize side effects [11–13]. Low-dose combination therapy may become a valuable option to initiate antihypertensive therapy [14].

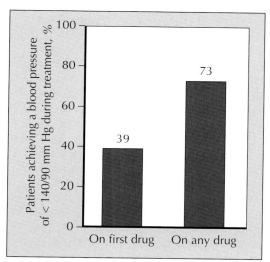

FIGURE 7-5. An example of sequential monotherapy. What can be achieved by applying the sequential monotherapy strategy, assuming that the aim is to decrease blood pressure to less than 140/90 mm Hg? The results of a recent four-way, crossover study provide some valuable information regarding this issue [15]. A total of 56 patients with essential hypertension received, in monthly cycles, four different treatments, consisting of the angiotensin-converting enzyme inhibitor lisinopril (20 mg/d), the β-blocker bisoprolol (5 mg/d), the fixed-dose combination hydrochlorothiazide (25 mg/d) plus triamterene (50 mg/d), and the long-acting formulation of the calcium antagonist nifedipine (30 mg/d). Each treatment phase was separated by a 1-month washout period. Only 36 patients completed the rotation through the four treatment periods. Of the 56 patients, 22 (39%) had their blood pressure controlled to less than 140/90 mm Hg during the first treatment phase, independently of the medication used as first drug, compared with 41 (73%) who achieved blood pressure control when the results of any of the four treatment periods were taken into consideration. It appears, therefore, that the obligatory rotation through the four classes of antihypertensive agents considerably increased the probability of bringing blood pressure under control in each patient. Almost one third of the patients could not, however, be treated with each of the four types of agents, mainly because one drug or another was contraindicated.

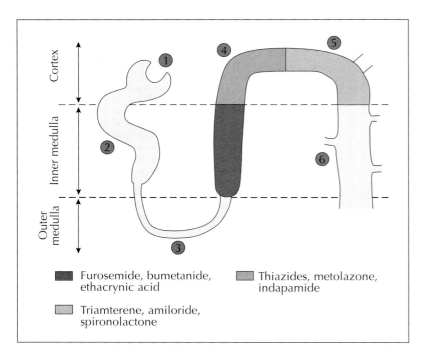

FIGURE 7-6. Site of action of diuretics. A common feature of all diuretics is their natriuretic action, which leads to a decrease in total body sodium [16,17]. The most potent diuretics (furosemide, bumetanide, and ethacrynic acid) decrease sodium resorption in the thick ascending loop of Henle. Urinary sodium excretion can be enhanced considerably with these agents by increasing the dose. Loop diuretics remain effective even in patients with severely impaired renal function. Thiazides, metolazone, and indapamide inhibit sodium resorption in the early portion of the distal convoluted tubule. The dose-response curve to these diuretics is rather flat. Furthermore, the natriuretic effect of thiazides and indapamide is lost when the glomerular filtration rate is reduced below a rate of approximately 40 mL/min, whereas metolazone is still active down to a glomerular filtration rate of approximately 20 mL/min. Triamterene, amiloride, and spironolactone act in the late portion of the distal convoluted tubule and the cortical collecting duct. Loop diuretics, thiazides, and metolazone as well as triamterene, amiloride, and spironolactone act in the late portion of the distal convoluted tubule and the cortical collecting duct. Triamterene and amiloride have weak natriuretic action. 1—glomerulus; 2—proximal convoluted tubule; 3—loop of Henle; 4—early portion of the distal convoluted tubule; 5—late portion of the distal convoluted tubule and cortical collecting tubule; 6— medullary collecting tubule.

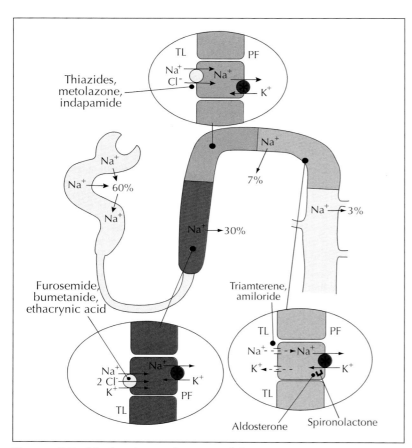

FIGURE 7-7. Mechanisms of action of diuretics. Sixty percent of filtered sodium is resorbed in the proximal convoluted tubule (obligatory resorption) [17]. The more distal segments of the nephron can modulate excretion of only a fraction of the total filtered sodium. Diuretics that impair sodium resorption in the thick ascending loop of Henle (furosemide, bumetanide, ethacrynic acid) interfere with the $Na^+,K^+,2Cl^-$ cotransport system located at the apical membrane of the renal tubule. These diuretics act at a site where a large quantity of sodium is normally resorbed. Thiazides, metolazone, and indapamide inhibit the apical Na^+,Cl^- cotransport system in the early portion of the distal convoluted tubule. Only a small fraction of filtered sodium is normally resorbed at this site of the nephron, which accounts for the limited natriuretic activity of the diuretics. In the late portion of the distal convoluted tubule and in the cortical collecting duct, sodium is transported at the apical level of the tubular cell through a sodium channel. Sodium is then exchanged against a potassium ion at the basal membrane due to the activity of Na^+,K^+ ATPase. The activity of this enzyme is enhanced by aldosterone, the mineralocorticoid hormone secreted by the adrenal glomerulosa. Spironolactone is a competitive antagonist of aldosterone and consequently inhibits pump activity. Amiloride and triamterene block the apical sodium transport. The elimination of potassium is reduced by diuretics acting in these most distal portions of the nephron because of decreased sodium-potassium exchange. In contrast, loop diuretics and diuretics acting in the early distal convoluted tubule increase kaliuresis and tend to cause hypokalemia. This is mainly because these agents enhance delivery of sodium downstream and subsequently accentuate the sodium-potassium exchange. As a result, an increased quantity of sodium is available for resorption in the late distal convoluted tubule and the cortical collecting tubule. Potassium-sparing diuretics must be avoided in patients with renal failure because they may cause life-threatening hyperkalemia. PF—peritubular interstitial fluid; TL—tubular lumen.

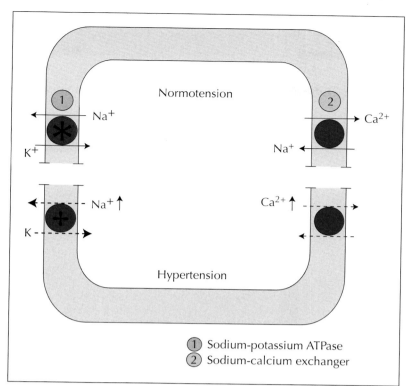

FIGURE 7-8. The link between sodium and calcium metabolism in vascular smooth muscle cells. Sodium loading enhances the vascular responsiveness to pressor stimuli. This effect may be mediated by an increase in intracellular free calcium [18]. In the wall of vascular smooth muscle cells is a sodium-calcium transport system, which allows extrusion of calcium ions in exchange for sodium ions. The entry of sodium into the cell is powered by a concentration gradient maintained in normal conditions by an energy-dependent Na^+,K^+ ATPase pump. In hypertensive patients, intracellular sodium seems to be elevated, perhaps partially because of suppressed Na^+,K^+ ATPase activity. This abnormality in turn reduces the propensity of calcium to move out of the cell, resulting in an increased concentration of intracellular free calcium and vasoconstriction. Diuretics, when reducing total body sodium, may reverse these intracellular ionic perturbations and facilitate relaxation of the vasculature.

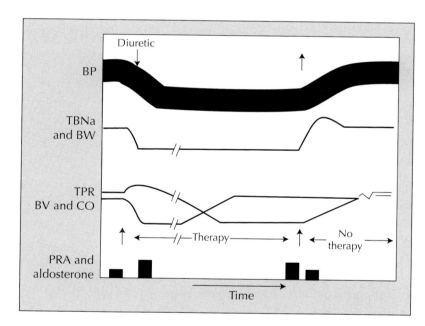

FIGURE 7-9. Hemodynamic and hormonal effects of diuretic therapy. At the initiation of treatment, diuretic-induced blood pressure (BP) reduction is associated with a reduction in total body sodium (TBNa), reflected by loss of body weight (BW), reductions in blood volume (BV) and cardiac output (CO), and an increase in total peripheral resistance (TPR). During chronic therapy, the antihypertensive effect persists together with the negative sodium balance, but both BV and CO return to pretreatment values. With time, however, a reduction in TPR occurs [19]. The initial BP response to diuretics is probably caused for the most part by the hemodynamic changes resulting from salt depletion, whereas the long-term response might depend more on progressive mobilization of sodium from the vascular smooth muscle cells and the ensuing reduction in intracellular calcium. The diuretic-mediated salt depletion is accompanied by a compensatory activation of the renin-angiotensin-aldosterone system. PRA—plasma renin activity.

MAIN RESPONSES MEDIATED BY β-ADRENOCEPTORS

	β-ADRENOCEPTER SUBTYPE	RESPONSE TO STIMULATION
Heart	β_1	Increase in heart rate, conduction velocity, excitability, and force of contraction
Blood vessels	β_2	Dilatation
Kidney	β_1	Stimulation of renin release
Lung	$\beta_2 > \beta_1$	Bronchodilatation
Skeletal muscle	β_2	Tremor
Uterine	β_2	Relaxation
Eye	β_1	Increase in intra-ocular pressure
Glucogenolysis	β_1 (heart) β_2 (skeletal muscle, liver)	Promoted
Lipolysis (white adipocytes)	$\beta_1 > \beta_2$	Promoted

FIGURE 7-10. Distribution and function of β-adrenoceptors. There are two types of β-adrenoceptors: β_1 and β_2 [20]. β-adrenoceptors are ubiquitous in tissues, and activation of these receptors causes a wide variety of responses. Both norepinephrine discharged by sympathetic nerve terminals and epinephrine released into the circulation by the adrenal medulla can stimulate β-adrenoceptors. The number of β_1-adrenoceptors relative to β_2-adrenoceptors varies greatly from one organ to another.

PROPERTIES OF β-BLOCKERS

	β_1-SELECTIVITY	INTRINSIC SYMPATHO-MIMETIC ACTIVITY	α-BLOCKADE
Acebutolol	+	+	-
Alprenolol	-	+	-
Atenolol	+	-	-
Betaxolol	+	-	-
Bisoprolol	+	-	-
Bopindolol	-	+	-
Carvedilol	+	-	+
Celiprolol	+	$+\beta_2$	-
Dilevolol	+	$+\beta_2$	-
Labetalol	-	-	+
Metoprolol	+	-	-
Nadolol	-	-	-
Nebivolol	+	-	-
Oxprenolol	-	+	-
Pindolol	-	+	-
Propranolol	-	-	-
Sotalol	-	-	-
Timolol	-	-	-

FIGURE 7-11. Pharmacologic characteristics of β-blockers. The β-blockers are competitive inhibitors of the effects of catecholamines at β-adrenergic receptors [21,22]. The so-called cardioselective β-blockers combine preferentially with β_1-receptors. This selectivity is progressively lost when the doses of the drugs are increased. Some β-blockers have partial agonist activity (intrinsic sympathomimetic activity [ISA]). These agents competitively block the effect of catecholamines but simultaneously maintain a stimulatory activity of their own. Celiprolol and dilevolol have a stimulatory effect on β_2-adrenoceptors, resulting in some degree of vasodilation. Carvedilol and labetalol have also α_1-blocking properties, accounting for a vasodilatory action. Nebivolol triggers the release of nitric oxide from the endothelium, which also leads to vasodilation. Labetalol and carvedilol have concurrent β- and α-adrenoceptor blocking properties. Sotalol, which possesses class III antiarrhythmic activity, is a racemate of d- and l-isomers, both of which block cardiac potassium channels; by this mechanism, the duration of the cardiac action potential is prolonged and cardiac refractoriness is increased. Only the l-isomer of sotalol has significant β-blocking activity.

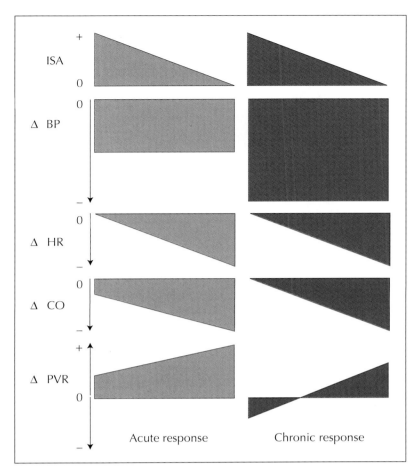

FIGURE 7-12. Hemodynamic response to β-adrenoceptor blockade. Blood pressure (BP) is determined by cardiac output (CO) multiplied by peripheral vascular resistance (PVR). Responses to β-adrenoceptor blockade, both acute and chronic, have been organized according to the amount of intrinsic sympathomimetic activity (ISA) shown by the individual agents. At initiation of treatment, heart rate (HR) and CO are reduced. This effect is most prominent in compounds with the least pronounced ISA [22]. These changes are accompanied by an increase in PVR that is inversely proportional to the degree of sympathomimetic activity. Although the BP decrease shortly after first administration (acute response) is modest, with continued treatment the BP decrease becomes substantially larger in many patients (chronic response). The magnitude of the decrease in heart rate and cardiac output and the reactive increase in PVR vary with the degree of ISA, as shown in this figure, but these responses do not account for the long-term decrease in BP.

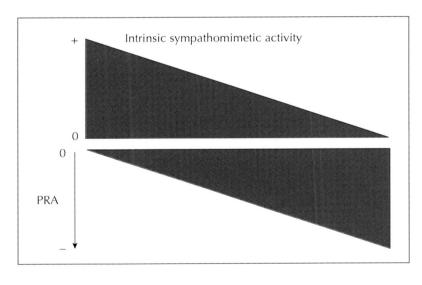

FIGURE 7-13. Effects of β-blockers on plasma renin activity (PRA). β-blockers inhibit renin secretion [22]. By analogy with the hemodynamic response shown in Figure 7-12, the magnitude of the inhibition and the consequent decrease in PRA vary with the degree of intrinsic sympathomimetic activity (ISA). Although renin inhibition might contribute to the depressor response, as is indicated in Figure 7-12, the depressor response to β-blockers with ISA is complete.

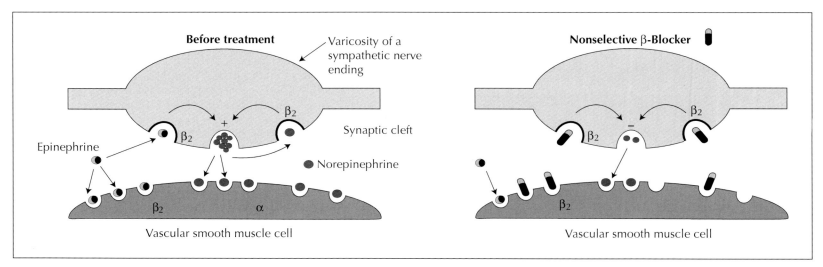

FIGURE 7-14. Reduced release of norepinephrine during blockade of presynaptic β-adrenoceptors. As shown on the *left panel*, β2-adrenoceptors are located on varicosities of sympathetic nerve endings. Activation of these receptors enhances the neurally induced release of norepinephrine. Blockade of presynaptic β2-receptors causes a decrease in norepinephrine discharge (*right panel*). This effect may be an important contributor to the antihypertensive action of β-blockers.

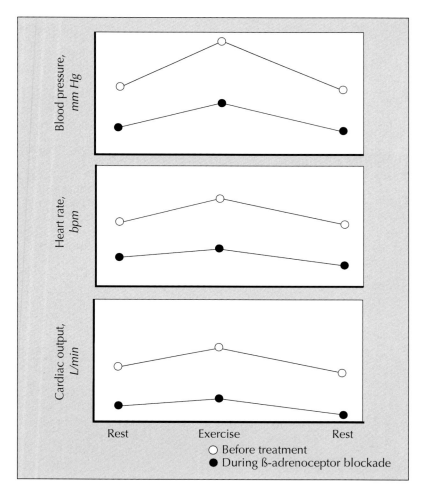

FIGURE 7-15. Effects of β-blockers on hemodynamic responses to exercise. Blockade of cardiac β1-adrenoceptors markedly attenuates the heart rate and cardiac output increase that occurs during physical exercise [23]. The rise in blood pressure (BP) is also blunted, most likely because BP at rest is lower. Decreased exercise capacity induced by β-blockers is dose-dependent.

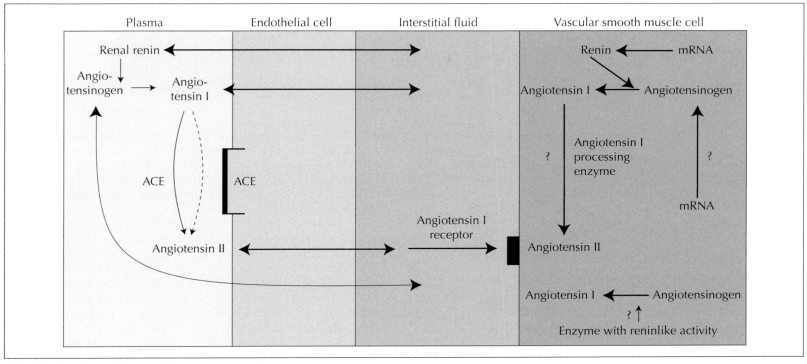

FIGURE 7-16. The renin-angiotensin system is an enzymatic cascade [24]. Renin released into the circulation by the renal juxtaglomerular cells cleaves the decapeptide angiotensin I from angiotensinogen, a protein substrate synthesized by the liver and present in the blood. Angiotensin I is devoid of vasoactive effects. It is metabolized to the octapeptide angiotensin II by angiotensin-converting enzyme (ACE). This enzyme is mostly a membrane-bound enzyme of the vascular endothelium but is also present in the circulation. Angiotensin II binds to specific receptors located on vascular smooth muscle cells to induce vascular contraction.

Some components of the renin-angiotensin system have been identified in the vascular wall, including mRNA for renin and angiotensinogen [25], but it remains uncertain whether renin, angiotensinogen, and angiotensin II are actually generated in the vasculature [26]. Renin of renal origin may be taken up from the circulation. Alternate pathways for the cleaving of angiotensinogen or the processing of angiotensin I might exist in vascular smooth muscle cells; however, the bulk of angiotensin II synthesis takes place in the lumen of the endothelium.

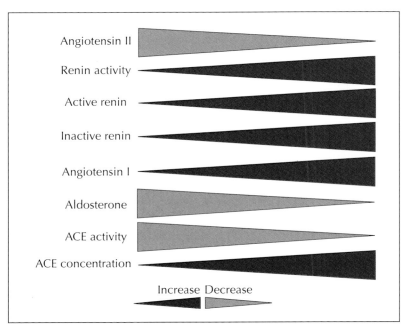

FIGURE 7-17. Effects of chronic angiotensin-converting enzyme (ACE) inhibition on the components of the renin-angiotensin system. Angiotensin II nearly disappears from the circulation during peak ACE inhibition [27]. Angiotensin II normally exerts a negative inhibitory feedback on renin secretion. During blockade of angiotensin II generation or angiotensin II receptor blockade, plasma renin activity as well as active and inactive renin concentrations increase. The hyperreninemia is accompanied by a rise in plasma angiotensin I levels. Angiotensin II is a physiologic stimulus of aldosterone secretion. The plasma levels of this salt-retaining hormone are reduced during ACE inhibition. There is an induction of ACE synthesis during long-term treatment with ACE inhibitors.

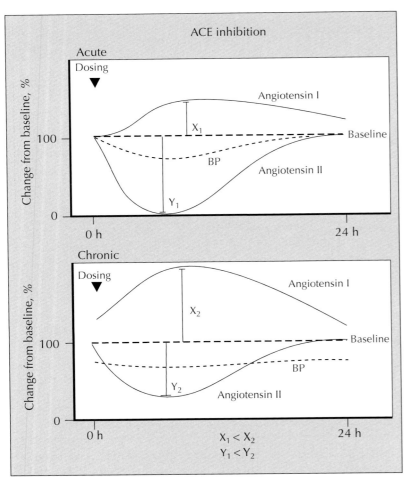

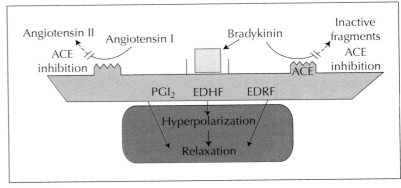

FIGURE 7-19. Effects of angiotensin-converting enzyme (ACE) inhibition on the kallikrein-kinin system. Activation of the kallikrein-kinin system results in the generation of bradykinin [28]. This peptide is derived from kininogen (an α_2-globulin) that has been exposed to active kallikreins or other kininogenases. Bradykinin is normally inactivated by ACE. Inhibition of this enzyme may thus lead to local accumulation of bradykinin. Bradykinin, by stimulating receptors on endothelial cells, can induce release of such vasodilators as endothelium-derived relaxing factor (nitric oxide or EDRF), endothelium-derived hyperpolarizing factor (EDHF), and prostacyclin (PGI_2) [29,30]. It is not yet clear, however, whether such a mechanism is actually involved in the blood pressure–lowering action of ACE inhibitors or has any effect on the microcirculation. Bradykinin accumulation may contribute to the genesis of cough, a typical side effect of ACE inhibitors.

FIGURE 7-18. Dissociation between antihypertensive effect and blockade of angiotensin II generation during angiotensin-converting enzyme (ACE) inhibition. At initiation of treatment with an ACE inhibitor, the changes in blood pressure (BP) usually parallel those in plasma angiotensin II levels [27]. During long-term therapy, however, it is not necessary to suppress angiotensin II generation continuously to keep BP normalized throughout the day. During chronic ACE inhibition, the reactive hyperreninemia becomes more pronounced, resulting in higher concentrations of angiotensin I. Consequently, for a given inhibition of ACE activity, more angiotensin II is formed during chronic treatment than during acute treatment.

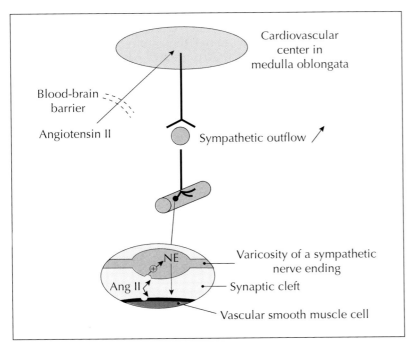

FIGURE 7-20. Interaction between angiotensin II and the sympathetic nervous system. Circulating angiotensin II can reach brain stem cardiovascular centers through areas devoid of a tight blood-brain barrier, thereby increasing sympathetic efferent activity. In the periphery, angiotensin II stimulates presynaptic receptors, thereby enhancing the release of norepinephrine (NE). The reduced synthesis of angiotensin II during angiotensin-converting enzyme (ACE) inhibition can therefore attenuate the neurogenic contribution to blood pressure maintenance via both a central and a peripheral mechanism [31]. The interaction between angiotensin II and the sympathetic nervous system is probably responsible for the lack of reflex heart rate acceleration when blood pressure is lowered with an ACE inhibitor.

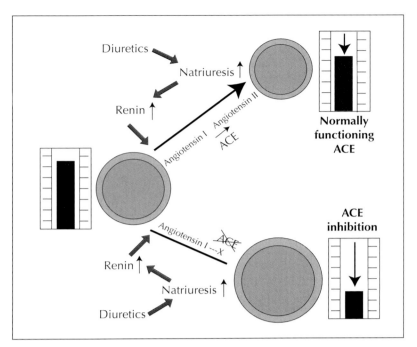

FIGURE 7-21. Interaction between the response to diuretics and to angiotensin-converting enzyme (ACE) inhibition. The use of diuretics alone leads to a natriuresis, a reduction in total body sodium, and thus to a reactive activation of the renin-angiotensin system. The reactive response of the renin system limits the decrease in blood pressure [32]. When the diuretic is combined with an ACE inhibitor, the generation of angiotensin II is limited, the natriuresis is more complete, and a more substantial decrease in blood pressure follows.

CALCIUM ANTAGONISTS

COMPARATIVE PHARMACOLOGIC PROPERTIES OF CALCIUM ANTAGONISTS

	PHENYL-ALKYLAMINES	BENZO-THIAZEPINES	DIHYDROPYRIDINES
	(verapamil)	(diltiazem)	(amlodipine, felodipine, isradipine, lacidipine, nicardipine, nitrendipine, nifedipine)
Vasodilation	+	++	+++
Negative inotropic effect	++	+	-
Negative chronotropic effect	++	+	-

FIGURE 7-22. Comparative pharmacologic properties of calcium antagonists. Calcium antagonists act by blocking the entry of calcium ions from the extracellular space into the cytoplasm of vascular smooth muscle cells and cardiac cells through voltage-dependent calcium channels [33,34]. There are three major classes of calcium antagonists: the phenylalkylamines, benzothiazepines, and dihydropyridines. These agents differ markedly in their potency on the vasculature versus the myocardium. The differential pharmacologic effects of the various classes of calcium antagonists are clinically relevant. For instance, verapamil should not be combined with a β-blocker, as both types of agents have a negative inotropic and chronotropic effect; verapamil or diltiazem are preferred for treating hypertensive patients with supraventricular tachycardia or sinus tachycardia; a dihydropyridine should be chosen for hypertensive patients with bradycardia or overt congestive heart failure. First-generation dihydropyridines are thought to have a measurable, albeit small, negative inotropic effect. Conversely, newer dihydropyridines, such as amlodipine and felodipine, are thought to have less of this influence.

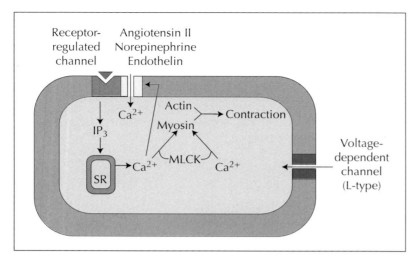

FIGURE 7-23. Mechanism of action of calcium antagonists. Increased free calcium in the cytoplasm of vascular smooth muscle cells leads to vasoconstriction [35,36]. The calcium ion, after binding to calcium-binding proteins, activates a myosin light-chain kinase (MLCK), causing phosphorylation of myosin filaments followed by an interaction of these filaments with actin filaments and finally cell contraction. The calcium ion can enter the vascular smooth muscle cell by two main channels. The receptor-regulated channels cause, upon activation with an agonist (*eg*, angiotensin II, norepinephrine, endothelin), the formation of inositol trisphosphate (IP_3). This intracellular messenger triggers the release of calcium from the sarcoplasmic reticulum (SR). The rapid calcium mobilization by this pathway stimulates then sustains entry of calcium through the channel. Calcium antagonists block voltage-dependent channels. These channels allow the entry of calcium in response to cell depolarization.

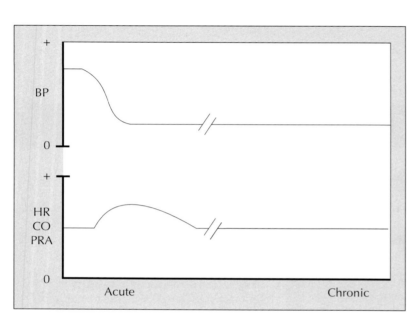

FIGURE 7-24. Reflex responses to the vasodilation induced by dihydropyridines. Dihydropyridines are potent vasodilators. The initial blood pressure (BP) reduction is sometimes accompanied by a reflex increase in sympathetic nerve activity, mainly with short-acting antagonists as reflected by an accelerated heart rate (HR), a rise in cardiac out-put (CO), and stimulation of the renin-angiotensin system. These reflex responses usually do not occur during chronic therapy, most likely because of a progressive resetting of the baroreceptor reflex at lower blood pressures, and can largely be prevented by concomitant β-adrenoreceptor blockade [11]. The different classes of calcium antagonists are equally effective during long-term treatment. Peripheral edema may develop in response to blockade of calcium entry. This side effect results from drug-induced changes in the microcirculation and not from renal sodium retention, as the calcium antagonists tend to have a natriuretic action. PRA—plasma renin activity.

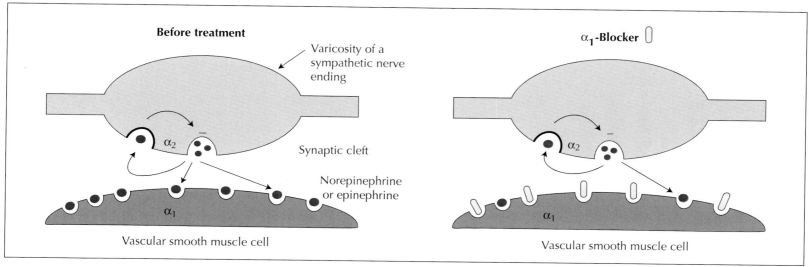

FIGURE 7-25. α_1-Adrenoceptor blocking agents. α_1-Blockers (doxazosin, prazosin, terazosin) lower blood pressure by preventing catecholamine-induced vasoconstriction [37]. In this illustration, norepinephrine released from the sympathetic nerve ending is depicted as *circles*, and the α_1-adrenergic blocking agent as *ovals*. The competitive action is confined to the vascular smooth muscle cell. These agents selectively block postsynaptic α_1-adrenoceptors. Catecholamines can still activate presynaptic α_2-receptors and thus exert an inhibitory action on norepinephrine release by the sympathetic nerve terminal. This probably accounts for the lack of reflex heart rate acceleration during α_1-adrenoceptor blockade. α_1-Blockers induce dilation of both arteries and veins. The effect on the capacitive system accounts for the prominent decrease in postural blood pressure that occurs in some patients; this effect often limits the utility of these agents. α_1-Blockers are effective in reducing the symptoms of benign prostatic hypertrophy, which makes them an attractive choice in hypertensive elderly men with that disorder.

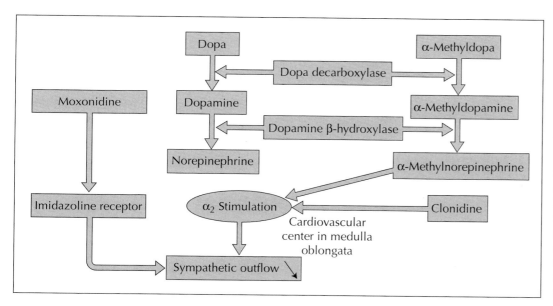

FIGURE 7-26. Centrally acting agents. α-Methyldopa and clonidine lower blood pressure predominantly via a central mechanism. Clinical use of these drugs is declining, however, principally because of the common occurrence of side effects such as sedation and dry mouth. α-Methyldopa is metabolized to α-methylnorepinephrine by the enzymes that are normally involved in the transformation of dopa to norepi-nephrine. α-Methylnorepinephrine and clonidine both stimulate α_2-adrenoceptors located in the cardiovascular center of the medulla oblongata, thereby decreasing sympathetic outflow. A new centrally acting drug (moxonidine) is currently available [38]. This drug reduces sympathetic nerve activity by activating central imidazoline receptors and seems to have a more favorable tolerability profile than older centrally acting agents.

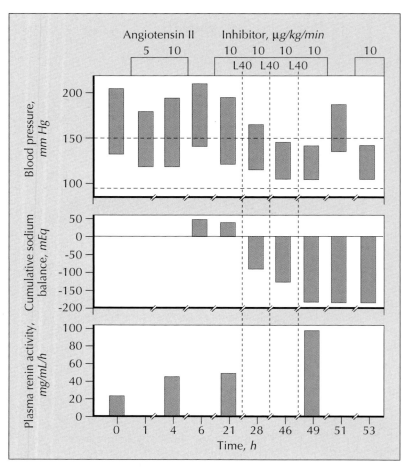

FIGURE 7-27. The first pharmacologic agent able to block the renin-angiotensin system was saralasin, an analogue of angiotensin II developed in the early 1970s. Because of its polypeptide nature, this compound was active only when administered parenterally. It also had an inherent partial agonistic property that could cause an increase in blood pressure in some patients, particularly those with low renin levels. However, saralasin was found to reduce blood pressure in patients with high renin values. A major observation was that the efficacy of angiotensin II blockade could be improved markedly by concomitant diuretic-induced salt depletion, which is exemplified in this 45-year-old male patient with bilateral renal artery stenosis who was given saralasin [39]. The drug produced a rapid decrease of 15 mm Hg in diastolic pressure, but the pressure did not fall below 120 mm Hg. However, when 40 furosemide (L40, Lasix) was administered intravenously during angiotensin blockade, blood pressure decreased to near normal values as cumulative sodium balance was reduced. (*Adapted from* Brunner *et al.* [39].)

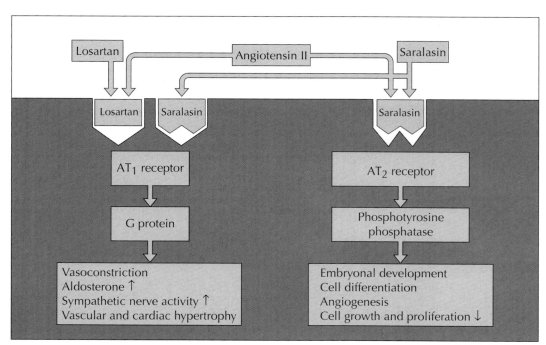

FIGURE 7-28. Angiotensin II antagonists. There now are available nonpeptide, orally active angiotensin II antagonists. Losartan represents the pioneer in this new class of agents [40]. The discovery of this compound led to the recognition of two functionally different angiotensin II receptors: AT_1 and AT_2. Losartan is a selective antagonist of the AT_1 receptor, whereas saralasin blocks both the AT_1 and AT_2 receptors.

The AT_1 receptor is a protein G–coupled receptor mediating the main physiologic effects of angiotensin II (vasoconstriction, stimulation of aldosterone secretion, stimulation of norepinephrine release from sympathetic nerve terminals, inhibition of renin release, vascular and cardiac hypertrophy). The transduction system for the AT_2 receptor is not well defined, but appears to involve phosphotyrosine phosphatase. The effects of AT_2 receptor stimulation in humans are still unclear. The AT_2 receptor might play a role in embryonal development and cell differentiation, promote angiogenesis, and inhibit cell growth and proliferation. Stimulation of this receptor may also lead to vasodilation and natriuresis [41,42]. During AT_1-receptor blockade, the interruption of the negative feedback that is exerted normally by angiotensin II on renin secretion leads to a reactive hyperreninemia. There is, however, no evidence to date that the increased circulating levels of angiotensin II observed during AT_1-receptor blockade have any undesirable effects. (*Adapted from* Timmermans *et al.* [40].)

POSSIBLE ROLE OF ANGIOTENSIN II IN THE PATHOGENESIS OF ATHEROSCLEROSIS

Oxidative stress
Oxidized LDL
Oxidized LDL receptor
Inactivation of NO
Vascular cell adhesion molecules
Inflammation
Fibrinolysis
Extracellular matrix
Migration of vascular smooth muscle cells

FIGURE 7-29. The role of angiotensin II in hypertension. In addition to its classic effects on the cardiovascular system, angiotensin II appears more and more to play a critical role in the pathogenesis of atherosclerosis [43–45]. For example, this peptide 1) increases the vascular oxidative stress and, by, this way, enhances the formation of oxidized low-density lipoprotein (LDL) and accelerates the inactivation of nitric oxide to generate peroxynitrite; 2) upregulates the receptor for oxidized LDL on endothelial cells and macrophages; 3) inactivates and enhances the expression of vascular cell adhesion molecules; 4) has a procoagulant activity by activating the plasminogen-activator inhibitor; 5) induces an inflammatory response in the vascular wall by triggering the release of cytokines and chemokines; 6) increases the extracellular matrix via activation of metalloproteinases; and 7) stimulates the migration of vascular smooth muscle cells from the media to the intima. Blockade of the renin-angiotensin system is therefore expected to be highly effective in the prevention of atherosclerosis and its complications.

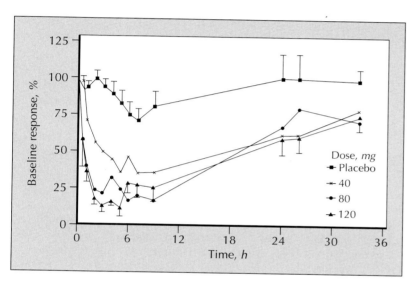

FIGURE 7-30. That losartan is an effective angiotensin II antagonist in humans can be demonstrated by assessing the effect of the drug on the pressor action of exogenous angiotensin II. This has been done in healthy volunteers [46]. The test dose of angiotensin II was selected to increase systolic blood pressure by about 30 mm Hg. This dose was used to define the baseline systolic blood pressure response to angiotensin and became the challenge dose for that given subject. The effect of losartan was established by serial intravenous bolus injections of this test dose of angiotensin II after oral intake of a single dose of losartan (40, 80, or 120 mg) or placebo. Losartan caused a dose-dependent increase in the degree of angiotensin blockade. Losartan is metabolized to EXP 3174, which exhibits a longer half-life and an approximately 10-fold higher affinity for the AT_1-receptor than does losartan. Losartan by itself has an uricosuric effect that manifests in hypertensive patients by a significant reduction of serum uric acid concentration [47]. (*Adapted from* Munafo *et al.* [46].)

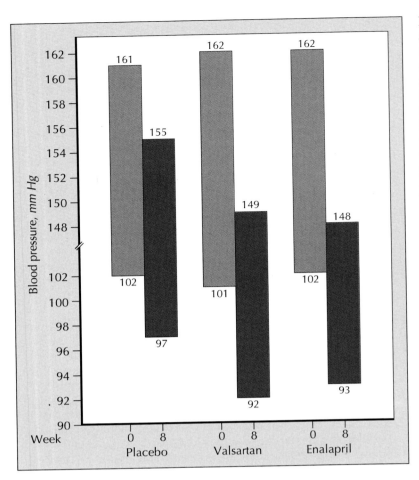

FIGURE 7-31. Comparison of valsartan with enalapril. Valsartan is a new long-acting selective antagonist of the AT_1 receptor. Its angiotensin II–blocking effect is at its maximum at 2 to 3 hours after oral administration and is maintained up to 24 hours after dosing [48]. The angiotensin-converting enzyme (ACE) is physiologically involved in the degradation of bradykinin, a peptide that can trigger the release of nitric oxide from the endothelium and, by this mechanism, cause vasodilation (*see* Fig. 7-19). Therefore, the blood pressure–lowering effect of ACE inhibitors may be due, to some extent, to an accumulation of bradykinin. Thus an important issue is the comparative antihypertensive efficacy of chronic ACE inhibition and chronic angiotensin II receptor blockade. This issue was tested in a randomized, double-blind study in which 348 patients with mild to moderate uncomplicated hypertension received an 8-week treatment of either valsartan (80 mg) once a day (*n* = 136), enalapril (20 mg) once a day (*n* = 69), or placebo (*n* = 142) [49]. There was no significant difference in blood pressure between the three groups at baseline (week 0). Both valsartan and enalapril were significantly superior to placebo in lowering systolic and diastolic blood pressure. However, there was no difference between the antihypertensive effects of the two blockers of the renin-angiotensin system.

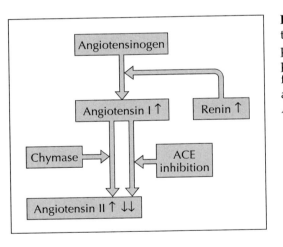

FIGURE 7-32. High renin levels might lead to generation of angiotensin II either by the traditional angiotensin-converting enzyme (ACE) pathway or by alternative enzymatic pathways that are not blocked by ACE inhibitors. For example, chymase, a chymotrypsin-like proteinase present in the heart and blood vessels, could play an important role in the tissue formation of angiotensin II [50]. Blocking the renin-angiotensin system using an AT_1-receptor antagonist allows inhibition of angiotensin II produced by both the ACE- and the non-ACE–dependent mechanisms. (*Adapted from* Urata *et al.* [50].)

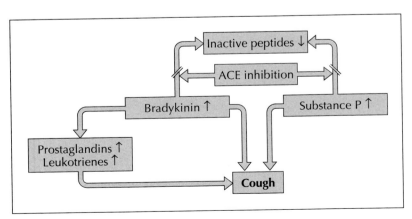

FIGURE 7-33. The most common side effect of angiotensin-converting enzyme (ACE) inhibitors as a class is a dry, irritating cough. The underlying mechanisms may involve pulmonary accumulation of bradykinin and substance P, two peptides normally inactivated by ACE and known to activate afferent sensory C fibers via type I receptors, thereby causing cough. Bradykinin is also a known stimulant of prostaglandin and leukotriene formation, two possible mediators of cough. (*Adapted from* Lacourcière *et al.* [51].)

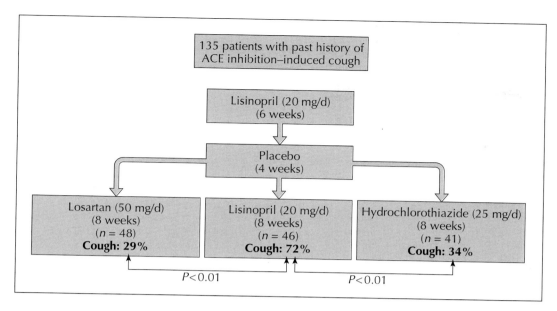

FIGURE 7-34. The profile of side effects of losartan is very similar to that of angiotensin-converting enzyme (ACE) inhibitors, with the exception of dry cough. A group of 135 hypertensive patients with a history of cough during ACE inhibition received the ACE inhibitor lisinopril (20 mg once daily) in single-blind fashion until they again developed cough [52]. This was followed by a 4-week placebo period. The patients were then randomized in a double-blind, parallel-group design to an 8-week treatment with either losartan (50 mg), lisinopril (20 mg), or hydrochlorothiazide (25 mg), each given once daily. The incidence of cough was 29% with losartan, 72% with lisinopril ($P < 0.01$), and 34% with hydrochlorothiazide. Thus, the angiotensin II antagonist is free of cough, an annoying and common side effect of ACE inhibition. (*Adapted from* Ramsay *et al.* [52].)

METABOLIC EFFECTS OF ANTIHYPERTENSIVE DRUGS

EFFECTS OF ANTIHYPERTENSIVE DRUGS ON CARBOHYDRATE METABOLISM

	INSULIN SENSITIVITY	GLUCOSE TOLERANCE
Thiazides	↓	↓
β-Blockers		
Nonselective	↓	↓
Selective	↓	↓
With ISA	→	→
Calcium antagonists	→	→
ACE inhibitors	↑	↑
Angiotensin II antagonists	→	→
α₁-Blockers	↑	↑
Moxonidine	↑	↑

↑ Increase; ↓ decrease; → neutral.

FIGURE 7-35. Effects on insulin sensitivity and glucose tolerance. Hypertension, obesity, hyperlipidemia, insulin resistance, and glucose intolerance are frequently associated with hypertension [53]. Some antihypertensive drugs may adversely alter insulin sensitivity and glucose tolerance, whereas others are neutral or may even have favorable effects [54,55]. The drug-induced reduction in insulin sensitivity and glucose tolerance is dose-dependent. ACE—angiotensin-converting enzyme; ISA—intrinsic sympathomimetic activity.

EFFECTS OF ANTIHYPERTENSIVE DRUGS ON BLOOD LIPIDS

	TOTAL CHOLESTEROL	LDL CHOLESTEROL	HDL CHOLESTEROL	TRIGLYCERIDES
Diuretics				
Thiazides	↑	↑	→	↑
Loop	↑	↑	→	↑
Spironolactone	→	→	→	→
β-Blockers				
Nonselective	→	→	⇓	⇑
Selective	→	→	⇓	⇑
With ISA	→	→	→	→
Calcium antagonists	→	→	→	→
ACE inhibitors	→	→	→	→
Angiotensin II antagonists	→	→	→	→
α_1-Blockers	↓	↓	↑	↓

↑ Increase; → neutral; ↓ decrease; ⇓ minimal decrease; ⇑ minimal increase.

FIGURE 7-36. Effects on lipid metabolism. Antihypertensive drugs may influence blood lipids in certain ways [54]. Duringprolonged therapy, however, deterioration of lipid metabolism is generally not a problem, particularly if a low dose is given. ACE—angiotensin-converting enzyme; ISA—intrinsic sympathomimetic activity; HDL—high-density lipoprotein; LDL—low-density lipoprotein.

REGRESSION OF VASCULAR AND CARDIAC HYPERTROPHY

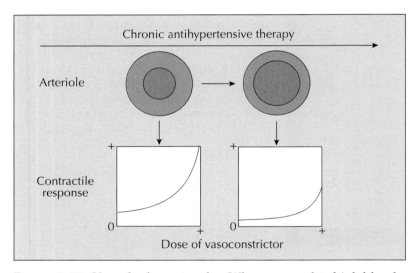

FIGURE 7-37. Vascular hypertrophy. When exposed to high blood pressure, resistant blood vessels undergo an adaptive hypertrophy that makes it possible to keep the wall stress constant but considerably amplifies the vascular responsiveness to all constrictors [56]. In addition to blood pressure, such growth factors as angiotensin II, norepinephrine, and endothelin may contribute to vascular hypertrophy. Regression of structural changes may be obtained by antihypertensive therapy, rendering the arteries less responsive to vasoconstrictors.

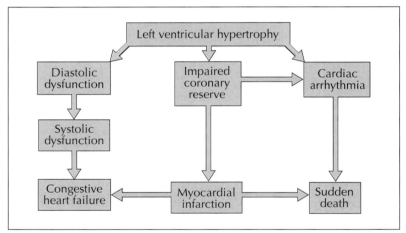

FIGURE 7-38. Cardiac hypertrophy. Left ventricular hypertrophy is an early complication of hypertension that initially leads to diastolic (impaired relaxation) and then to systolic (impaired contractility) dysfunction of the heart. The increased cardiac mass is associated with a diminished coronary reserve, an enhanced propensity to life-threatening cardiac arrhythmia, and sudden death [2]. Lowering blood pressure leads to regression of left ventricular hypertrophy. Although this effect apparently can be obtained with all types of antihypertensive drugs, it is believed that some classes of drugs are more effective in this regard [57]. The reduction in cardiac mass can improve both systolic and diastolic function of the heart.

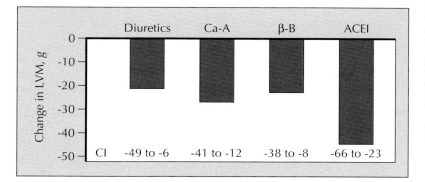

FIGURE 7-39. Results of a meta-analysis evaluating the effect of antihypertensive treatment on left ventricular structure. This figure reports the findings of 109 studies [57]. A total of 2357 patients were included. Overall left ventricular mass (LVM) measured by echocardiography was reduced by 11.9%. ACE inhibitors (ACEI) were more effective than the other first-line therapies (studies involving AT_1-receptor blockers were not yet available at the time the meta-analysis was performed). β-B—β-blockers; Ca-A—calcium antagonists.

REFERENCES

1. Mac Mahon S, Peto R, Cutler J, *et al.*: Blood pressure, stroke, and coronary heart disease. Part I. Prolonged differences in blood pressure: prospective observational studies corrected for the regression, dilution bias. *Lancet* 1990, 335:765–777.

2. Frohlich ED, Apstein C, Chobanian AV, *et al.*: The heart in hypertension. *N Engl J Med* 1992, 327:998–1007.

3. Whelton PK, Klag MJ: Hypertension as a risk factor for renal disease: review of clinical and epidemiological evidence. *Hypertension* 1989, 13(suppl 1):19–27.

4. Collins R, Peto R, Mac Mahon S, *et al.*: Blood pressure, stroke and coronary heart disease. Part 2. Short-term reductions in blood pressure: overview of randomized drug trials in their epidemiological context. *Lancet* 1990, 335:827–838.

5. Mac Mahon S, Rodgers A: The effects of blood pressure reduction in older patients: an overview of five randomized controlled trials in elderly hypertensives. *Clin Exp Hypertens* 1993, 15:967–978.

6. The Sixth Report of the Joint National Committee on Prevention, Detection, Evaluation, and Treatment of High Blood Pressure. *Arch Intern Med* 1997, 157:2413–2446.

7. Chalmers J: The 1999 WHO-ISH guidelines for the management of hypertension. *Med J Aust* 1999, 171: 458–459.

8. Brunner HR, Gavras H: Clinical implications of renin in the hypertensive patient. *JAMA* 1975, 233:1091–1093.

9. Folkow B: Sympathetic nervous control of blood pressure: role in primary hypertension. *Am J Hypertens* 1989, 2:103S–111S.

10. Muntzel M, Drueke T: A comprehensive review of the salt and blood pressure relationship. *Am J Hypertens* 1992, 5:1S–42S.

11. Chalmers J: The place of combination therapy in the treatment of hypertension in 1993. *Clin Exp Hypertens* 1993, 15:1299–1313.

12. Brunner HR, Ménard J, Waeber B, *et al.*: Treating the individual hypertensive patient: considerations on dose, sequential monotherapy and fixed-dose combinations. *J Hypertens* 1990, 8:3–11.

13. Ménard J: Critical assessment of combination therapy development. *Blood Pressure* 1993, 2(suppl 1):5–9.

14. Waeber B: Treatment strategy to control blood pressure optimally in hypertensive patients. *Blood Pressure* 2001, 10:62–73.

15. Dickerson CJE: Optimisation of antihypertensive treatment by rotation of four major classes. *Lancet* 1999, 353:2008–2013.

16. Johnston CI: The place of diuretics in the treatment of hypertension in 1993: can we do better? *Clin Exp Hypertens* 1993, 15:1239–1255.

17. Puschett JB: Diuretics in hypertension. In *Cardiovascular Pharmacology and Therapeutics*. Edited by Singh BN, Dzau VJ, Vanhoutte PM, Woosley RL. New York: Churchill Livingstone; 1994:885–908.

18. Blaustein MP: Sodium ions, calcium ions, blood pressure regulation and hypertension: a reassessment of a hypothesis. *Am J Physiol* 1977, 232:165–173.

19. Tarazi RC, Dustan HP, Frohlich ED: Long-term thiazide therapy in essential hypertension. *Circulation* 1970, 41:709–717.

20. Lefkowitz RJ: β-adrenergic receptors: recognition and regulation. *N Engl J Med* 1976, 295:323–328.

21. Franca G, Nies AS: β-Adrenergic blockers in the treatment of hypertension. In *Cardiovascular Pharmacology and Therapeutics*. Edited by Singh BN, Dzau VJ, Vanhoutte PM, Woosley RL. New York: Churchill Livingstone; 1994:945–956.

22. Man in't Veld AJ, van den Meiracker A, Schalekamp MADH: The effect of β-blockers on total peripheral resistance. *J Cardiovasc Pharmacol* 1986, 8(suppl 4):49–60.

23. Lund-Johansen P: Hemodynamic changes at rest and during exercise in long-term clonidine therapy of essential hypertension. *Acta Med Scand* 1974, 195:111–115.

24. Oparil S, Haber E: The renin-angiotensin system. *N Engl J Med* 1974, 291:389–401.

25. Dzau VJ, Re R: Tissue angiotensin system in cardiovascular medicine. *Circulation* 1994, 89:493–498.

26. van Lutterotti N, Catanzaro DF, Sealy JE, Laragh JH: Renin is not synthesized by cardiac and extrarenal vascular tissues: a review of experimental evidence. *Circulation* 1994, 89:458–470.

27. Waeber B, Nussberger J, Juillerat L, Brunner HR: Angiotensin converting enzyme inhibition: discrepancy between antihypertensive effect and suppression of enzyme activity. *J Cardiovasc Pharmacol* 1989, 14(suppl 4):53–59.

28. Carretero OA, Scicli AG: Local hormonal factors (intracrine, autocrine, and paracrine) in hypertension. *Hypertension* 1991, 18(suppl I):58–69.

29. Moncada S, Palmer RMJ, Higgs EA: Nitric oxide: physiology, pathophysiology and pharmacology. *Pharmacol Rev* 1991, 43:109–142.

30. Vanhoutte PM: Other endothelium-derived vasoactive factors. *Circulation* 1993, 87(suppl V):9–17.

31. Zimmerman BG, Sybert EG, Wong PC: Interaction between sympathetic and renin-angiotensin system. *J Hypertens* 1984, 2:581–588.

32. Brunner HR, Gavras H, Waeber B: Enhancement by diuretics of the antihypertensive action of long-term angiotensin converting enzyme blockade. *Clin Exp Hypertens* 1980, 2:639–657.

33. Luft FC, Haller H: Calcium channel blockers in current medical practice: an update for 1993. *Clin Exp Hypertens* 1993, 15:1263–1276.

34. Weber MA, Graettinger WF: Calcium channel blockers as hypotensive agents. In *Cardiovascular Pharmacology and Therapeutics*. Edited by Singh BN, Dzau VJ, Vanhoutte PM, Woosley RL. New York: Churchill Livingstone; 1994:931–943.

35. Tonyz RM, Schiffrin EL: Signal transduction in hypertension: part I. *Curr Opin Nephrol Hypertens* 1993, 2:5–16.

36. Tonyz RM, Schiffrin EL: Signal transduction in hypertension: part II. *Curr Opin Nephrol Hypertens* 1993, 2:17–26.

37. Grimm RH: α_1-Antagonists in the treatment of hypertension. *Hypertension* 1989, 13(suppl I):131–136.

38. Bousquet P, Feldman J: Drugs acting on imidazoline receptors: a review of their pharmacology, their use in blood pressure control and their potential interest in cardioprotection. *Drugs* 1999, 58:799–812.

39. Brunner HR, Gavras H, Laragh JH, Keenan R: Hypertension in man: exposure of the renin and sodium components using angiotensin II blockade. *Circ Res* 1974, 34 (suppl 1):35–43.

40. Timmermans BM, Wong WMPC, Chiu AT, *et al.*: Angiotensin II receptors and angiotensin II receptor antagonists. *Pharmacol Rev* 1993, 45:205–251.

41. Chung O, Stoll M, Unger T: Physiologic and pharmacologic implications of AT1 versus AT2 receptors. *Blood Pressure* 1996 (suppl 2):47–52.

42. Siragy HM, Bedigian M: Mechanism of action of angiotensin-receptor blocking agents. *Curr Hypertens Rep* 1999, 1:289–295.

43. Weiss D, Sorescu D, Taylor WR: Angiotensin II and atherosclerosis. *Am J Cardiol* 2001, 87:25C–32C.

44. Vaughan DE: Angiotensin, fibrinolysis, and vascular homeostasis. *Am J Cardiol* 2001, 87:18C–24C.

45. Ruiz-Ortega M, Lorenzo O, Suzuki Y, *et al.*: Proinflammatory actions of angiotensins. *Curr Opin Nephrol Hypertens* 2001, 10:321–329.

46. Munafo A, Christen Y, Nussberger J, *et al.*: Drug concentration response relationships in normal volunteers after oral administration of losartan (DuP 753, MK 954), an angiotensin II receptor antagonist. *Clin Pharmacol Ther* 1992, 51:513–521.

47. Nakashima M, Uematsu T, Kosuge K, Kanamur M: Pilot study of the uricosuric effect of DuP 753, a new angiotensin II receptor antagonist, in healthy subjects. *Eur J Clin Pharmacol* 1992, 42:333–335.

48. Morgan JM, Palmisano M, Piraino A, *et al.*: The effect of valsartan on the angiotensin II pressor response in healthy normotensive male subjects. *Clin Pharmacol Ther* 1997, 61:35–44.

49. Holwerda NJ, Fogari R, Angeli P, *et al.*: Valsartan, a new angiotensin II antagonist for the treatment of essential hypertension: efficacy and safety compared with placebo and enalapril. *J Hypertens* 1996, 14:1147–1151.

50. Urata H, Strobel F, Ganten D: Widespread tissue distribution of human chymase. *J Hypertens* 1994, 12 (suppl 9):17–22.

51. Lacourcière Y, Lefebvre J, Nakhle G, *et al.*: Association between cough and angiotensin converting enzyme inhibitory versus angiotensin II antagonists: the design of a prospective, controlled study. *J Hypertens* 1994, 12:549–553.

52. Ramsay LE, Yeo WS, on behalf of the Losartan Cough Study Group: Double-blind comparison of losartan, lisinopril and hydrochlorothiazide in hypertensive patients with a previous angiotensin converting enzyme inhibitor-associated cough. *J Hypertens* 1995, 13(suppl 1):73–76.

53. De Fronzo RA: Insulin resistance, hyperinsulinemia, and coronary artery disease: a complex metabolic web. *J Cardiovasc Pharmacol* 1992, 20(suppl 11):1–16.

54. Lithell HOL: Effect of antihypertensive drugs on insulin, glucose and lipid metabolism. *Diabetes Care* 1991, 14:203–209.

55. Krentz AJ, Evans AJ: Selective imidazoline receptor agonists for metabolic syndrome. *Lancet* 1998, 351:152–153.

56. Folkow B: Physiological aspects of primary hypertension. *Physiol Rev* 1982, 62:347–504.

57. Dahlöf B, Pennert K, Hansson L: Reversal of left ventricular hypertrophy in hypertensive patients: a meta-analysis of 109 treatment studies. *Am J Hypertens* 1992, 5:95–110.

Recent Therapeutic Trials

Kenneth A. Jamerson

The trials reviewed in this chapter evaluate the long-term effects of reducing blood pressure in preventing the morbidity and mortality associated with hypertension. Clinical trials have established the value of treatment by defining the level of elevated blood pressure above which treatment is warranted. The most recent trials helped to delineate specific agents for target organ protection (*see* Fig. 8-1).

Coming to a conclusion shortly are ongoing trials for identifying the optimal drug class for overall cardiovascular protection in essential hypertension. With the availability of effective anti-hypertensive agents, any method of reducing blood pressure became lifesaving in malignant and accelerated hypertension. For less severe hypertension, it was necessary to use clinical trials to demonstrate the value of therapy. The landmark trial by the Veterans Administration, published in 1967, was the first to demonstrate the value of treating elevated blood pressure (diastolic blood pressure > 110 mm Hg) in preventing morbidity and mortality. Subsequent trials have treated blood pressure at less severe levels; benefit is best in diabetic subjects and others at high risk for cardiovascular disease. Although these groups of high-risk subjects demonstrated the largest effect from treatment of hypertension, lowering blood pressure confers benefit on the general hypertensive population, including most ethnic and gender groups in the United States.

Two fundamental questions are guiding hypertension clinical trials at this point: Is specific antihypertensive medication able to provide cardiovascular benefits beyond lowering blood pressure? Is there an ideal blood pressure target that confers maximal cardiovascular protection? In November 1997, when the Sixth Joint National Committee on Prevention, Detection, Evaluation, and Treatment of High Blood Pressure (JNC-VI) issued its recommendations, there existed few data suggesting that antihypertensive agents other than diuretics and β-blockers could provide such benefits. However, clinical trials involving hundreds of thousands of subjects have been conducted during the 5 years since that report, yielding new data. This chapter summarizes those data.

Ultimately, the findings suggest that targeting interventions that will lower blood pressure below the conventional goal of 140/90 (≈ 138/85) mm Hg is advantageous, particularly for hypertensive diabetic patients. The benefit of achieving more aggressive targets has yet to be demonstrated.

As the inquiry into the "best" antihypertensive drug class continues, it appears that diuretics, angiotensin-converting enzyme inhibitors, β-blockers, angiotensin II receptor blockers, and calcium channel blockers (excluding their use in patients with impaired renal function) are still contenders. It is likely that multiple drugs will be necessary for controlling blood pressure to a target systolic blood pressure less than 140 mm Hg. Clinical trials of lifestyle modification have confirmed this intervention as an important tool in reducing the number of medications required for achieving blood pressure control.

During the past three decades, the number of hypertensive patients who have control of their blood pressure to the target of less than 140/90 mm Hg has increased threefold. The mortality rates from cardiovascular disease have been substantially reduced. The evidence from clinical trials suggests that the many therapeutic options for the treatment of hypertension should help sustain the trend in improving cardiovascular morbidity and mortality.

TARGET ORGAN PROTECTION

RECENT CLINICAL TRIALS DEMONSTRATING TARGET ORGAN PROTECTION

DISEASE STATE	TRIAL	OUTCOME
Diabetic nephropathy	IDNT, RENAAL	ARB is preferred (to regimen with or without ARB)
Hypertensive nephropathy	AASK	ACE-based regimen is preferred to BB- or CCB-based regimen
Stroke	PROGRESS, SCOPE	Unable to identify a specific preferred drug class
Coronary artery disease, myocardial infarction	LIFE, PROGRESS, STOP-II, NORDIL, CONVINCE	Unable to identify a preferred drug class
Left ventricular hypertrophy	LIFE	ARB preferred to BB

FIGURE 8-1. Recent clinical trials demonstrating target organ protection. AASK— African American Study of Kidney (disease); ACE—angiotensin-converting enzyme; ARB—angiotensin II receptor blocker; BB—β-blocker; CCB—calcium channel blocker; CONVINCE—Controlled Onset Verapamil Investigation of Cardiovascular Endpoints; IDNT—Irbesartan Diabetic Nephropathy Trial; LIFE—Lifestyle Intervention, Food and Exercise (program); NORDIL—Nordic Diltiazem (study); PROGRESS—Perindopril Protection Against Recurrent Stroke Study; RENAAL—Reduction of Endpoints in NIDDM with the Angiotensin II Antagonist Losartan; SCOPE—Surveillance and Control Of Pathogens of Epidemiologic (importance); STOP-II—Swedish Trial in Old Patients with Hypertension 2 (ongoing trial).

TRENDS IN CARDIOVASCULAR DISEASE

HYPERTENSION AWARENESS, TREATMENT, AND CONTROL

	BLOOD PRESSURE ≥140/90 mm Hg, %	BLOOD PRESSURE ≥160/95 mm Hg, %
Aware	65	84
Treated	49	73
Controlled	21	55

FIGURE 8-2. Public awareness of hypertension has increased to the point where mass screening is no longer cost-effective or necessary. Nevertheless, the percentage of patients treated and controlled indicates that there is still considerable room for improvement, especially for those with the mildest degree of hypertension, of whom nearly 80% are not controlled. (Adapted from the Fifth Report of the Joint National Committee on Detection, Evaluation, and Treatment of High Blood Pressure [1].)

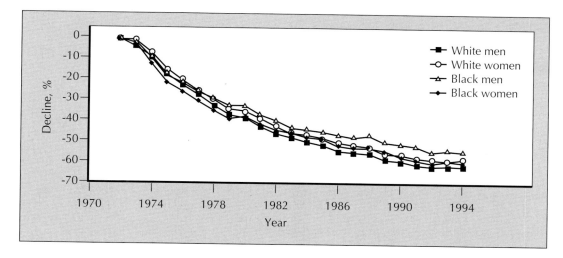

FIGURE 8-3. Decline in age-adjusted (to the 1940 US census population) mortality rates for stroke by sex and race in the United States (1972 to 1994). The decline in age-adjusted mortality for stroke in the total population is 59.0%.

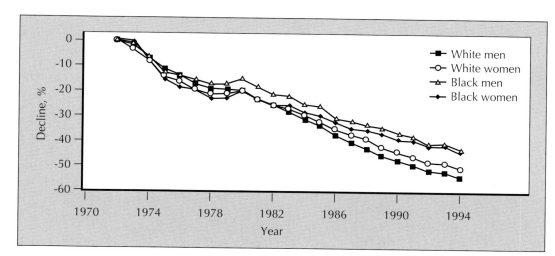

FIGURE 8-4. Decline in age-adjusted (to the 1940 US census population) mortality rates for congestive heart disease (CHD) by sex and race in the United States (1972 to 1994). The decline in age-adjusted mortality for CHD in the total population is 53.2%.

EARLY TRIALS

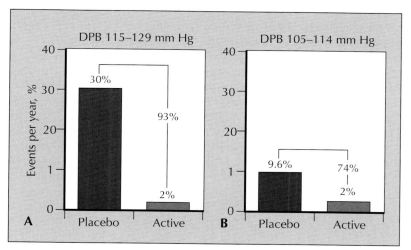

FIGURE 8-5. The 1967 Veterans Administration Study. The early trials covered in this section demonstrate the cardiovascular benefit of lowering blood pressure in hypertensive patients and the importance of specific drug regimens. The 1967 Veterans Administration Study [2] was the first major therapeutic trial to establish the value of treating hypertension compared with placebo by demonstrating a 93% reduction in mortality and cardiovascular events. This study firmly established the value of treatment for patients with diastolic blood pressure (DBP) of 115 to 129 mm Hg (**A**). For patients with DBP of 105 to 114 mm Hg (**B**) a 74% reduction in events per year was observed after 5 years of follow-up. No statistically proven benefit for DBP in the range of 90 to 105 mm Hg was seen in these studies, nor did there appear to be any benefit in preventing coronary heart disease. (*Adapted from* the Veterans Administration Cooperative Study Group on Antihypertensive Agents [3].)

AUSTRALIAN THERAPEUTIC TRIAL: FATAL AND NONFATAL ENDPOINTS

	ACTIVE TREATMENT (n = 1721)		PLACEBO (n = 1706)	
	TRIAL ENDPOINTS, n	RATE*	TRIAL ENDPOINTS, n	RATE*
Fatal				
Cardiovascular	4	0.8	13	2.5[†]
Noncardiovascular	5	0.9	6	1.2
Total	9	1.7	19	3.7[‡]
Nonfatal	82	15.5	108	20.8[†]
All endpoints	91	17.2	127	24.5[§]

*Rates per 1000 person-years exposure to risk.
[†]$P<0.05$.
[‡]$P<0.025$.
[§]$P<0.01$.

FIGURE 8-6. The Australian National Blood Pressure Trial [4] treated patients with diastolic blood pressures of 95 to 109 mm Hg (mild hypertension). There was a significant reduction in fatal and nonfatal cardiovascular events as well as in all trial endpoints. This study established the value of treatment for patients with diastolic blood pressure greater than 95 mm Hg. (*Adapted from* the Australian National Blood Pressure Management Committee [4].)

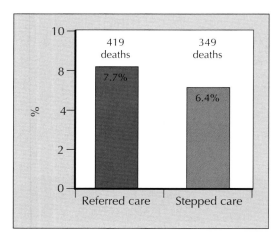

FIGURE 8-7. The Hypertension Detection and Follow-up Program [5] differed from previous studies in that patients were randomly assigned either to special centers for vigorous antihypertensive treatment (stepped care; n = 5485) or back to community physicians (referred care; n = 5455). A greater reduction in diastolic blood pressure (5 mm Hg) was achieved in stepped care, resulting in a 16.9% reduction in mortality (5-year mortality from all causes). This benefit understates the value of treatment because patients in referred care also were treated. (*Adapted from* the Hypertension Detection and Follow-up Program Cooperative Group [5].)

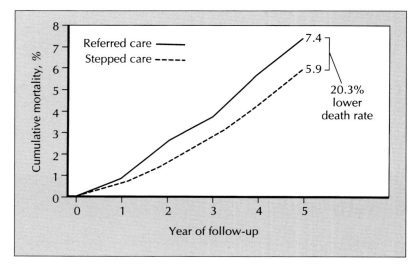

FIGURE 8-8. The life table for the mildly hypertensive patient (diastolic blood pressure 90 to 104 mm Hg) in the Hypertension Detection and Follow-up Program reveals diverging trends in mortality. It is clear that little benefit can be shown in the first year or so of treatment. Had the study been carried out beyond 5 years, even greater benefit could have been anticipated. The longer hypertension control is sustained, the greater the benefit. (*Adapted from* the Hypertension Detection and Follow-up Program Cooperative Group [5].)

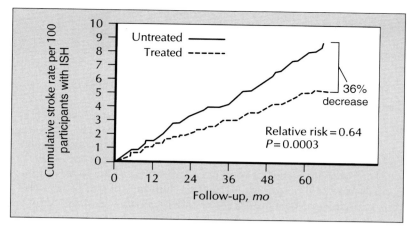

FIGURE 8-9. Cumulative stroke rate per 100 participants with isolated systolic hypertension (ISH) in the Systolic Hypertension in the Elderly Program (SHEP). This life-table analysis showed a 36% reduction in fatal and nonfatal stroke. The benefit was not statistically significant until 2 years of therapy had been received because of the small number of events. (*Adapted from* the SHEP Cooperative Research Group [6].)

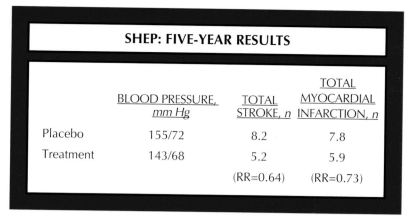

SHEP: FIVE-YEAR RESULTS

	BLOOD PRESSURE, *mm Hg*	TOTAL STROKE, *n*	TOTAL MYOCARDIAL INFARCTION, *n*
Placebo	155/72	8.2	7.8
Treatment	143/68	5.2	5.9
		(RR=0.64)	(RR=0.73)

FIGURE 8-10. The rates of stroke and coronary heart disease (a secondary endpoint) in the Systolic Hypertension in the Elderly Program (SHEP) trial revealed significant reductions of 36% and 27%, respectively. Whether these results in isolated systolic hypertension apply to confirmed systolic and diastolic high blood pressure for coronary heart disease in the elderly is unknown. RR—relative risk. (*Adapted from* the SHEP Cooperative Research Group [6].)

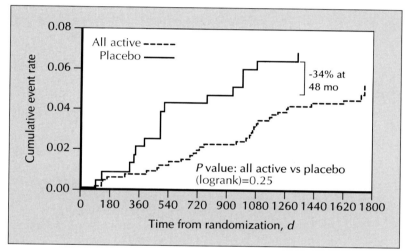

FIGURE 8-11. Major clinical events in the Treatment of Mild Hypertension Study (TOMHS), which was designed to test the efficacy of five different classes of antihypertensive agents versus placebo in preventing the complications of hypertension. All patients received hygienic measures of weight loss, salt and alcohol restriction, and increased physical activity. Because this was a pilot study with an inadequate number of subjects, the five active treatments were pooled. Compared with placebo there was a 34% reduction in major events. (*Adapted from* Neaton *et al.* [7].)

META-ANALYSIS OF PRE-1990 TRIALS

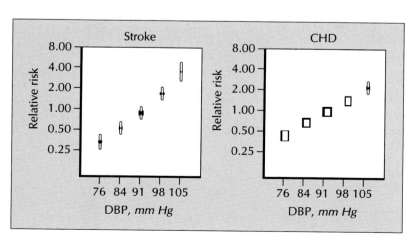

FIGURE 8-12. Diastolic blood pressure (DBP) versus relative risk of coronary heart disease (CHD) and stroke. The relationship between increasing levels of DBP and the risk of stroke and CHD is log-linear, based on observational studies of 420,000 individuals [18]. In these data there is no evidence of an increased risk associated with low levels of blood pressure (J curve). The risk of both stroke and CHD is substantially increased well below the conventional cut-point of 90 mm Hg. Stroke patients included seven prospective studies (843 events); CHD patients included nine prospective studies (4856 events). The slope of the curve for stroke is steep, confirming the fact that high blood pressure is the major risk factor for stroke. The slope of the curve for CHD is less steep because there are multiple risk factors for CHD. The data points in both curves show ± 2 SE on the vertical axis and the blood pressure range on the horizontal axis. (*Adapted from* MacMahon *et al.* [8].)

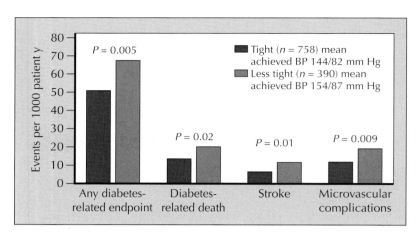

FIGURE 8-13. The UK Prospective Diabetes Study (UKPDS) examined whether relatively tight control of blood pressure would prevent microvascular and macrovascular sequelae in 1148 hypertensive patients with type 2 diabetes. The participants in this study, aged 25 to 65 years (mean age, 56.4 years), had a mean blood pressure of 160/94 mm Hg. Participants were randomly assigned to undergo tight control (< 150/85 mm Hg) or less tight control (< 180/105 mm Hg). The data demonstrated a prominent reduction in cardiovascular risk, death, and complications due to diabetes among the patients who were randomly assigned to tight control. Moreover, blood pressure control was more important than glycemic control in preventing cardiovascular events in this cohort. The study, however, was not able to recommend aggressive blood pressure targets below 140/90 mm Hg because the tight blood pressure control group on average achieved a systolic blood pressure (SBP) of 144 mm Hg [9].

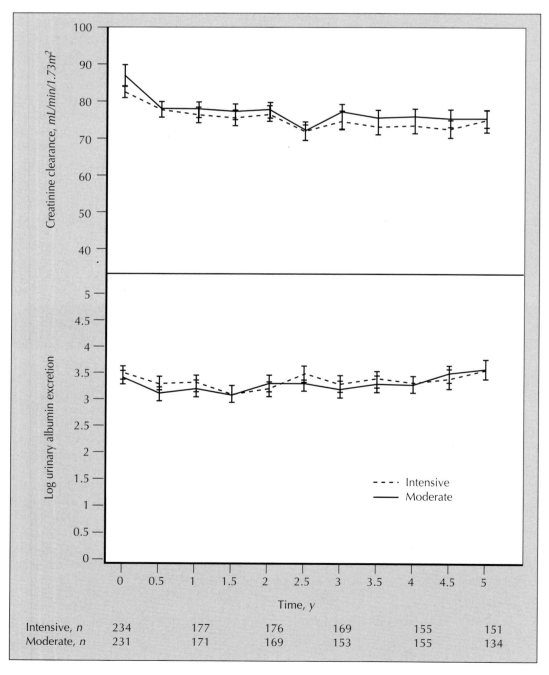

FIGURE 8-14. The Appropriate Blood Pressure Control in Diabetes trial (ABCD) compared the effects of intensive blood pressure control (goal diastolic blood pressure [DBP], 75 mm Hg) with those of moderate control (goal DBP, 80–89 mm Hg) in 480 normotensive patients and 470 hypertensive patients with type 2 diabetes. The patients in this study were aged 40 to 74 years. Among patients without gross albuminuria, there was no difference between intensive and moderate control in the progression of microvascular disease. The incidence of all-cause mortality was lower in patients who received intensive blood pressure control than in those who received moderate control. (*Adapted from* Estacio *et al.* [10].)

CAPPP TRIAL RESULTS IN HIGH-RISK HYPERTENSION

EVENT	CAPTOPRIL GROUP, N	CONVENTIONAL GROUP, N
Fatal myocardial infarction	27	35
Fatal stroke	20	22
Other cardiovascular deaths	23	24
Sudden death	6	14
Nonfatal myocardial infarction	137	128
Nonfatal stroke	173	127
Ischemic heart disease	258	251
Atrial fibrillation	117	135
Congestive heart failure	75	66
Diabetes mellitus	337	380
Transient ischemic attacks	31	25

FIGURE 8-15. Results from the Captopril Prevention Project (CAPPP) regarding high-risk hypertension. The CAPPP randomized trial examined the incidence of cardiovascular events in 10,985 patients randomly assigned to receive an angiotensin-converting enzyme inhibitor, captopril, or conventional treatment with β-blockers or diuretics. The results demonstrated that captopril did not significantly reduce the number of cardio-vascular deaths when compared with conventional treatment (76 vs 95; $P = 0.092$; RR = 0.77). The rates of fatal and nonfatal myocardial infarction (MI) did not differ according to therapy; however, the rate of fatal and nonfatal stroke was greater with captopril than with conventional treatment (189 vs 148; $P = 0.044$; RR = 1.25) [11].

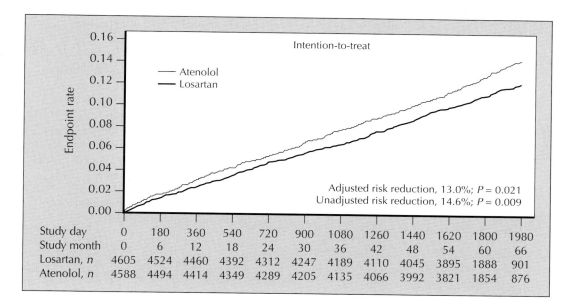

FIGURE 8-16. The recently completed Losartan Intervention for Endpoint reduction in hypertension study (LIFE) randomly assigned 9110 patients to receive either a β-blocker or angiotensin II receptor blocker (ARB) as the baseline therapy (diuretics were allowed as add-on therapy). In this cohort of primarily older Scandinavian hypertensive subjects with left ventricular hypertrophy (LVH), there was an overall 16% reduction in combined cardiovascular disease (CVD) events over the 4 years of follow-up. Interestingly, despite these subjects' having higher risk of coronary events (all had LVH), the benefit was driven by reduction in stroke rather than heart disease [12].

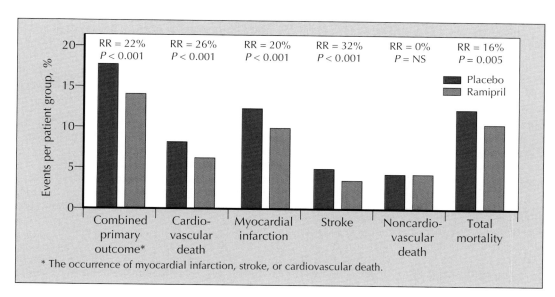

* The occurrence of myocardial infarction, stroke, or cardiovascular death.

FIGURE 8-17. The Heart Outcomes Prevention Evaluation study (HOPE) assessed the role of angiotensin-converting enzyme (ACE) inhibition versus matching placebo in 9297 patients (≥ 55 years of age) who were at high risk for cardiovascular events, but who did not have left ventricular dysfunction or heart failure. Treatment with ramipril significantly reduced the rates of death from cardiovascular causes (6.1% vs 8.1%; $P < 0.001$), myocardial infarction (9.9% vs 12.3%; $P < 0.001$), heart failure (9% vs 11.5%; $P < 0.001$), and complications related to diabetes (6.4% vs 7.6%; $P = 0.03$). The HOPE study also found that improved outcome from ramipril treatment was observed when patients were also treated with combination therapy. β-Blockers, diuretics, calcium channel blockers (CCBs), lipid-lowering drugs, and aspirin were most commonly used safely and effectively [13].

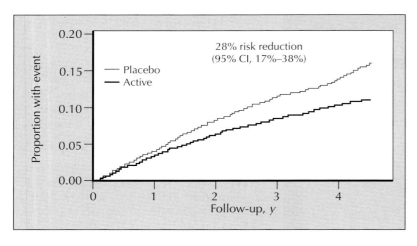

FIGURE 8-18. The Perindopril Protection Against Recurrent Stroke Study (PROGRESS) was started by an independent collaborative research group to determine the effects of a flexible blood pressure lowering regimen, involving an angiotensin-converting enzyme inhibitor and a diuretic on the risk of stroke and other major vascular events among individuals with a history of stroke or transient ischemic attack. A total of 6105 (aged 63 to 65 years of age) individuals were randomly assigned to active treatment versus placebo. Of those assigned active treatment, the regimen comprised combination therapy with perindopril plus indapamide and single-dose therapy with perindopril alone. Of those assigned placebo, the regimen comprised double and single placebo. A total of 307 individuals assigned to active treatment suffered a stroke compared with 420 assigned to placebo. Combination therapy with perindopril plus indapamide reduced blood pressure by 12/5 mm Hg and stroke risk by 43%. Single-drug therapy reduced blood pressure by 5/3 mm Hg and produced no discernible reduction in the risk of stroke [14].

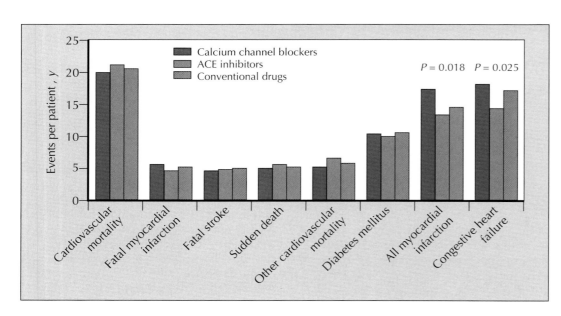

FIGURE 8-19. In the Swedish Trial in Old Patients with Hypertension-2 study (STOP-2), 6614 patients aged 70 to 84 years, with a systolic blood pressure (SBP) of 180 mm Hg and diastolic blood pressure of 105 mm Hg, or both, were randomly assigned to receive treatment with newer antihypertensive agents (enalapril, lisinopril, felodipine, isradipine), or conventional antihypertensive agents (atenolol, metoprolol, pindolol, hydrochlorothiazide, amiloride). The results showed similar decreases in blood pressure among all the treatment groups, with the newer and conventional antihypertensive agents equally effective in preventing cardiovascular morbidity and mortality [15].

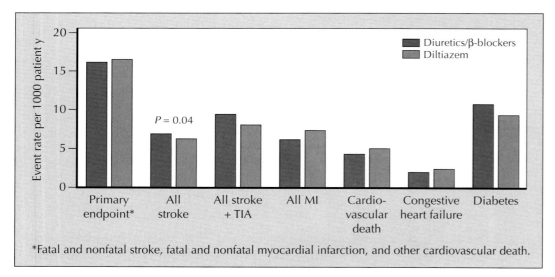

*Fatal and nonfatal stroke, fatal and nonfatal myocardial infarction, and other cardiovascular death.

FIGURE 8-20. In the Nordic Diltiazem study (NORDIL), 10,881 patients were randomly assigned to receive diltiazem, or diuretics and β-blockers, or both. The patients were aged 50 to 74 years and had a diastolic blood pressure of 100 mm Hg. The primary outcomes were fatal and nonfatal stroke, myocardial infarction (MI), and other cardiovascular death. The two regimens were identical for the primary endpoint (preventing stroke, MI, and other cardiovascular death). In a secondary analysis of a few hundred participants, diltiazem was slightly more effective than diuretic or β-blocker therapy in preventing stroke (159 vs 196; $P = 0.04$; RR = 0.80) [16].

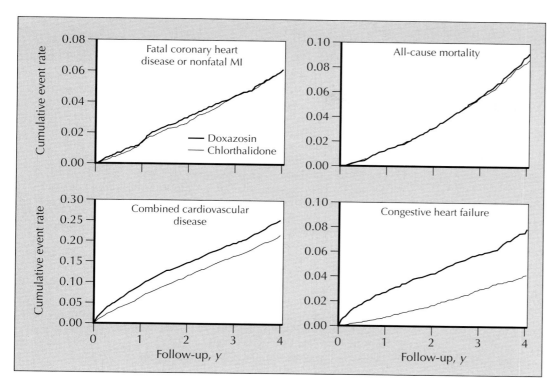

FIGURE 8-21. The Antihypertensive and Lipid Lowering Treatment to Prevent Heart Attack Trial (ALLHAT) is evaluating 40,389 high-risk patients with hypertension, aged 55 years or older. The study is comparing chlorthalidone, a diuretic; amlodipine, a calcium channel blocker (CCB); lisinopril, an angiotensin-converting enzyme inhibitor; and doxazosin, an α-adrenergic blocker. The primary outcome is a composite of fatal coronary heart disease (CHD) and nonfatal myocardial infarction (MI). The trial is ongoing, but the doxazosin arm was discontinued because patients demonstrated a 25% increase in cardio-vascular events driven primarily by a twofold greater hospitalization rate for heart failure when compared with the participants in the diuretic arm [17].

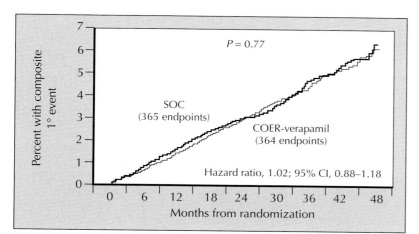

FIGURE 8-22. The Controlled Onset Verapamil Investigation of Cardiovascular Endpoints (CONVINCE) trial randomly assigned 16,602 patients internationally to receive controlled-release verapamil versus a physician-selected regimen that was diuretic or β-blocker based. The primary aim of the study was to test whether a calcium channel blocker (COER verapamil)–based regimen with control of the early morning rise in blood pressure would decrease fatal and nonfatal stroke and myocardial infarction or cardiovascular death when compared to diuretic beta blocker–based regimen (SOC). The investigators achieved excellent blood pressure control (on average 138/80) but could not demonstrate a benefit with either the CCB-based strategy or the lowering of blood pressure in the early morning. (Black H, Presented at the European Society of Hypertension meeting, Milan, 2002.)

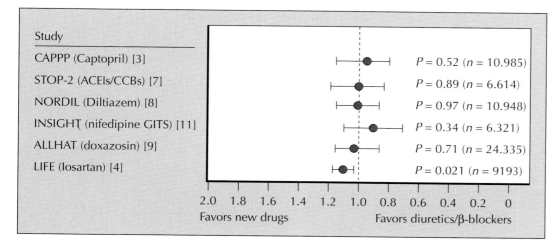

FIGURE 8-23. Several clinical trials have attempted to determine if newer drugs should be preferred to older ones (approximately 80,000 patients have been randomized). Thus far only the angiotensin II receptor blocker (ARB) class has demonstrated an advantage over the older class. The VALUE trial will compare valsartan to amlodipine to determine if the ARB drug class has an advantage over newer antihypertensive drugs in high-risk hypertension. The soon to be released ALLHAT trial will provide a more comprehensive answer to the question of best initial therapy for the treatment of hypertension because its trial population is larger than the sum total of all of the other previous trials [18].

1. The Fifth Report of the Joint National Committee on Detection, Evaluation, and Treatment of High Blood Pressure. *Arch Intern Med* 1993, 153:154–183.

2. Veterans Administration Cooperative Study Group on Antihypertensive Agents: Effects of treatment on morbidity in hypertension. I. Results in patients with diastolic blood pressures average 115 through 129 mm Hg. *JAMA* 1967, 202:1028–1034.

3. Veterans Administration Cooperative Study Group on Antihypertensive Agents: Effects of treatment on morbidity in hypertension. II. Results in patients with diastolic blood pressure averaging 90 through 114 mm Hg. *JAMA* 1970, 213:1143–1252.

4. Australian National Blood Pressure Management Committee: The Australian National Therapeutic trial in mild hypertension. *Lancet* 1980, 1:1261–1267.

5. Hypertension Detection and Follow-up Program Cooperative Group: Five-year findings of the Hypertension Detection and Follow-up Program. I. Reductions in mortality in persons with high blood pressure including mild hypertension. *JAMA* 1979, 242:2562–2571.

6. SHEP Cooperative Research Group: Prevention of stroke by antihypertensive treatment in older persons with isolated systolic hypertension: final results of the Systolic Hypertension in the Elderly Program (SHEP). *JAMA* 1991, 265:3255–3264.

7. Neaton JD, Grumm RH, Prineas RJ, *et al.*: Treatment of Mild Hypertension Study (TOMHS): final results. *JAMA* 1993, 270:713–724.

8. MacMahon S, Peto S, Cutter J, *et al.*: Blood pressure, stroke and coronary heart disease: part I. Prolonged differences in blood pressure: prospective observational studies corrected for the regression dilution bias. *Lancet* 1990, 335:765–774.

9. UK Prospective Diabetes Study Group: Tight blood pressure control and risk of macrovascular and microvascular complications in type 2 diabetes: UKPDS 38. *BMJ* 1998, 317:703–713.

10. Estacio RO, Jeffers BW, Gifford N, Schrier RW: Effect of blood pressure control on diabetic microvascular complications in patients with hypertension and type 2 diabetes. *Diabetes Care* 2000, 23(suppl 2):B54–B64.

11. Hansson L, Lindholm LH, Niskanen L, *et al.* for the Captopril Prevention Project (CAPPP) Study Group: Effect of angiotensin-converting enzyme inhibition compared with conventional therapy on cardiovascular morbidity and mortality in hypertension: the Captopril Prevention Project (CAPPP) randomised trial. *Lancet* 1999, 353:611–616.

12. Dahlöf B, Devereux RB, Kjeldsen SE, *et al.*for the LIFE study group: Cardiovascular morbidity and mortality in the Losartan Intervention For Endpoint reduction study (LIFE): a randomised trial against atenolol. *Lancet* 2002, 359:995–1003.

13. Yusuf S, Sleight P, Pogue J, *et al.* for the Heart Outcomes Prevention Evaluation Study Investigators: Effects of an angiotensin-converting-enzyme inhibitor, ramipril, on cardio-vascular events in high-risk patients. *N Engl J Med* 2000, 342:145–153.

14. PROGRESS Collaborative Group: Randomised trial of a perindopril-based blood-pressure-lowering regimen among 6,105 individuals with previous stroke or transient ischaemic attack. *Lancet* 2001, 358:1033–1041.

15. Hansson L, Lindholm LH, Ekbom T, *et al.* for the STOP-Hypertension-2 Study Group: Randomized trial of old and new antihypertensive drugs in elderly patients: cardiovascular mortality and morbidity, the Swedish Trial in Old Patients with Hypertension-2 study. *Lancet* 1999, 354:1751–1756.

16. Hansson L, Hedner TM, Lund-Johansen P, *et al.* for the NORDIL Study Group: Randomized trial effects of calcium antagonists compared with diuretics and β-blockers on cardiovascular morbidity and mortality in hypertension: the Nordic Diltiazem (NORDIL) study. *Lancet* 2000, 356:359–365.

17. The ALLHAT Officers and Coordinators for the ALLHAT Collaborative Research Group: Major cardiovascular events in patients randomized to doxazosin vs. chlorthalidone: the Antihypertensive and Lipid-Lowering Treatment to Prevent Heart Attack Trial (ALLHAT). *JAMA* 2000, 283:1967–1975.

18. Kjeldsen SE, Westheim A, Os I: INSIGHT and NORDIL. International Nifedipine GITS study: Intervention as a goal in hypertension treatment. Nordic Diltiazem Study. *Lancet* 2000, 356:1929–1930.

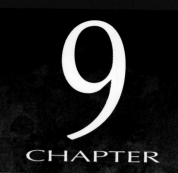

ANTIHYPERTENSIVE THERAPY: PATIENT SELECTION AND SPECIAL PROBLEMS

Barry J. Materson

Antihypertensive therapy clearly is effective in reducing the overall incidence of morbidity and mortality from cerebrovascular and cardiovascular disease. Hypertension, whether systolic, diastolic, or isolated systolic, is a major risk factor for vascular and target organ damage. Increased systolic blood pressure, increased pulse rate, and high baseline heart rate are definite cardiovascular risk factors. Recent data support the concept that even very mildly elevated blood pressure is associated with a substantial risk. Nonpharmacologic therapy alone may not be as effective as drug therapy superimposed on nonpharmacologic therapy in reducing that risk. Nevertheless, the milder the elevation in the average blood pressure of the treatment group, the greater the number of people who must be treated in order to prevent a stroke or myocardial infarction. In an increasingly cost-conscious society, the emphasis is on targeting effective single-drug, low-cost therapy for patients who are at the highest risk. We have progressed only a little in this regard. We do not yet have sophisticated markers of enzyme and receptor genotypes, which may someday increase our specificity of whom we treat and how we treat them. Nevertheless, we can no longer justify decerebrate "shotgun" antihypertensive therapy. Conversely, we are a long way from achieving 100% therapeutic precision. Well-informed, thoughtful caregivers now have the data to approach that ideal goal.

New data allow us to target the treatment of our patients at a level better than random. In those with additional risk factors, hypertension needs to be detected rapidly, evaluated efficiently, and treated aggressively. Information on the interaction of race and age as predictors of response to various antihypertensive medications has also helped to improve drug selection. Knowledge of the efficacy (or lack of), and adverse reactions to, previously used drugs constitutes critical data. Perhaps as many as one half of all patients with hypertension who are managed by primary caregivers have one or more disease processes concomitant with their hypertension. These disease processes need to be considered as specific indicators or contraindicators for the use of antihypertensive drugs. Hypertension concomitant with diabetes or benign prostatic hypertrophy has become a powerful indicator for the need to prescribe an angiotensin-converting enzyme inhibitor or an α_1-antagonist, respectively. Finally, we cannot ignore the costs of drugs to the patient, to the third-party insurer, or, in the long-term analysis, to the American public.

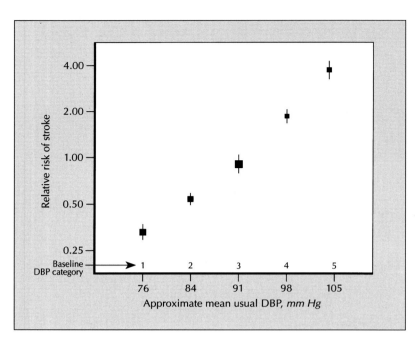

FIGURE 9-1. Stroke risk according to approximate mean usual diastolic blood pressure (DBP). Treating everyone who has hypertension is not cost-effective because only a few in the patient cohort will actually develop a target organ event. In fact, 57% of all heart attacks and almost half of all strokes occur in people with normal blood pressure. Nevertheless, the risk of both stroke and coronary heart disease does have a direct relationship to blood pressure. These data were compiled from prospective, observational studies. The five categories of DBP are defined by baseline DBP. Estimates of the usual DBP in each category are taken from mean DBP values 4 years after baseline in the Framingham study. This figure shows that each increase of 7.5 mm Hg in diastolic blood pressure is associated with 46% more strokes , but it does not indicate who will suffer the stroke. (*Adapted from* Alderman [1].)

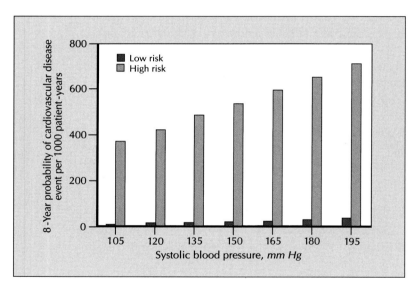

FIGURE 9-2. Absolute and relative risk of a cardiovascular disease event in a high-risk 55-year-old man and a low-risk 55-year-old man according to systolic blood pressure. *Relative risk* describes the increase or decrease in the likelihood of an event in one population compared with that of a reference population. *Absolute risk* quantifies the probability of an event occurring in a population. The risk factors for the high-risk patient are left ventricular hypertrophy, cigarette smoking, glucose intolerance, and cholesterol above 310 mg/dL (8.02 mmol/L). Clearly, there appears to be more benefit in treating the high-risk patient. (*Adapted from* Alderman [1].)

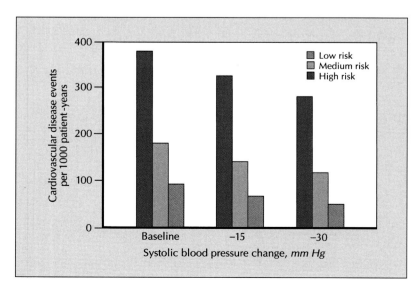

FIGURE 9-3. Cardiovascular disease events by systolic blood pressure change for high-, medium-, and low-risk men. High risk includes systolic blood pressure of 135 mm Hg, cholesterol at 8.02 mmol/L, glucose intolerance, and left ventricular hypertrophy (LVH). Medium risk includes systolic blood pressure of 165 mm Hg, cholesterol at 6.72 mmol/L, glucose intolerance, and no LVH. Low risk includes systolic blood pressure of 195 mm Hg, cholesterol at 4.78 mmol/L, no glucose intolerance, and no LVH. LVH, glucose intolerance, and hyperlipidemia are more powerful risk factors than the blood pressure elevation alone. In each group, a similar reduction in blood pressure confers about the same degree (30%) of risk reduction. (*Adapted from* Alderman [1].)

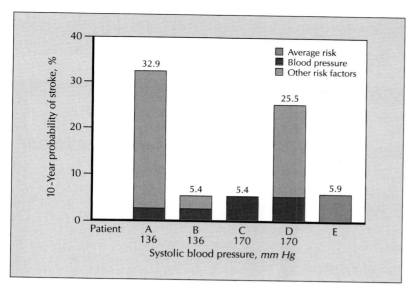

FIGURE 9-4. Ten-year probability of stroke by systolic blood pressure for four 55-year-old, white men with different risk profiles. Patient A was previously treated, has a history of cardio-vascular disease and diabetes, smokes cigarettes, and has left ventricular hypertrophy (LVH); patient B smokes cigarettes; patient C has no other risk factors; patient D has a history of diabetes, smokes cigarettes, and has LVH; and patient E is of average risk. Patients with clearly different blood pressures (such as patients B and C) can have the same absolute risk because of the other risk factors. Because a given reduction in blood pressure can be expected to produce a roughly equivalent percentage decrease in risk of events, it is probable that with the same degree of blood pressure reduction, more persons at greater absolute risk, such as patients A and D, would benefit than would patients such as B and C. (*Adapted from* Alderman [1].)

NNT TO AVOID A CARDIOVASCULAR EVENT BY RISK PROFILE

Profile	MEN		WOMEN	
	A	C	A	C
NNT	30	11	54	13

FIGURE 9-5. Another way of viewing the potential benefit of anti-hypertensive therapy is to estimate the number of patients who need to be treated (NNT) for 5 years to avoid one cardiovascular event. This differs for hypertensive patients with low (profile A) or high (profile C) cardiovascular risk profiles. The patient with profile A is a 65-year-old nonsmoker who has a blood pressure of 160/85 mm Hg, a serum cholesterol level of 250 mg/dL, and no ischemic changes on electrocardiography. The patient with profile C is a 75-year-old smoker who has a blood pressure of 190/110 mm Hg, a serum cholesterol level of 250 mg/dL, and ischemic changes on electrocardiography. (*Adapted from* Ménard and Chatellier [2] and MRC Working Party [3].)

BENEFITS OF HYPERTENSION TREATMENT

	INITIAL ABSOLUTE RISK, %	RELATIVE RISK REDUCTION, %	ODDS RATIO	NNT
Strokes				
Older	7.0	36	0.64	39
Younger	2.3	44	0.56	98
CHD				
Older	6.8	19	0.81	77
Younger	3.8	14	0.86	187

FIGURE 9-6. The benefits of hypertension treatment are dependent both on the magnitude of the absolute cardiovascular risk and on the relative reduction achieved. Because the initial risk is lower in younger patients, the number needed to treat (NNT) for 5 years to avoid one cardiovascular event is higher. CHD—coronary heart disease. (*Adapted from* Ménard and Chatellier [2].)

TRIAL RESULTS ON EFFICACY OF INTERVENTIONS FOR PRIMARY PREVENTION OF HYPERTENSION

DOCUMENTED EFFICACY	LIMITED OR UNPROVEN EFFICACY
Weight loss	Stress management
Reduced sodium intake	Potassium (pill supplementation)
Reduced alcohol consumption	Fish oil (pill supplementation)
Exercise	Calcium (pill supplementation)
	Magnesium (pill supplementation)
	Macronutrient alteration
	Fiber supplementation

FIGURE 9-7. Trial results on the efficacy of interventions for the primary prevention of hypertension. It is ideal to prevent hypertension from becoming clinically evident in genetically susceptible people. We have not yet learned how to select our own genes, but it is possible to manipulate our environment. Not surprisingly, the methods for primary prevention of hypertension are quite similar to those for nonpharmacologic treatment of established hypertension. (*Adapted from* the National High Blood Pressure Education Program Working Group [4].)

NONPHARMACOLOGIC THERAPY

Weight reduction

Ethanol intake reduction
(≤ 1 alcohol drink per day)

Sodium intake reduction
(to 68–103 mmol/d)

Aerobic exercise

Avoidance of vasopressor drugs
(*eg*, nasal decongestants) and
antivasodepressor drugs
(nonsteroidal anti-inflammatory
drugs)

Stress management

Increase calcium and
potassium intake

FIGURE 9-8. Given that hypertension is a life-long disorder of intra-arterial pressure regulation, it follows that treatment protocols should also be designed to be life-long. All individuals who have a genetic susceptibility to hypertension should, ideally, undergo lifestyle modification in order to reduce the risk of clinical hypertension. Such nonpharmacologic therapy may reduce blood pressure sufficiently to avoid drug treatment, but must be monitored in order to prevent or detect breaks in the routine.

WEIGHT LOSS

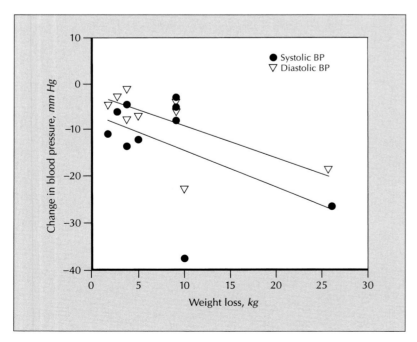

FIGURE 9-9. Regression of blood pressure (BP) following weight loss. Excellent studies have demonstrated that weight reduction, even without sodium restriction, is generally associated with substantial reductions in BP. Either the BP normalizes or the amount of drug required for normalization is reduced. The regressions of systolic and diastolic BP on weight loss from 10 studies were reviewed by Johnston [5]. Although there is a great deal of scatter, greater weight loss does seem to correlate with greater reduction in BP ($r = 0.50$ and $r = 0.66$ for systolic and diastolic BP, respectively). The regression lines for systolic (lower) and diastolic (upper) pressures are nearly parallel.

RESULTS OF DIETARY APPROACHES TO STOP HYPERTENSION DIET

Product of NIH-funded research

DASH combination diet is rich in fruits, vegetables, low-fat dairy foods, dietary fiber, potassium, calcium, magnesium, and protein; it is low in saturated and total fat and cholesterol

The DASH diet reduced blood pressure significantly even in normotensive patients, but was especially effective in hypertensives and blacks

Modest sodium restriction achieved a substantial additional reduction in blood pressure

FIGURE 9-10. Results of the Dietary Approaches to Stop Hypertension (DASH) diet. The federal government sponsored a very carefully controlled study of different diets for the purpose of improving overall health of the population. Following a 3-week control period, subjects were randomly allocated to 8 weeks of a usual control diet, a diet similar to control but rich in fruits and vegetables, or a combination diet rich in fruits, vegetables, low-fat dairy products, whole grains, fish, poultry, and nuts and with reduced amounts of fat, red meat, sweets, and sugar-containing beverages. Sodium intake and weight were held constant. After 8 weeks, 23% of these stage 1 hypertensives attained normal blood pressure on the control diet, 45% on the fruit and vegetable supplemented diet, and 70% on the combination diet [6,7]. Subjects were further allocated to modification of sodium intake: 144 mmol/d (high), 107 mmol/d (intermediate), or 67 mmol/d (low). The low- sodium diet effected a significant further reduction of blood pressure in subjects consuming the control diet and further reduced the blood pressure in those taking the DASH diet [8].

DASH DIET: DAILY SERVINGS FOR EACH FOOD GROUP

Grains and grain products: 7 to 8
Vegetables: 4 to 5
Fruits: 4 to 5
Low-fat or nonfat dairy foods: 2 to 3
Meats, poultry, fish: ≤ 2
Nuts, seeds, legumes: 4 to 5 per week
Reduction of sodium intake to 1.5 to 2.5 g/d greatly enhances the benefit

FIGURE 9-11. Daily servings for each food group in the Dietary Approaches to Stop Hypertension (DASH) diet. The components of the DASH diet are really quite simple and easy to achieve by motivated patients. Reasonable sodium restriction was especially effective in blacks [8]. The diet can be found in greater detail on the Joint National Committee (JNC)-VI web site: http://www.nhlbi.nih.gov/guidelines/hypertension/jncintro.htm.

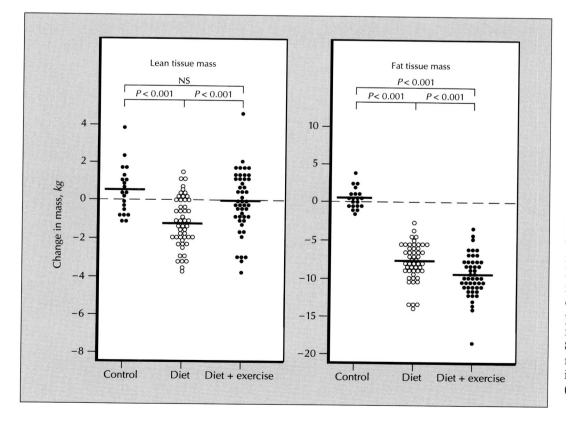

FIGURE 9-12. The interaction of diet and exercise on blood pressure reduction is demonstrated by this study of postmenopausal women. The experimental diet was an obligatory artificial diet plus a carefully defined amount of additional food. Considerable attention to detail by the patients was required. There were favorable changes in lean and fat tissue mass after 12 weeks of diet alone (*open circles, n = 50*) and additional improvement with diet plus exercise (*closed circles, n = 48*) for reduction of body mass index, total cholesterol, and systolic blood pressure. Exercise helped preserve lean tissue mass while enhancing loss of fat tissue mass. Even most women already at or less than 140 mm Hg systolic blood pressure at baseline had a further reduction in blood pressure with diet or diet plus exercise. Average blood pressure reductions were -2 ± 11 (SD)/-4 ± 7 mm Hg for 20 control patients, -13 ± 12/-7 ± 8 mm Hg for diet only, and -11 ± 11/-9 ± 8 mm Hg for diet plus exercise. *Thick bars* indicate mean values. NS—not significant. (*Adapted from* Svendsen *et al.* [9].)

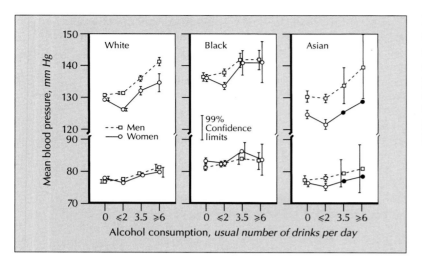

FIGURE 9-13. The consumption of more than two alcohol drinks per day has long been associated with an increase in systolic and diastolic blood pressure irrespective of race or gender. The closed circles in the right panel only represent data based on less than 30 persons. Mean blood pressure data are age-adjusted. The entire cohort included 83,947 members of the Kaiser-Permanente Medical Care Program. Alcohol intake reduction may be one of the most rapidly effective forms of nonpharmacologic treatment of hypertension. (*Adapted from* Klatsky *et al.* [10].)

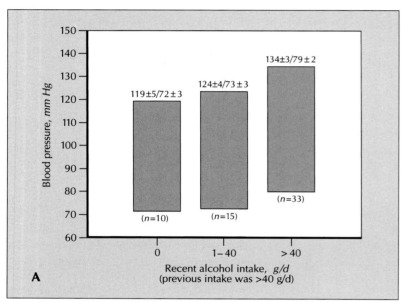

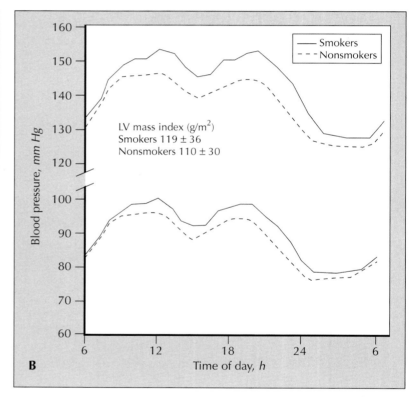

FIGURE 9-14. A, A detailed study of the alcohol consumption habits correlated with blood pressure (BP) in 577 factory workers suggested that recent alcohol intake (1 to 3 days prior to BP measurement) elevated the BP, but that previous alcohol intake (4 to 6 days prior to BP measurement) did not [11]. This figure depicts a subset of 58 men whose previous alcohol intake was more than 40 g/d. These data not only confirm the immediate pressor effect of alcohol, but also support the concept of rapid offset of the pressor effect. Reduction of excess alcohol intake, therefore, can have as rapid a beneficial effect on BP as do many drugs. **B,** Twenty-four-hour BP profile in 115 smokers and 460 age-, sex-, and BP-matched nonsmokers with essential hypertension. *Continuous lines* denote smokers; *broken lines* denote nonsmokers. BP was higher in the smokers than in the nonsmokers

during the day; however, the difference between the two groups was smaller and not statistically significant during the night. Smokers had a significantly higher left ventricular (LV) mass index (mean ± SD; $P < 0.005$) than did nonsmokers. It is not yet known whether smoking cessation will reverse either the daytime BP differential or the left ventricular hypertrophy. (Part B *adapted from* Verdecchia *et al.* [12].)

SODIUM RESTRICTION AND BLOOD PRESSURE

POOLED RESULTS

23 randomized trials of sodium reduction

1536 subjects with blood pressure outcome data

Urine sodium excretion reduced 50–100 mmol/d

SIGNIFICANT BLOOD PRESSURE–LOWERING EFFECTS

-5/-3 mm Hg in hypertensive subjects

-2/-1 mm Hg in normotensive subjects

FIGURE 9-15. Sodium restriction and blood pressure. Data pooled and analyzed by Cutler *et al.* [13] show a small but highly statistically significant effect of sodium restriction on blood pressure. High sodium intake by overweight persons (but not nonoverweight) is strongly and independently associated with an increased risk of cardiovascular disease and all-cause mortality [14].

RESPONSES TO STRESS

Elevation of systolic blood pressure

Elevation of diastolic blood pressure

Increase in circulating levels of catecholamines, cortisol, vasopressin, endorphins, and aldosterone

Decrease in urinary sodium excretion

FIGURE 9-16. Documented responses to acute stressful stimuli. The effects on blood pressure may be particularly marked in those individuals who are exposed to stress but are unable to control their environment in order to manage or avoid stressful situations. This may be particularly relevant in people with lower levels of education or income (markers of socioeconomic status).

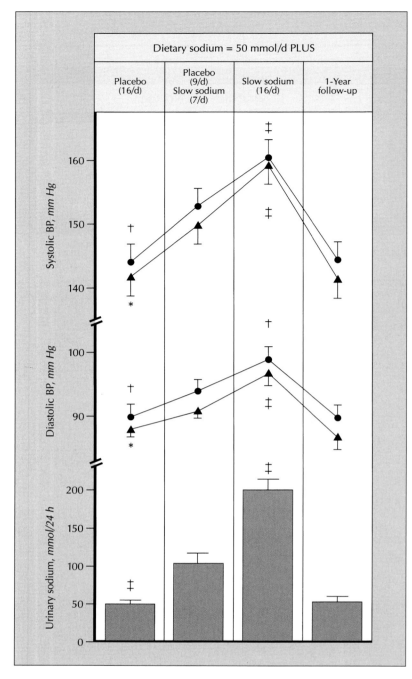

FIGURE 9-17. Data from one of many studies demonstrating the pressor effect of additional dietary sodium. These patients were placed on a sodium-restricted diet (about 50 mmol/d) to which either placebo or slow-release sodium tablets were added. Both systolic and diastolic blood pressures (BP) increased with the addition of sodium and returned to baseline when the supplement was discontinued. Patient samples included 19 patients (*closed circles*), 3 of whom required the addition of antihypertensive medications, and 16 patients (*closed triangles*) who were not taking medications. *Asterisks* indicate $P < 0.05$; *daggers* indicate $P < 0.01$; and *double daggers* indicate $P < 0.001$ compared with the phase of seven slow-release tablets per day. *T bars* indicate standard error. (*Adapted from* MacGregor *et al.* [15].)

POTASSIUM SUPPLEMENTATION

IN FAVOR

Natriuretic and antihypertensive effects in sodium-replete subjects

Helps correct dietary excess sodium: potassium ratio

Decreases risk of ventricular ectopy in susceptible patients

Has a long-term protective effect against strokes

May have vasculoprotective properties

AGAINST

High cost

Poor patient compliance

Ineffective if dietary sodium is restricted and potassium intake normal

FIGURE 9-18. Supplemental potassium appears to reduce blood pressure slightly in sodium-replete patients, probably by its facilitative natriuretic effect [16] and partial correction of excess dietary sodium to potassium intake [17]. It can be therapeutic in hypokalemic patients with documented organic heart disease and ventricular ectopy [18]. Long-term protection against strokes and other vasculoprotective properties have been demonstrated [19]. Conversely, almost any form of potassium supplementation is expensive, and patients tend to be noncompliant because of the cost, bad taste, and inconvenience of the products [20]. It is interesting that if the basic dietary inadequacy is corrected, potassium supplementation is neither necessary nor effective [21].

HOW MUCH LOWER WOULD POPULATION SYSTOLIC PRESSURE BE WITH IMPROVED LIFESTYLE?

	INTERSALT MEDIAN	IMPROVED LEVEL	PREDICTED DIFFERENCE, MM HG
Urinary sodium, mmol/24 h	170.0	70	-2.2
Urinary potassium, mmol/24 h	55.0	70	-0.7
Sodium:potassium	3.1	1	-3.4 ⎤
Body mass index	25.0	23	-1.6 ⎦ -5

FIGURE 9-19. Predicted differences in blood pressure that would result from decreasing sodium intake, increasing potassium intake, and decreasing body mass index. The combination of improving the sodium:potassium ratio and weight loss should decrease systolic blood pressure by 5 mm Hg. *INTERSALT median* refers to the median values derived for these variables in the INTERSALT Cooperative Study. (*Adapted from* Stamler [22].)

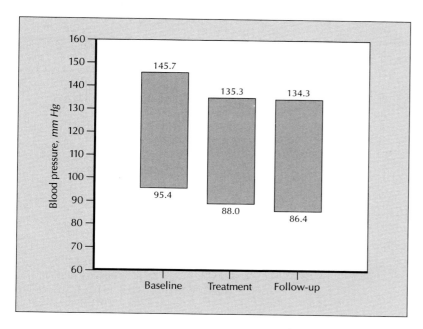

FIGURE 9-20. Various behavioral modifications ranging from stress management counseling to biofeedback to meditation can achieve clinically important reductions in blood pressure. These average data are based on 24 studies of 526 subjects collected by Johnston [5]. Because the studies are very different, this cannot be considered a formal meta-analysis. On average, patients with mildly elevated blood pressure (146/95 mm Hg) achieved an average decrement of -10.4/7.4 mm Hg after the intervention. Follow-up of 422 subjects at widely varying intervals suggested that the effect persisted if the intervention was continued (-11.4/-9.0 mm Hg). Job strain characterized by high demand associated with low control is one mechanism for blood pressure increase. Job modification has the potential for reducing blood pressure [23].

STRESS

POTENTIAL FOR LOWERING MORTALITY WITH LOWER AVERAGE POPULATION SYSTOLIC PRESSURE

AMOUNT SUBTRACTED FROM SBP, MM HG	DEATHS, %			POTENTIAL LIVES SAVED PER YEAR, N*
	CORONARY	STROKE	ALL	
2	-4	-6	-3	12,000
3	-5	-8	-4	16,000
5	-9	-14	-7	28,000

*Based on number of US deaths in 1985 from all causes for men and women aged 45–64 years.

FIGURE 9-21. Even small reductions in blood pressure can be translated into substantial decreases in death, particularly from coronary disease and stroke. The potential number of lives saved per year resulting from a 5 mm Hg reduction in blood pressure (achieved by improving the sodium:potassium ratio and body mass index) is 28,000. Values are based on systolic blood pressure (SBP) and mortality in five large-population follow-up studies. (*Adapted from* Stamler [22].)

FIGURE 9-22. Calcium supplementation can reduce blood pressure in low-renin, salt-sensitive individuals. These people are most likely to be elderly or black, which is also the group most likely to have lactose intolerance. Calcium from nondairy foods and antacid tablets is more palatable and may have an additional benefit of protecting against osteoporosis. Possible mechanisms of action focus on changes in vascular tone mediated by suppression of parathyroid hormone and 1,25 $(OH)_2$-D–induced increases in intracellular calcium, and calcium-induced natriuresis. (*Adapted from* Sowers *et al.* [24].)

NONPHARMACOLOGIC VERSUS DRUG THERAPY

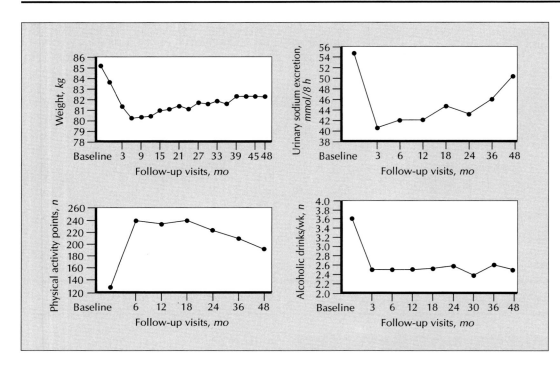

FIGURE 9-23. Does nonpharmacologic therapy have a favorable impact on cardiovascular and cerebrovascular morbidity and mortality? The Treatment of Mild Hypertension Study [24] addressed this question by randomizing 902 patients with very mild hypertension (140.4/90.5 mm Hg) to intensive nutritional-hygienic therapy alone (placebo) or nutritional-hygienic therapy plus one of five drugs. The results of the intensive therapy are shown here. Maximum weight loss occurred at 6 months, but weight then began to creep upward. Physical activity increased with training, but slacked off with time. Sodium intake was effectively reduced at first, but was heading toward baseline at 4 years. Only the reduction in alcohol intake was sustained in these patients, who were very moderate drinkers. (*Adapted from* Neaton *et al.* [25].)

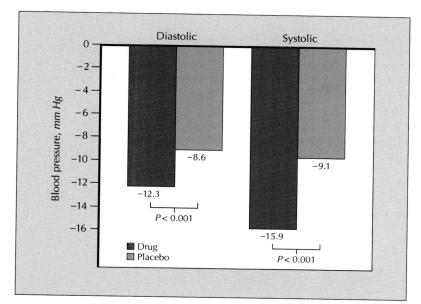

FIGURE 9-24. Patients in the Treatment of Mild Hypertension Study protocol were randomly allocated to treatment with nutritional-hygienic measures alone (placebo) or nutritional-hygienic methods plus one of five drugs [24]. The placebo group had a striking reduction of blood pressure (-9.1/-8.6 mm Hg) based only on the intensive nutritional-hygienic interventions. The addition of active antihypertensive medication effected a reduction of -15.9/-12.3 mm Hg from baseline (140.4/90.5 mm Hg). There were no significant differences in efficacy among the drugs.

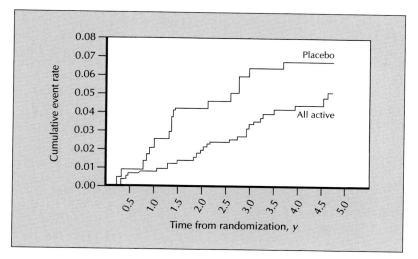

FIGURE 9-25. Cumulative percentage of major clinical events for the Treatment of Mild Hypertension Study participants randomly assigned to drug treatment and nutritional-hygienic intervention (all active) or to nutritional-hygienic intervention alone (placebo). The difference was not statistically significant. Nevertheless, even in this very mildly hypertensive group of patients who had a substantial response to the nonpharmacologic therapy alone, the addition of drug treatment had a clinically important effect. Major clinical events were death from coronary heart disease or other cardiovascular disease including stroke, death from other causes, nonfatal myocardial infarction or stroke, congestive heart failure, surgery for aortic aneurysm, coronary artery bypass surgery or angioplasty, thrombolytic therapy, or hospitalization for unstable angina. (*Adapted from* Neaton *et al.* [25].)

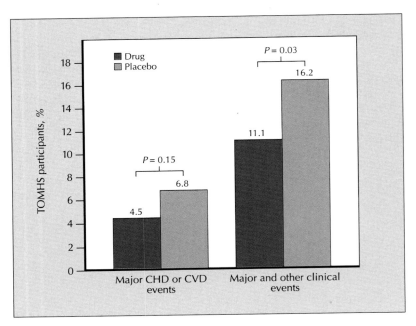

FIGURE 9-26. Despite the substantial reduction in blood pressure (-9.1/-8.6 mm Hg) achieved in the Treatment of Mild Hypertension Study (TOMHS) patients with nutritional-hygienic intervention alone, the greater reduction achieved by the addition of drug therapy to nutritional-hygienic intervention (-15.9/-12.3 mm Hg) was sufficient to reduce major coronary heart disease (CHD) and cerebrovascular disease (CVD) events more than that achieved by nutritional-hygienic intervention alone [25]. This difference did not achieve statistical significance, but when major and all other clinical events were combined, drug treatment was significantly more effective than was nonpharmacologic therapy alone. Other clinical events included hospitalization for cerebral transient ischemic attacks, definite angina or intermittent claudication, and peripheral arterial occlusive disease.

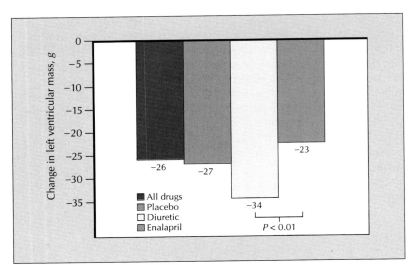

FIGURE 9-27. The reduction in left ventricular mass achieved in the Treatment of Mild Hypertension Study patients treated with nutritional-hygienic intervention alone was no different from that achieved with drug therapy superimposed on the nutritional-hygienic intervention [25]. This suggests that reduction of blood pressure, per se, has an important effect on reversing left ventricular hypertrophy. The drugs were generally similar in their effect on left ventricular mass with the exception of the diuretic, chlorthalidone, and the angiotensin-converting enzyme inhibitor, enalapril. Interestingly, the diuretic was significantly more effective in reducing left ventricular mass. It must be noted, however, that the diuretic group had a left ventricular mass 5.4 g higher at baseline than did the enalapril group.

FIGURE 9-28. Nonpharmacologic (nutritional-hygienic) therapy is of great potential value. However, there are disadvantages to its use as well.

NONPHARMACOLOGIC (NUTRITIONAL-HYGIENIC) THERAPY

ADVANTAGES

May reduce blood pressure substantially without drugs

Enhances efficacy of drug therapy

May prevent or mitigate adverse drug effects
  (*eg*, hypokalemia, hyperlipidemia)

May effect regression of left ventricular hypertrophy

DISADVANTAGES

Labor-intensive, expensive

Requires high patient and provider motivation

Requires continuous monitoring and reinforcement

May not protect against coronary artery disease and
  cardiovascular disease, including stroke, as well
  as does the addition of drugs

RACE AND AGE

FACTORS THAT INFLUENCE THE SELECTION OF ANTIHYPERTENSIVE DRUGS

Race
Age
Prior medication history
Concomitant diseases
Severity of hypertension
Quality of life
Cost

FIGURE 9-29. If nonpharmacologic therapy does not normalize blood pressure, drug therapy must be added. Several factors should be considered in the selection of antihypertensive drug therapy, particularly if the patient has sufficiently mild hypertension to be likely to respond to the appropriate single drug. Race and age are simple factors to determine. Prior medication history should include both efficacy and adverse drug reactions. If the adverse drug reactions are multiple or bizarre, the clinician should be alert to the possibility of panic attacks or some other psychiatric problem. Severity of hypertension does not dictate the choice of drug (or drugs) per se, but the higher the blood pressure the more likely that two or more drugs will be required to achieve control. Quality-of-life effects are crucial, especially in young and fully employed people. Cost of treatment is of major national concern.

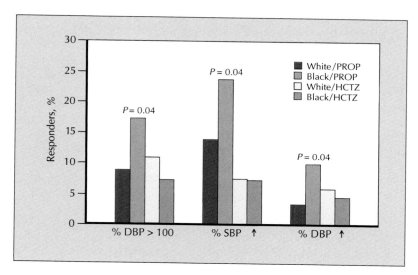

FIGURE 9-30. An effect of race on drug efficacy was noted in this study of 683 men who were randomly allocated to treatment with either propranolol (PROP) or hydrochlorothiazide (HCTZ). There was no difference in systolic blood pressure (SBP) reduction between the two drugs in white patients, but HCTZ was highly superior in blacks (-20.3 vs -8.2 mm Hg). PROP reduced diastolic blood pressure (DBP) by 12.6 mm Hg compared with -10.9 mm Hg for HCTZ in whites. In contrast, HCTZ reduced DBP in blacks by 13 mm Hg compared with 9.5 mm Hg for PROP. More blacks achieved goal blood pressure with HCTZ than with PROP. PROP in blacks was associated with a significant number of patients whose blood pressure *increased* with treatment. (*Adapted from* the Veterans Administration Cooperative Study Group on Antihypertensive Agents [26].)

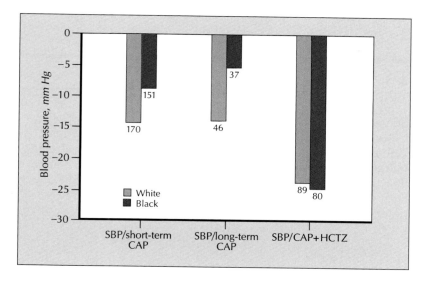

FIGURE 9-31. The effect of race on the response of patients to captopril (CAP) was also observed. In a Veterans Administration study, 495 patients were randomly allocated to CAP (37.5 to 150 mg/d in divided doses), hydrochlorothiazide (HCTZ) alone (50 mg), or CAP plus HCTZ. The short-term was 7 weeks, and the long-term 14 weeks with CAP alone. Blacks responded better to HCTZ than did whites. The combination of the drugs abolished the racial difference in response. The numbers below each bar represent the total number of patients in each group. SBP— systolic blood pressure. (*Adapted from* the Veterans Administration Cooperative Study Group on Antihypertensive Agents [27].)

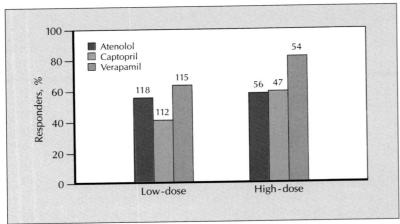

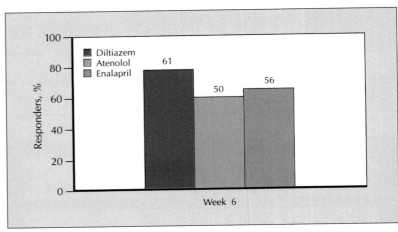

FIGURE 9-32. The Veterans Administration data were confirmed and extended to calcium channel blockers in a study of 394 black men and women who were randomly allocated to treatment with atenolol, 50 to 100 mg/d, captopril, 25 to 50 mg/12 h, or verapamil-SR, 240 to 360 mg/d [28]. After washout, patients were treated for 4 weeks at the lower dose, after which half were randomly assigned to treatment with the higher dose. Patients treated with verapamil responded better than those treated with captopril and, at the higher doses, atenolol. Note that although the response to captopril was less than with verapamil, there was still a substantial effect. The numbers over each bar represent the number of patients in each group.

FIGURE 9-33. The Veterans Administration studies included only men. A study of 244 women 65 years or older (20% black) confirmed that the prior data were not gender-specific [29]. Diltiazem-SR, 60 to 180 mg twice daily, was more effective in the older women at week 16 than was atenolol, 50 to 100 mg/d, or enalapril, 5 to 20 mg/d. The numbers above each bar represent the number of patients in each group.

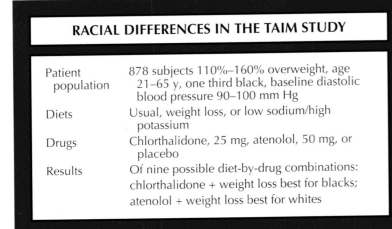

RACIAL DIFFERENCES IN THE TAIM STUDY

Patient population	878 subjects 110%–160% overweight, age 21–65 y, one third black, baseline diastolic blood pressure 90–100 mm Hg
Diets	Usual, weight loss, or low sodium/high potassium
Drugs	Chlorthalidone, 25 mg, atenolol, 50 mg, or placebo
Results	Of nine possible diet-by-drug combinations: chlorthalidone + weight loss best for blacks; atenolol + weight loss best for whites

FIGURE 9-34. The Trial of Antihypertensive Interventions and Management (TAIM) Study [30] was a complex trial that focused on nonpharmacologic interventions such as weight reduction and a diet that was both sodium-restricted and potassium-replete. Patients were randomly allocated to one of the two experimental diets or to their usual diet. They were also randomly allocated to treatment with chlorthalidone, 25 mg/d, atenolol, 50 mg/d, or placebo; therefore, nine drug-by-diet combinations were possible.

SINGLE-DRUG THERAPY FOR HYPERTENSION STUDY

VETERANS AFFAIRS SINGLE-DRUG THERAPY FOR HYPERTENSION STUDY

Randomized, prospective, double-blind

15 VA medical centers

Entry blood pressure 95–109 mm Hg

Compared one representative drug from each of six major classes plus placebo

Randomized 1292 patients (all men)

FIGURE 9-35. Race, age, and race-by-age interactions were studied by the Department of Veterans Affairs (VA) Cooperative Study Group on Antihypertensive Agents to determine how these factors influenced the efficacy of various classes of antihypertensive drugs [31]. In keeping with their usual policy, the study was designed to be as close as practical to what could be achieved and used in an office practice setting.

OBJECTIVES OF VETERANS AFFAIRS SINGLE-DRUG THERAPY FOR HYPERTENSION STUDY

Determine efficacy of each drug in lowering blood pressure
Determine the ability of each drug to control blood pressure over time
Compare the drugs' efficacy in the short-term and long-term control of blood pressure according to age and race
Compare the incidences of medical terminations from the study

FIGURE 9-36. The study size was calculated to provide enough randomized patients in each of the subgroups to permit statistically valid comparisons of the drugs with each other and with placebo [31]. During the study, more patients responded to treatment and fewer dropped out than had been calculated, so that the numbers in each cell were actually higher than required.

DRUGS AND DOSES USED IN VETERANS AFFAIRS SINGLE-DRUG THERAPY FOR HYPERTENSION STUDY

DRUG, mg	LOW DOSE	MEDIUM DOSE	HIGH DOSE
Hydrochlorothiazide	12.5	25.0	50.0
Atenolol	25.0	50.0	100.0
Clonidine*	0.2	0.4	0.6
Captopril*	25.0	50.0	100.0
Prazosin*†	4.0	10.0	20.0
Diltiazem-SR*	120.0	240.0	360.0

*Given in divided doses twice daily.
†Started at 1 mg twice daily for 2 days.

FIGURE 9-37. After a 4- to 8-week washout period, patients who met the criteria for randomization received one of six drugs or the placebo double-blind. The blind was maintained by a double-dummy system in which each patient took medication from both of two bottles, one containing placebo, and the other active drug. (For those allocated to placebo, both bottles contained placebos). The titration period lasted 4 to 8 weeks and required that the drug be titrated to a blood pressure of less than 90 mm Hg for two consecutive visits without adverse effects. (*Adapted from* Materson *et al.* [31].)

VETERANS AFFAIRS SINGLE-DRUG THERAPY FOR HYPERTENSION STUDY BASELINE PATIENT CHARACTERISTICS

Mean blood pressure: 152±14/99±3 mm Hg
Younger patients (<60 y): *n*=546; age 50±8 y
Older patients (≥60 y): *n*=746; age 66±4 y
Racial mix: 52% white, 48% black
Age by race subgroups, *n(%)*
　Younger blacks　　291(22)
　Older blacks　　　330(26)
　Younger whites　　246(19)
　Older whites　　　408(32)

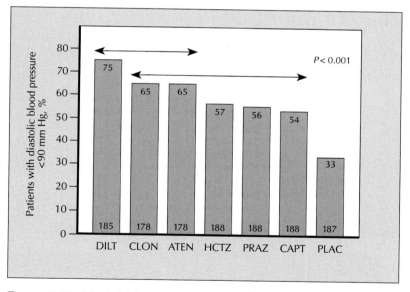

FIGURE 9-38. The randomization scheme was effective in that there were no important statistically significant differences across the drug groups. These patients had mild to moderate hypertension. The results of a single-drug therapy cannot be extrapolated to more severe levels of hypertension. The subgroup numbers do not total 100% because 17 patients were neither black nor white (mostly Asian). (*Adapted from* Materson *et al.* [31].)

FIGURE 9-39. The initial results at the end of the titration phase. The horizontal arrows group drugs whose effects were not significantly different from each other. A drug or drugs not under an arrow are significantly different from those that are. Note that these are overall data without consideration for age or race and are, therefore, skewed by the racial and age mix that is not indicative of the population at large. The numbers at the top of the bars indicate the percentage of patients with the response shown; the numbers at the bottom of the bars indicate the numbers of patients in each group. ATEN—atenolol; CAPT—captopril; CLON—clonidine; DILT—diltiazem-SR; HCTZ—hydrochlorothiazide; PLAC—placebo; PRAZ—prazosin. (*Adapted from* Materson *et al.* [31].)

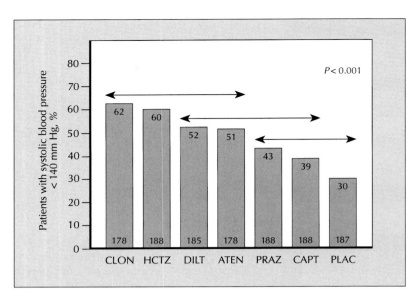

FIGURE 9-40. The Department of Veterans Affairs Study was not designed to look specifically at systolic blood pressure. Randomization was based on diastolic blood pressure criteria, and the systolic blood pressure at randomization was mildly elevated. Nevertheless, the data are of interest. The horizontal arrows group drugs that are not statistically different from each other. The numbers at the top of the bars indicate the percentage of patients with the response shown; the numbers at the bottom of the bars indicate the numbers of patients in each group. ATEN—atenolol; CAPT—captopril; CLON—clonidine; DILT—diltiazem-SR; HCTZ—hydrochlorothiazide; PLAC—placebo; PRAZ—prazosin. (*Adapted from* Materson *et al.* [31].)

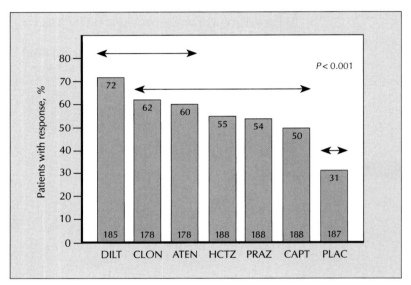

FIGURE 9-41. Overall data for the percentage of patients who responded to each drug. *Response* was defined as having achieved goal blood pressure (< 90 mm Hg) at the end of the short-term titration period *and* maintaining a diastolic blood pressure of less than 95 mm Hg at the end of 1 year. Analysis was by intention to treat. The horizontal arrows group drugs that were not statistically different from each other. Note that all drugs were superior to placebo despite a fairly high placebo response rate. This is an excellent example of why study results should be reported by age and race. These overall data do not give a true picture of the results for specific subsets of patients. The numbers at the top of the bars indicate the percentage of patients with the response shown; the numbers at the bottom of the bars indicate the numbers of patients in each group. ATEN—atenolol; CAPT—captopril; CLON—clonidine; DILT—diltiazem-SR; HCTZ—hydrochlorothiazide; PLAC—placebo; PRAZ—prazosin. (*Adapted from* Materson *et al.* [31].)

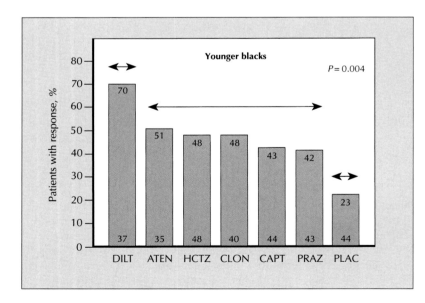

FIGURE 9-42. Success rates (diastolic blood pressure < 90 mm Hg at the end of titration and < 95 mm Hg at the end of at least 1 year of treatment) for each drug and placebo in younger (< 60 years) blacks. The horizontal arrows group drugs that were not more than 15% different from each other. This was deemed to be a clinically important difference during the design of the study. Note that this is *not* the same as statistically significantly different, although pairwise analysis did demonstrate that there were statistically significant differences. Analysis was by intention to treat. Diltiazem-SR (DILT) was most effective, while captopril (CAPT) was not clinically importantly different from placebo. The numbers at the top of the bars indicate the percentage of patients with the response shown; the numbers at the bottom of the bars indicate the numbers of patients in each group. ATEN—atenolol; CLON—clonidine; HCTZ—hydrochlorothiazide; PLAC—placebo; PRAZ—prazosin. (*Adapted from* Materson *et al.* [31].)

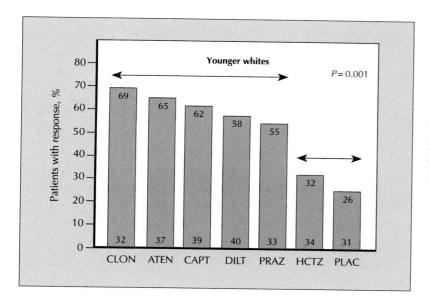

FIGURE 9-43. Younger whites had a pattern of drug efficacy almost exactly the opposite of that of younger blacks. Captopril (CAPT), the least effective drug for the younger blacks, was the most effective for the younger whites. Atenolol (ATEN), another drug thought to be most effective in younger patients, was next in line. The calcium channel blocker, diltiazem-SR (DILT), and diuretic, hydrochloro-thiazide (HCTZ), were least effective. The numbers at the top of the bars indicate the percentage of patients with the response shown; the numbers at the bottom of the bars indicate the numbers of patients in each group. CLON—clonidine; PLAC—placebo; PRAZ—prazosin. (*Adapted from* Materson *et al.* [31].)

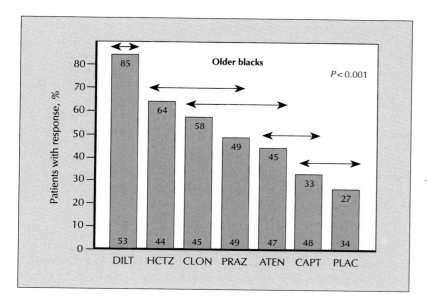

FIGURE 9-44. Older (≥ 60 y) black patients fared best with diltiazem-SR (DILT) and hydrochlorothiazide (HCTZ). The angiotensin-converting enzyme inhibitor, captopril (CAPT), was less effective than placebo (PLAC) in this group. DILT was associated with more terminating adverse effects than was HCTZ and is also much more costly. The diuretic, then, is a legitimate first-line drug in this subgroup. The numbers at the top of the bars indicate the percentage of patients with the response shown; the numbers at the bottom of the bars indicate the numbers of patients in each group. ATEN—atenolol; CLON—clonidine; PRAZ—prazosin. (*Adapted from* Materson *et al.* [31].)

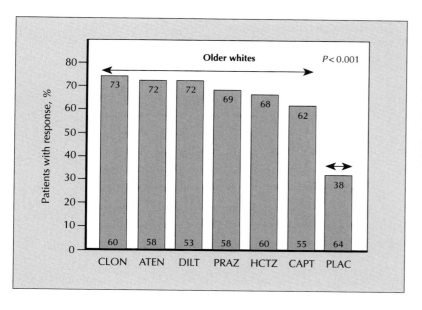

FIGURE 9-45. Older white patients seem to respond well to almost anything, including the placebo (PLAC). Their pattern was a combination of characteristics for white race and age. Clonidine (CLON; 17.7%) and prazosin (PRAZ; 19%) were associated with considerably more adverse drug effect terminations than atenolol (ATEN) and hydrochlorothiazide (HCTZ; both 1.7%). The numbers at the top of the bars indicate the percentage of patients with the response shown; the numbers at the bottom of the bars indicate the numbers of patients in each group. CAPT—captopril; DILT—diltiazem-SR. (*Adapted from* Materson *et al.* [31].)

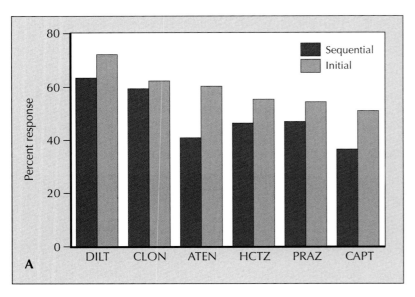

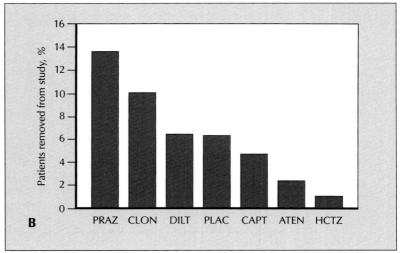

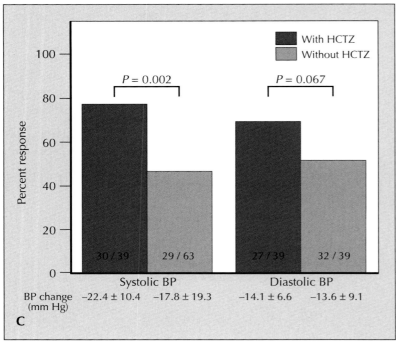

FIGURE 9-46. A, Sequential single-drug therapy as a treatment strategy. These data validate the concept of sequential single-drug

therapy. Unlike this study, which required random allocation of patients to each treatment group, the clinician would be able to select an alternative drug based on age-by-race interactions plus the knowledge of the response achieved with the first drug. **B,** Adverse drug effects tending to termination of treatment. A total of 194 patients were removed from the study because of medical reasons, but only 84 (6.5%) were removed for adverse drug reactions. The overall data show that prazosin (PRAZ) and clonidine (CLON) were the least well tolerated and that hydrochlorothiazide (HCTZ), atenolol (ATEN), and captopril (CAPT) were the best tolerated drugs. The rate for placebo (PLAC; 6.4%) underscores the need for doing placebo-controlled trials in order to put drug-related adverse effects into perspective. In fact, there was a termination for proteinuria in all drug groups (including placebo) except clonidine. Proteinuria certainly was not specific to the angiotensin-converting enzyme inhibitor. **C,** In the Veteran's Administration (VA) study, patients with diastolic blood pressure (BP) greater than 100 mm Hg at baseline were less likely to respond to a single drug than were those with a baseline diastolic BP less than 100 mm Hg. When a single drug was not sufficient to achieve a therapeutic BP goal, the results of the VA study showed that the two drugs that were not effective when given alone were often effective when combined. This was especially true if one of the two drugs was HCTZ. DILT—diltiazem hydrochloride (sustained release). (Part A *adapted from* Materson *et al.* [28]; part B *adapted from* Materson *et al.* [32]; and part C *adapted from* Materson *et al.* [33].)

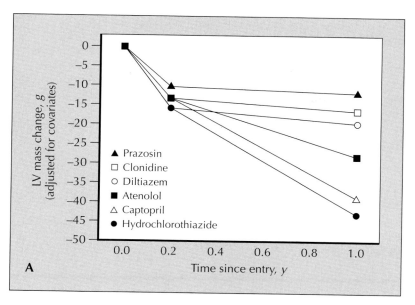

FIGURE 9-47. **A**, Highest tertile of baseline left ventricular (LV) mass. Hydrochlorothiazide effected a significant reduction of LV mass as did captopril and atenolol in this upper tertile of LV mass [34]. This unexpected beneficial effect of hydrochlorothiazide has been replicated with chlorthalidone. **B**, Selected plasma lipid levels at end titration and at 1-year maintenance. Neither hydrochlorothiazide nor atenolol had a long-term (1-year) adverse effect on plasma lipids. Only those nonresponders to hydrochlorothiazide who were forced to the highest titration level of 50 mg had any significant effect [35]. **C**, Response rate and changes in systolic blood pressure and diastolic blood pressure using Renin Profile vs Age–Race Subgroup Methods for choice of an initial antihypertensive agent. When response rates predicted by the age–race paradigm were compared with those predicted by the renin profile, there was no significant difference. Obviously, the cost of determining age and race is virtually zero. HDL—high-density lipoprotein; LDL—low-density lipoprotein. (*Adapted from* Preston *et al.* [36].)

B. SELECTED PLASMA LIPID LEVELS AT END TITRATION AND AT 1–YEAR MAINTENANCE*

VARIABLE	HYDROCHLOROTHIAZIDE	ATENOLOL	CAPTOPRIL	CLONIDINE	DILTIAZEM	PRAZOSIN	PLACEBO	P
Total cholesterol, ≥240 mg/dL								
End titration	25.3	16.5	18.5	14.2	17.6	13.2	13.2	0.06
1-year maintenance	16.3	19.4	14.0	16.7	26.6	15.6	16.3	0.31
LDL cholesterol, ≥160 mg/dL								
End titration	23.5	22.7	22.2	18.4	22.6	18.8	17.6	0.14
1-year maintenance	18.6	19.8	23.5	22.5	29.3	23.4	16.7	0.55
HDL cholesterol, <35 mg/dL								
End titration	10.2	13.9	13.0	8.1	13.2	11.1	5.7	0.18
1-year maintenance	15.1	16.7	8.3	12.4	11.3	13.0	8.3	0.63

*Values are percentages. To convert total cholesterol values in millimole equivalents multiply, by 0.02586.

C. RESPONSE RATE AND CHANGES IN SYSTOLIC BLOOD PRESSURE AND DIASTOLIC BLOOD PRESSURE USING RENIN PROFILE VS AGE–RACE SUBGROUP METHODS FOR CHOICE OF AN INITIAL ANTIHYPERTENSIVE AGENT

RENIN PROFILE METHOD	AGE–RACE SUBGROUP METHOD		
	CORRECT	INCORRECT	COMBINED
	RESPONSE RATE, %		
Correct	74.9	58.7	64.5
Incorrect	63.1	55.4	57.5
Combined	71.6	57.5	

VETERANS AFFAIRS SINGLE-DRUG THERAPY FOR HYPERTENSION STUDY SUBGROUP TERMINATIONS

SUBGROUP	RESULT
Younger blacks	≤ 6.8%; no significant difference between drugs
Younger whites	Prazosin (15.2%) > hydrochlorothiazide (2.9%) and captopril (2.6%)
Older whites	Prazosin (19%) and clonidine (16.7%) > atenolol (1.7%) and hydrochlorothiazide (1.7%)
Older blacks	Diltiazem (12.2%) and prazosin (11.3%) > placebo (0%)

FIGURE 9-48. Just as the overall blood pressure data may be misleading, so it may be with adverse drug effect data [31]. Younger blacks seemed to handle all of the drugs well, whereas younger whites were bothered by prazosin. Older whites had problems with both prazosin and clonidine, but tolerated atenolol and hydrochlorothiazide very well. Although older blacks responded well to diltiazem-SR, they had more adverse drug reactions from it than they did from hydrochlorothiazide, to which they responded equally well.

DIFFERENCES IN RACIAL RESPONSE

POSSIBLE EXPLANATIONS FOR RACIAL DIFFERENCES IN RESPONSE TO ANTIHYPERTENSIVE AGENTS

GENETIC FACTORS	There is clear evidence of racial differences in drug metabolism based on hepatic and other enzyme systems; pharmacogenetics is a growing field; renal sodium handling may be genetically determined
SOCIOECONOMIC FACTORS	Low income and poor education are established measures of low socioeconomic status and correlate well with poor health, stress, and hypertension
ETHNIC FACTORS	Diet, particularly if high in sodium and low in potassium and calcium; cultural attitudes toward disease and its treatment

FIGURE 9-49. There is no single answer to differences in racial response. White, black, and Asian people have been demonstrated to have different rates of metabolism of different drugs. These differences may also be found within races and are under genetic control. The stress of low socioeconomic status may lead to excessive alcohol use, a setting in which prazosin may be more effective. Less efficient renal sodium excretion mechanisms coupled with culturally determined high sodium/low potassium intake could cause volume expansion, release of ouabain, influx of sodium into cells, increased intracellular calcium as a compensatory mechanism, and resultant increased vascular smooth muscle contractility.

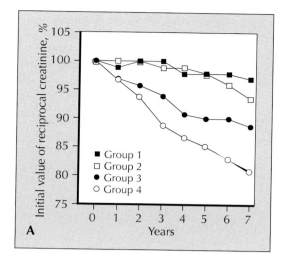

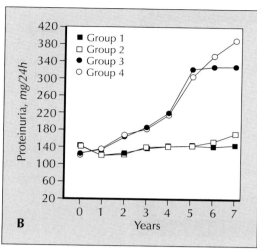

increase of urinary albumin excretion leveled off in contrast with the patients in group 4, who refused to take the active drug; their urinary protein excretion continued to increase, and their renal function continued to decline. Therefore, patients with hypertension and concomitant diabetes mellitus, either type 1 or type 2, should be treated with an ACE inhibitor (*see* Chapter 10). **A,** The decline of reciprocal creatinine expressed as the percentage of the initial value, in the four groups of patients. Patients in group 1 received enalapril treatment in years 1 to 7; patients in group 2 received enalapril treatment in years 1 to 5 and no treatment in years 6 and 7; patients in group 3 received a placebo in years 1 to 5 and enalapril treatment in years 6 and 7; and patients in group 4 received a placebo in years 1 to 5 and no treatment in years 6 and 7. **B,** Evolution of urinary albumin excretion rate during 7 years in the four groups of patients. (*Adapted from* Ravid *et al.* [37].)

FIGURE 9-50. It is now clear that angiotensin-converting enzyme (ACE) inhibitors do reduce the urinary albumin excretion rate and slow the rate of progression toward end-stage renal disease in patients with diabetes mellitus with or without concomitant hypertension. Patients in groups 1 and 2, who received the ACE inhibitor enalapril, did very well compared with those in the groups who received placebo. When group 2 patients refused to continue the enalapril after 5 years of the blinded study, they began to excrete more urinary albumin, and their renal function began to worsen. When the patients in group 3 agreed to be treated with enalapril instead of placebo, their rate of

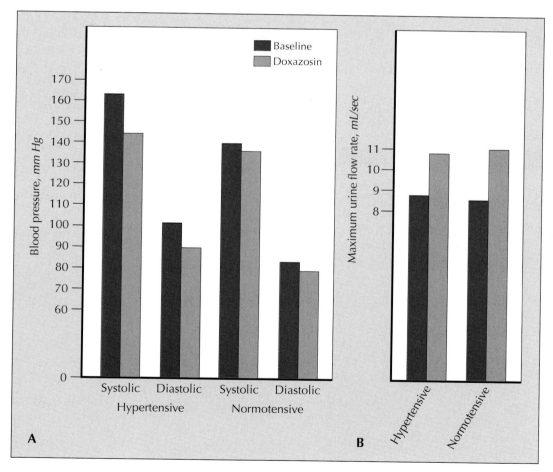

FIGURE 9-51. α_1-Antagonists not only reduce blood pressure but also relax prostatic and urinary sphincter smooth muscle. In this study, doxazosin reduced blood pressure in the hypertensive patients being treated for benign prostatic hypertrophy, but not in the normotensive patients (**A**). Both hypertensive and normotensive patients benefited by an equal increase in urinary flow rate (**B**). Therefore, hypertension with concomitant prostatic hypertrophy is a good indication for the use of an α_1-antagonist. Improvement in symptoms actually is substantially greater than what might have been predicted by measures of maximum flow rate. (*Adapted from* Kirby [38].)

RELATIVE RISK OF HYPERTENSION IN MIDDLE-AGED MEN*

TENSION LEVEL[†]	n	RELATIVE RISK	95% CI
0.00	124	1.00	
0.14	52	1.10	0.63–1.94
0.29	46	1.25	0.74–2.13
0.43	40	1.16	0.64–2.08
0.57	25	1.29	0.69–2.43
0.70–1.00	27	2.19	1.22–3.94

*Model includes age, initial systolic blood pressure, initial heart rate, relative weight, alcohol intake, glucose intolerance, smoking, and education.

[†]The psychologic scale is scored from 0 to 1.0, with higher scores associated with greater evidence of the trait.

FIGURE 9-52. Relative risk of hypertension in middle-aged men. Numerous studies have demonstrated that stress can play a role in hypertension. Hypertension also can be a feature of panic attacks. "White coat" hypertension can confound the office measurement of blood pressure. In the Framingham Study, men who expressed high tension levels on psychometric testing were more likely to develop fixed hypertension than were those with no tension; this did not apply to women. When hypertension is concomitant with panic attacks or anxiety, the underlying problem must be recognized and treated. Antihypertensive drugs will not resolve these problems alone, and their use is frequently associated with adverse drug reactions. Bizarre or pharmacologically improbable adverse drug reactions are good clues to an underlying psychiatric problem. β-Blockers and central α_2-agonists can be very useful in treatment of hypertensive patients with concomitant mild anxiety. (*Adapted from* Markovitz et al. [39].)

COMPARISON OF METABOLIC EFFECTS OF LOW-DOSE HYDROCHLOROTHIAZIDE AND LISINOPRIL IN OBESE HYPERTENSIVE PATIENTS

VARIABLE	HCTZ		LISINOPRIL	
	BEFORE	AFTER	BEFORE	AFTER
SSPG, *mg/dL*	254 ± 11	252 ± 17	272 ± 9	280 ± 9
SSPI, *µU/mL*	60 ± 6	58 ± 6	65 ± 9	64 ± 6
TG, *mg/dL*	182 ± 19	196 ± 29	172 ± 18	164 ± 15
VLDL-TG, *mg/dL*	142 ± 19	158 ± 30	130 ± 16	124 ± 14
Cholesterol, *mg/dL*	200 ± 7	193 ± 8	193 ± 15	200 ± 12
VLDL-C, *mg/dL*	38 ± 4	35 ± 6	37 ± 4	37 ± 4
LDL-C, *mg/dL*	108 ± 8	105 ± 9	101 ± 10	108 ± 9
HDL-C, *mg/dL*	43 ± 2	43 ± 3	44 ± 2	43 ± 2

FIGURE 9-53. In a study of obese hypertensive patients treated for 3 months with lisinopril, 20 mg, or hydrochlorothiazide (HCTZ), 12.5 mg, there was "little or no untoward effect on multiple aspects of glucose, insulin, and lipoprotein metabolism that increase risk of coronary heart disease, although these metabolic variables did increase somewhat in HCTZ-treated patients" [33]. Although dietary reduction of weight reduces blood pressure in most obese hypertensive patients, drug therapy provides the most rapid and, often, the most long-lasting results. Obesity and hypertension are linked to hyperinsulinemia, decreased tissue sensitivity to insulin, and dyslipidemia. Angiotensin-converting enzyme inhibitors improve insulin sensitivity in contrast to diuretics and β-blockers, which reduce insulin sensitivity. This has created some reluctance to use diuretics in treatment of obese hypertensive patients, even though such patients tend to be volume replete and respond well to diuretic therapy. Low-dose thiazide diuretic therapy alone or in combination with other antihypertensive agents should be considered along with dietary treatment of obese hypertensive patients. Chol—cholesterol; HDL—high-density lipoprotein; LDL—low-density lipoprotein; SSPG—steady-state plasma glucose concentration; SSPI—steady-state plasma insulin concentration; TG—triglyceride; VLDL—very low density lipoprotein. (*Adapted from* Reaven et al. [40].)

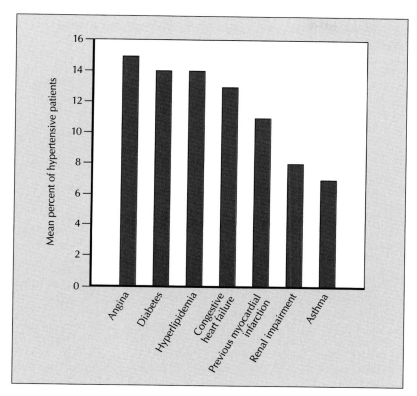

FIGURE 9-54. A survey of primary care physicians showed that 47% of their patients making office visits for management of hypertension had one or more concomitant diseases. This must be considered in drug selection. β-Blockers are now known to have a secondary preventive effect on myocardial infarction. Angiotensin-converting enzyme inhibitors may limit infarct size, and may help slow the rate of progression toward end-stage renal disease (at least in diabetics). α-Blockers may be beneficial in patients with urinary outflow obstruction. Patients with painful rheumatologic disorders may be taking nonsteroidal anti-inflammatory drugs that can interfere with their drug treatment. α-Blockers may be particularly effective in patients with heavy alcohol intake. Anxiety and depression, both extremely common in the general population, must be considered as well. Often treatment of the primary psychiatric problem normalizes blood pressure or reduces the amount of antihypertensive medication required. (*Adapted from* Materson [41].)

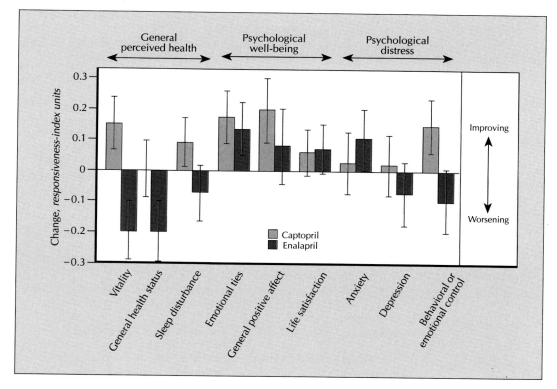

FIGURE 9-55. Considerable literature supports the concept that there is a difference among drug classes in their impact on patient quality of life. Croog *et al.* [42] developed instruments for measuring several parameters of quality of life and were able to show differences between captopril, propranolol, and methyldopa. This study of 379 men [43] lasted 24 weeks and demonstrated for the first time important differences between two drugs of the same class that had equal antihypertensive effects and were otherwise equal by the usual clinical measures. The negative impact of enalapril was greatest on patients who had the highest quality of life at baseline. These data suggest that it may not be quite so easy to designate therapeutic equivalents from the same drug class. *T bars* represent standard error. (*Adapted from* Testa *et al.* [43].)

1. Alderman MH: Blood pressure management: individualized treatment based on absolute risk and the potential for benefit. *Ann Intern Med* 1993, 119:329–335.

2. Ménard J, Chatellier G: Mild hypertension: the mysterious viability of a faulty concept. *J Hypertens* 1995, 13:1071–1077.

3. Medical Research Council Working Party: MRC trial of treatment of hypertension in older adults: principal results. *BMJ* 1992, 304:405–412.

4. National High Blood Pressure Education Program Working Group: National High Blood Pressure Education Program Working Group report on primary prevention of hypertension. *Arch Intern Med* 1993, 153:186–208.

5. Johnston DW: The behavioral control of high blood pressure. *Curr Psychol Res Rev* 1987, 6:99–114.

6. Appel LJ, Moore TJ, Obarzanek E, *et al.*: A clinical trial of the effects of dietary patterns on blood pressure. *N Engl J Med* 1997, 336:1117–1124.

7. Conlin PR, Chow D, Miller ER III, *et al.*: The effect of dietary patterns on blood pressure control in hypertensive patients: results from the Dietary Approaches to Stop Hypertension (DASH) trial. *Am J Hypertens* 2000, 13:949–955.

8. Sacks FM, Svetkey LP, Vollmer WM, *et al.*: Effects on blood pressure of reduced dietary sodium and the dietary approaches to stop hypertension (DASH) diet. *N Engl J Med* 2001, 344:3–10.

9. Svendsen OL, Hassager C, Christiansen C: Effect of an energy-restrictive diet, with or without exercise, on lean tissue mass, resting metabolic rate, cardiovascular risk factors, and bone in overweight postmenopausal women. *Am J Med* 1993, 95:131–140.

10. Klatsky AL, Friedman GD, Siegelaub AB, *et al.*: Alcohol consumption and blood pressure: Kaiser-Permanente Multiphasic Health Examination Data. *N Engl J Med* 1977, 296:1194–1200.

11. Maheswaran R, Gill JS, Davies P, *et al.*: High blood pressure due to alcohol: a rapidly reversible effect. *Hypertension* 1991, 17:787–792.

12. Verdecchia P, Schillaci G, Borgioni, *et al.*: Cigarette smoking, ambulatory blood pressure and cardiac hypertrophy in essential hypertension. *J Hypertens* 1995, 13:1209–1215.

13. Cutler JA, Follmann D, Elliott P, *et al.*: An overview of randomized trials of sodium reduction and blood pressure. *Hypertension* 1991, 17(suppl I):27–33.

14. He J, Ogden LG, Vupputuri LA, *et al.*: Dietary sodium intake and subsequent risk of cardiovascular disease in overweight adults. *JAMA* 1999, 282:2027–2034.

15. MacGregor GA, Markandu ND, Sagnella GA, *et al.*: Double-blind study of three sodium intakes and long-term effects of sodium restriction in essential hypertension. *Lancet* 1989, 2:1244–1247.

16. Tabuchi Y, Ogihara T, Gotoh, *et al.*: Hypotensive mechanism of potassium supplementation in salt-loaded patients with essential hypertension. *J Clin Hypertens* 1985, 2:145–152.

17. Veterans Administration Cooperative Study Group on Antihypertensive Agents: Urinary and serum electrolytes in untreated black and white hypertensives. *J Chronic Dis* 1987, 40:839–847.

18. Materson BJ: Diuretic-associated hypokalemia. *Arch Intern Med* 1985, 145:1966–1967.

19. Khaw K-T, Barrett-Connor E: Dietary potassium and stroke-associated mortality: a 12-year prospective population study. *N Engl J Med* 1987, 316:235–240.

20. Harrington JT, Isner JM, Kassirer JP: Our national obsession with potassium. *Am J Med* 1982, 73:155–159.

21. Grimm RH Jr, Neaton JD, Elmer PJ, *et al.*: The influence of oral potassium chloride on blood pressure in hypertensive men on a low-sodium diet. *N Engl J Med* 1990, 322:569–574.

22. Stamler R: Implications of the INTERSALT study. *Hypertension* 1991, 17(suppl I):I-16–I-20.

23. Steptoe A, Fieldman G, Evans O, *et al.*: Control over work place, job strain and cardiovascular responses in middle-aged men. *J Hypertens* 1993, 11:751–759.

24. Sowers JR, Zemel MB, Zemel PC, *et al.*: Calcium metabolism and dietary calcium in salt sensitive hypertension. *Am J Hypertens* 1991, 4:557–563.

25. Neaton JD, Grimm RH, Prineas RJ, *et al.*: The Treatment of Mild Hypertension Study Research Group. *JAMA* 1993, 270:713–724.

26. Veterans Administration Cooperative Study Group on Antihypertensive Agents: Comparison of propranolol and hydrochlorothiazide for the initial treatment of hypertension: I. Results of short-term titration with emphasis on racial differences in response. *JAMA* 1982, 248:1996–2003.

27. Veterans Administration Cooperative Study Group on Anti-hypertensive Agents: Racial differences in response to low-dose captopril are abolished by the addition of hydrochlorothiazide. *Br J Clin Pharmacol* 1982, 14(suppl 2):97–101.

28. Saunders E, Weir MR, Kong BW, *et al.*: A comparison of the efficacy and safety of a beta-blocker, a calcium channel blocker, and a converting enzyme inhibitor in hypertensive blacks. *Arch Intern Med* 1990, 150:1707–1713.

29. Applegate WB, Phillips HL, Schnaper H, *et al.*: A randomized controlled trial of the effects of three antihypertensive agents on blood pressure control and quality of life in older women. *Arch Intern Med* 1991, 151:1817–1823.

30. Wassertheil-Smoller S, Oberman A, Blaufox MD, *et al* : The Trial of Antihypertensive Interventions and Management (TAIM) Study: final results with regard to blood pressure, cardiovascular risk, and quality of life. *Am J Hypertens* 1992, 5:37–44.

31. Materson BJ, Reda DJ, Cushman WC, *et al.*: Single drug therapy for hypertension in men: a comparison of six antihypertensive agents with placebo. *N Engl J Med* 1993, 328:914–921.

32. Materson BJ, Reda DJ, Preston RA, *et al.*: Response to a second single antihypertensive agent used as monotherapy for hypertension after failure of the initial drug. *Arch Intern Med* 1995, 55:1757–1762.

33. Materson BJ, Reda DJ, Cushman WC, *et al.*: Results of combination anti-hypertensive therapy after failure of each of the components. *J Human Hypertens* 1995, 9:791–795.

34. Gottdiener JS, Reda DJ, Massie BM, *et al.*:Effect of single-drug therapy on reduction of left ventricular mass in milde to moderate hypertension: comparison of six antihypertensive agents. The Departmetn of Veterans Affirs Cooperative Study Group on Antihypertensive Agents. *Circulation* 1997, 95:2007–2014.

35. Lakshman MR, Reda DJ, Materson BJ, *et al.*:Diuretics and beta-blockers do not have adverse effects at 1 year on plasma lipid and lipoprotein profiles in men with hypertension. Department of Veterans Affirs Cooperative Study Group on Antihypertensive Agents. *Arch Intern Med* 1999, 159:551–558.

36. Preston RJ, Materson BJ, Reda DJ, *et al.*:Age–subgoup compared with renin profile as predictors of blood pressure response to antihy-pertensive therapy. Department of Veterans Affirs Cooperative Study Group on Antihypertensive Agents. *JAMA* 1998, 280:1168–1172.

37. Ravid M, Lang R, Rachmani R, Lishner M: Long-term renoprotective effect of angiotensin-converting enzyme inhibition in non–insulin-dependent diabetes mellitus. A 7-year follow-up study. *Arch Intern Med* 1996, 156:286–289.

38. Kirby RS: Doxazosin in benign prostatic hyperplasia: effects of blood pressure and urinary flow in normotensive and hypertensive men. *Urology* 1995, 46:182–186.

39. Markovitz JH, Matthews KA, Kannel WB, *et al.*: Psychological predictors of hypertension in the Framingham Study. Is there tension in hypertension? *JAMA* 1993, 270:2439–2443.

40. Reaven GM, Clinkingbeard C, Jeppesen J, *et al.*: Comparison of the hemodynamic and metabolic effects of low-dose hydrochlorothiazide and lisinopril treatment in obese patients with high blood pressure. *Am J Hypertens* 1995, 8:461–466.

41. Materson BJ: Hypertension and concomitant disease: guidelines for treatment. *Drug Therapy* 1985, 15:177–188.

42. Croog SH, Levine S, Testa MA, *et al.*: The effects of antihypertensive therapy on the quality of life. *N Engl J Med* 1986, 314:1657–1664.

43. Testa MA, Anderson RB, Nackley JF, *et al.* and the Quality-of-Life Hypertension Study Group: Quality of life and antihypertensive therapy in men: a comparison of captopril with enalapril. *N Engl J Med* 1993, 328:907–913.

ANTIHYPERTENSIVE THERAPY: PROGRESSION OF RENAL INJURY

Matthew R. Weir

Although traditional antihypertensive therapies are effective in controlling blood pressure (BP), deaths from hypertensive sequelae such as coronary artery disease and renal disease have not been prevented [1,2]. Our ability to prevent hypertensive nephropathy through traditional methods of lowering BP may not be as effective as once thought, particularly in high-risk patients [3–6]. One reason for this may be our inability to adequately control glomerular capillary pressure. The autoregulation of glomerular capillary pressure through selective vasoconstriction of the afferent and efferent glomerular arterioles is tightly regulated within a narrow range of approximately 5 mm Hg [7]. The main function of the afferent arteriole is to vasoconstrict and step down systemic pressure to ideal glomerular capillary pressure, which is approximately one half to two thirds of systemic BP [8]. The efferent arteriole vasoconstricts during states of diminished effective arterial blood volume in order to maintain the glomerular capillary pressures necessary for ultrafiltration. With injury of the afferent arteriole, the glomerulus becomes more vulnerable to the effects of systemic BP due to inadequate vasoconstriction. This frequently occurs in patients with diabetes or vascular disease. Thus, injury to the glomerulus may occur even with "normal" BPs [9–11].

Two classes of vasodilators, the ACE inhibitors [12–16] and the angiotensin II receptor blockers [12–16], have been demonstrated not only to lower systemic BP but also to reduce proteinuria and attenuate the rate of progression of renal disease in both experimental models and humans. By inhibiting the renin angiotensin system, these drugs not only lower systemic BP but also glomerular capillary pressure by attenuating the vasoconstrictor effects of angiotensin II on the efferent glomerular arteriole. This effect also reduces urinary albumin and protein excretion.

Other antihypertensive medications have not been demonstrated to be as effective in protecting against progressive renal injury when compared with drugs that block the renin-angiotensin system. Despite this, these drugs maintain their importance in clinical therapy because they facilitate better control of systemic BP, which becomes more important as renal autoregulation begins to fail.

Patients with hypertension and renal parenchymal disease frequently require as many as three to four drugs to reduce systemic BP to below 130/85 mm Hg, which is the recommended target. BP reduction to below 125/75 mm Hg is recommended in patients with clinical proteinuria [17]. Thus, the use of drugs that block the renin-angiotensin system, sometimes even both classes, may be necessary as part of a multidrug strategy to facilitate better BP control and reduce the likelihood of progression of renal injury. This chapter reviews the evidence that antihypertensive therapy can modify the natural history of progressive renal injury as well as the specifics of the individual agents that have been used.

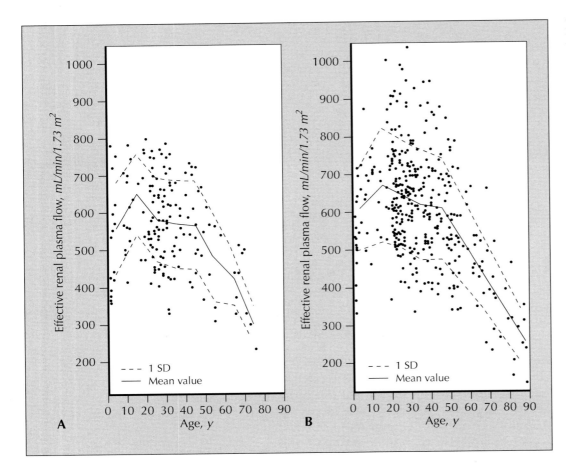

FIGURE 10-1. Hypertension and aging can lead to a progressive deterioration of renal function. Both normal normotensive women (**A**) and men (**B**) have age-associated declines in effective renal plasma flow [18]. (*Adapted from* Wesson [18].)

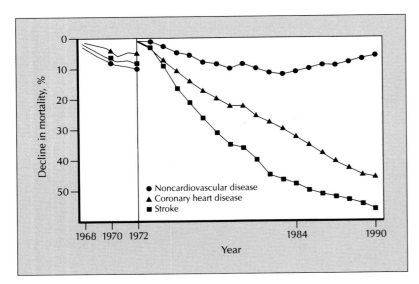

FIGURE 10-2. Since 1972, when the National High Blood Pressure Education Program was initiated, there has been a significant reduction in mortality related to both stroke and coronary heart disease. This is related in part to the reduction in systemic arterial pressure. Noncardiovascular disease has not benefited as much, and there is little evidence to suggest that beneficial results similar to those that have occurred for both the brain and the heart have also occurred for the kidney. Mortality rates are age-adjusted from 1968 to 1972. Data are provisional for 1990. (*Adapted from* the Joint National Committee on Detection, Evaluation, and Treatment of High Blood Pressure [19].)

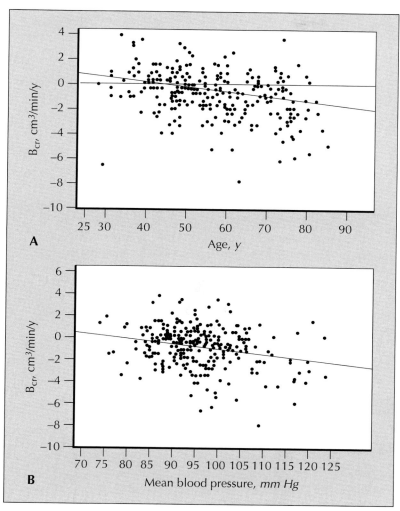

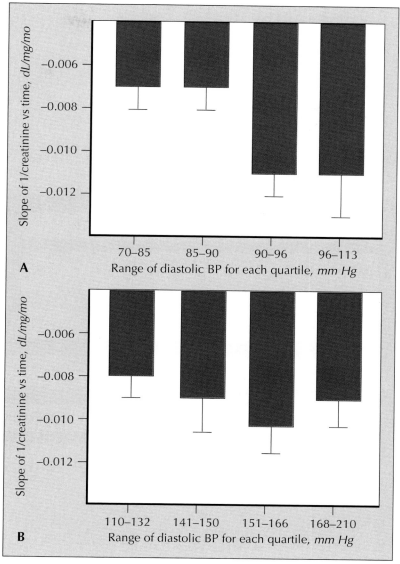

FIGURE 10-3. Results of two recent, large-scale, long-term, retrospective studies confirm that hypertension is a risk factor for declining renal function. Lindeman *et al.* [20] reported data from the Baltimore Longitudinal Study of Aging (BLSA). **A,** Regression coefficient plotting change in creatinine clearance over time in years (B_{cr}). Mean creatinine clearance was found to decline over time. **B,** The correlation between mean blood pressure and an increase in mean serum creatinine over time was significant ($P < 0.001$). Multiple regression analysis demonstrated that mean blood pressure and age are independent variables for declining renal function. A second study by Rosansky *et al.* [21], with a mean follow-up of 9.8 years, included both normotensives and hypertensives. When race, age, and body mass index were controlled for, hypertensive patients had a significantly greater increase in serum creatinine over time ($P = 0.038$). The authors concluded that hypertensive patients without clinically detectable renal disease will have a greater future decline in renal function than will nonhypertensive subjects. (*Adapted from* Lindeman *et al.* [20].)

FIGURE 10-4. Brazy *et al.* [22] studied the effect of high blood pressure (BP) on renal insufficiency in a group of 86 patients who eventually required dialysis. Patients were stratified into quartiles by mean diastolic (**A**) and systolic (**B**) BP. The authors noted that there was an association between control of diastolic BP and a slower rate of decline of renal function. However, they did not see a statistically significant difference for systolic BP reduction. *T bars* represent mean plus or minus standard error of slope for reciprocal creatinine versus time plot for 21 patients. (*Adapted from* Brazy *et al.* [22].)

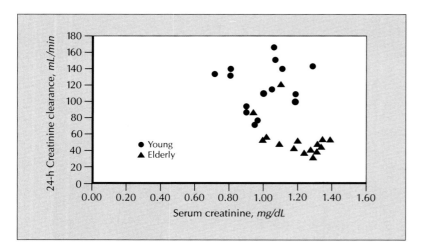

FIGURE 10-5. Renal function progressively declines with age [20,21]. However, the speed of this decline is not always predictable. The routine clinical measurements in which we place the most faith may not be the most accurate indicators of the true level of renal function [23]. Each point in this graph represents a pairing of a serum creatinine and a simultaneously determined inulin clearance. There is a distinct clustering of points for inulin clearance that exists between 40 and 80 mL/min, all of which have a matched serum creatinine below the usual upper limits of normal (1.4 mg/dL). The lower serum creatinine relative to the glomerular filtration rate reflects reduced creatinine production due to muscle atrophy. In this study, young patients were 19 to 35 years of age; elderly patients were 67 to 93 years of age. (*Adapted from* Friedman *et al.* [23].)

MULTIPLE RISK FACTOR INTERVENTION TRIAL

Renal function was retrospectively evaluated over 6 years in 5260 men with diastolic blood pressure of < 90 mm Hg at entry

Negative slopes in Δ (1/Cr)t, suggesting a decline in renal function, were identified in 33% of participants

FIGURE 10-6. A retrospective analysis of the Multiple Risk Factor Intervention Trial (MRFIT) assessed the influence of antihypertensive therapy on renal function in 5260 men over a 6-year period [6]. The average patient age was 46.5 years; the average systolic/diastolic blood pressure was 143/97 mm Hg, and serum creatinine was 1.1 mg/dL. Negative slopes by plotting 1 over serum creatinine (1/Cr) versus time (t) were observed in approximately one third of the participants, suggesting a progressive loss of renal function.

DEMOGRAPHIC FACTORS RESULT IN AN INVERSE SLOPE OF CREATININE

INDEPENDENT VARIABLE	COEFFICIENT	P VALUE
Age, *y*	-0.00023	<0.001
Race (black)	-0.00458	<0.001
Creatinine at entry, *mg/dL*	0.02600	<0.001
Systolic blood pressure, *mm Hg*	0.00009	<0.001
Body mass index, *kg/m²*	0.00004	NS
LDL cholesterol, *mg/dL*	0.00000	NS
HDL cholesterol, *mg/dL*	0.00004	0.06

FIGURE 10-7. A multiple regression summary of the demographic factors of the men in the Multiple Risk Factor Intervention Trial (MRFIT) demonstrated that increasing age, black race, and higher systolic blood pressure were risk factors for an inverse slope of creatinine. These data suggest that despite the use of antihypertensive therapy (*eg*, diuretic, β-blocker, vasodilator) in all study patients, there remains a risk of hypertensive renal injury in certain groups of patients. HDL—high-density lipoprotein; LDL—low-density lipoprotein; NS—not significant.

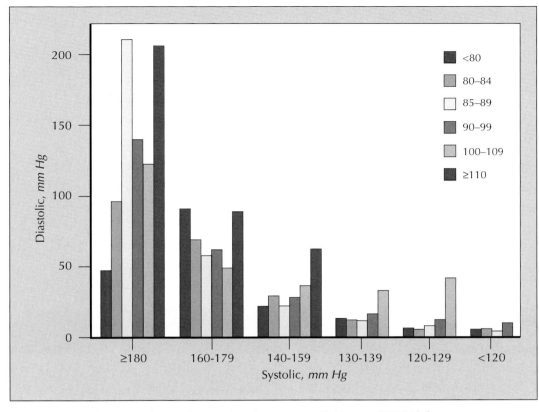

FIGURE 10-8. The age-adjusted rate of end-stage renal disease (ESRD) from any cause per 100,000 person-years, according to systolic and diastolic blood pressure (BP). Klag *et al.*

[24] assessed the risk factors for the development of ESRD through the year 1990 in 332,544 men, aged 35 to 57 years, who were screened between 1973 and 1975 for entry into the Multiple Risk Factor Intervention Trial. A strong, graded relationship between both systolic and diastolic BP and development of renal failure was observed independent of other factors, including age, race, income, coronary artery disease, serum cholesterol, cigarette smoking, and the use of medication for diabetes mellitus. The estimated risk of ESRD was greater for elevation of systolic BP than it was for diastolic BP when both variables were considered together. The study did have limitations in that no women were included, BP was measured only once (during screening), information on antihypertensive therapy did not exist, and renal function was not assessed at baseline. The lack of baseline measurement of renal function interferes with the determination of whether the strong association between higher levels of BP and renal failure is due to initiation of renal disease or worsening of pre-existing disease. (*Adapted from* Klag *et al.* [24].)

RENAL INSUFFICIENCY IN TREATED ESSENTIAL HYPERTENSION

94 patients with normal renal function
  (serum creatinine < 1.1 mg/dL) followed up for 58±34 months
Blood pressure normalized with therapy (< 140/90 mm Hg)
15% developed progressive renal insufficiency despite therapy

FIGURE 10-9. Rostand *et al.* [4] studied 94 patients with normal renal function over a follow-up period of approximately 5 years. Blood pressure was reduced to less than 140/90 mm Hg in these patients with traditional antihypertensive therapy. Despite this intervention, 15% developed progressive renal insufficiency (serum creatinine increase of 0.4 mg/dL or more). Older patients and blacks were at greater risk for hypertensive renal injury.

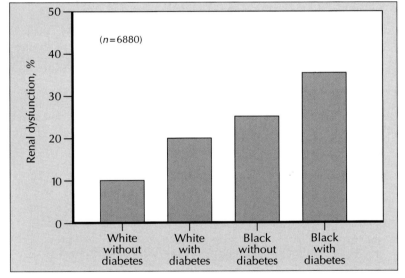

FIGURE 10-10. The prevalence of renal dysfunction according to race and the presence or absence of diabetes [5]. In this patient population, 72% were black and 41% were diabetic (type 2 diabetes in 95% of cases). All patients received antihypertensive therapy, and most received traditional therapies (*eg,* diuretics, β-blockers). Approximately one third of black diabetic patients developed decreased renal dysfunction (serum creatinine ≥ 2 mg/dL), more than 1.5 times that found in white diabetic patients. A similar trend was seen in nondiabetic patients.

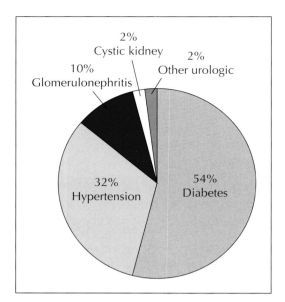

FIGURE 10-11. Preliminary data for the distribution of patients with new end-stage renal disease (ESRD) by primary disease in 2001 [25]. Diabetes and hypertension are the leading causes of ESRD. The majority of diabetic ESRD cases are related to type 2 diabetes. Both diabetic and hypertensive causes of ESRD are increased relative to other causes. (*Adapted from* National Institute of Diabetes and Digestive Kidney Diseases [25].)

NEUROHORMONAL RESPONSES

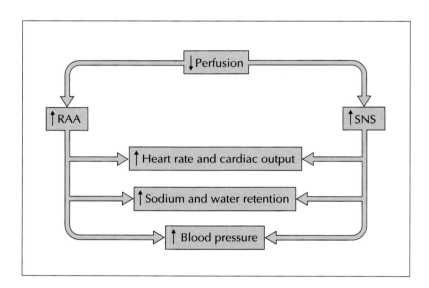

FIGURE 10-12. When cardiac output fails, systemic neurohormonal events are triggered, primarily the activity of the renin-angiotensin-aldosterone (RAA) system and the sympathetic nervous system (SNS). These two systems regulate the activity of the heart, the kidneys, and the blood vessels in various ways to acutely affect and restore blood pressure and ultimately the adequacy of perfusion [26].

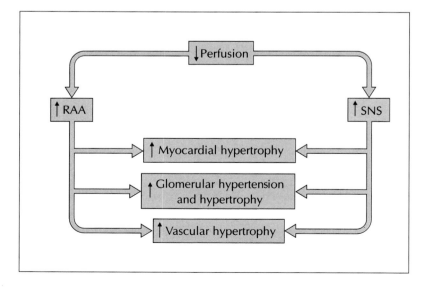

FIGURE 10-13. Although the acute homeostatic effects of the renin-angiotensin-aldosterone (RAA) system and sympathetic nervous system (SNS) are important for blood pressure stability, the trade-off in relying on these systems is that they may lead to remodeling and hypertrophy of various cardiovascular tissues, including those in the kidney [26].

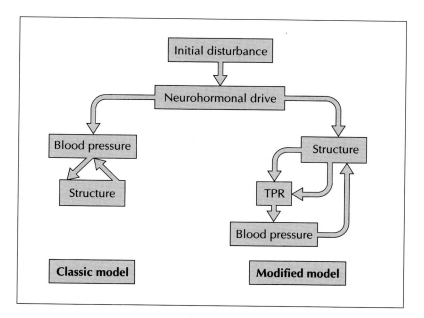

FIGURE 10-14. Classic teaching dictates that higher levels of arterial pressure lead to restructuring, which contributes to greater vascular resistance and consequently higher levels of blood pressure (BP). A vicious cycle then ensues. Alternatively, genetic or environmental influences may lead to cardiovascular restructuring, with consequent alterations and total peripheral resistance (TPR), which result in an increase in BP. Subsequently, a vicious cycle could propagate structural injury [27,28]. Thus a central question is whether higher BP levels accelerate the loss of renal function or, conversely, whether more rapidly progressing renal disease leads to higher BP.

CLINICAL CONSIDERATIONS

APPROACH TO HYPERTENSION WITH COEXISTING RISK OF NEPHROPATHY

Reduce arterial pressure

Maintain renal blood flow and glomerular filtration rate

Preserve nephrons and renal function, perhaps by reducing intraglomerular pressures or neurohormonal stimulation at the vascular level

FIGURE 10-15. An ideal approach to the patient with hypertension and coexisting risk of nephropathy would be to reduce not only arterial pressure but also the effect of aging and hypertension on renal blood flow. Therapies that maintain or enhance renal perfusion may be preferable because they may lessen neurohormonal activation within the kidney, which may be critical to avoiding glomerular capillary hypertension.

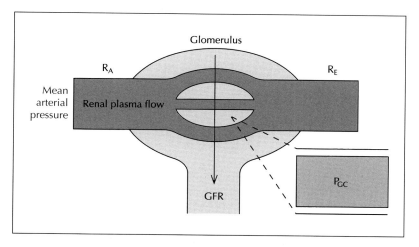

FIGURE 10-16. Normal microcirculation. Normal renal microcirculation is unique in that the afferent and efferent glomerular vascular supply is arterial. The regulation of vascular tone in both the pre- and postglomerular vascular beds allows proper balance between glomerular capillary pressure (P_{GC}) and glomerular filtration rate (GFR) [29]. R_A—afferent resistance; R_E—efferent resistance. (*Adapted from* Bauer and Reams [30].)

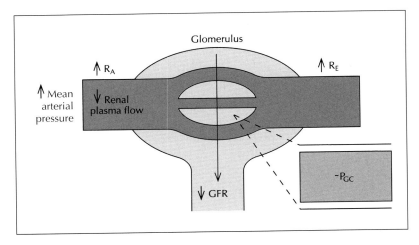

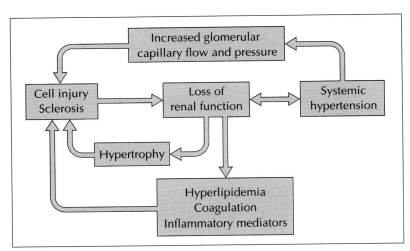

FIGURE 10-17. Essential hpertension. The glomerular microcirculation responds to an increase in arterial blood pressure with preglomerular vasoconstriction, which is likely a protective mechanism to limit glomerular capillary hypertension. However, the associated decrease in renal plasma flow and glomerular capillary pressure (P_{GC}) activates the renin-angiotensin system, which causes postglomerular vasoconstriction and restores P_{GC} and glomerular filtration rate (GFR) to baseline values. The net result of hypertension is intrarenal vasoconstriction as a result of augmented neurohormonal activity [29]. In situations of renal disease with diminishing nephron numbers, elevated P_{GC} occurs as a result of failure of adequate preglomerular vasoconstriction, thus allowing the transmission of higher pressures to the glomerular capillary network with subsequent injury [10,11]. R_A—afferent resistance; R_E—efferent resistance. (*Adapted from Bauer and Reams [30].*)

FIGURE 10-18. Antihypertensive therapies that maintain renal perfusion and diminish the neurohormonal influence (particularly angiotensin II–mediated postglomerular vasoconstriction) are likely to be beneficial in patients at risk of nephropathy. Interruption of the renin-angiotensin-aldosterone system in patients with essential hypertension reduces renal vascular resistance (RVR), enhances renal perfusion, facilitates sodium and water clearance, and diminishes urinary albumin excretion. These responses probably contribute to limiting progressive renal injury [30]. GFR—glomerular filtration rate.

INTERRUPTION OF THE RENIN-ANGIOTENSIN-ALDOSTERONE AXIS

Lower RVR

Enhanced renal blood flow or redistribution toward the outer renal cortex

Enhanced GFR

Acute natriuresis and antikaliuresis, not sustained during prolonged therapy

Higher free water clearance

Lower urinary protein excretion

POSSIBLE FACTORS IN PROGRESSIVE NEPHRON INJURY

Glomerular capillary hypertension with associated hyper-filtration-induced epithelial cell injury

Glomerular hypertrophy

Intraglomerular platelet aggregation

Hypermetabolism of remaining nephrons

Complement-dependent, nucleophile-initiated tubulointerstitial injury

Mesangial cell-matrix overload

Hyperlipidemia-associated cellular injury

FIGURE 10-19. Many factors may be involved in progressive nephron injury. The different effects of various antihypertensive agents on the progressive nature of renal disease may be related to their influence on one, some, or all of these putative factors, which have been demonstrated experimentally to be important in leading to progressive glomerulosclerosis [31].

FIGURE 10-20. Pathways relating systemic hypertension and loss of renal function [32]. Specific therapies may better control glomerular capillary pressure, diminish glomerular hypertrophy, and control the influence of hyperlipidemia and other mediators of both coagulation and inflammation, thus reducing the risk of nephron injury.

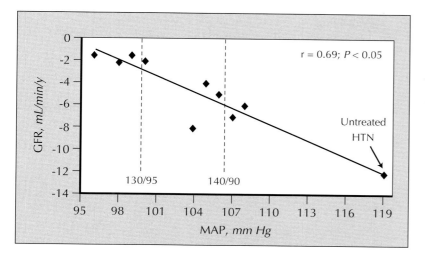

FIGURE 10-21. The relationship between achieved mean arterial pressure (MAP) with antihypertensive therapy and declines in glomerular filtration rate (GFR) in clinical trials of patients with diabetic and nondiabetic renal disease. Note that reducing MAP below 100 (130/85 mm Hg) provides an approximate threefold slowing of loss of renal function compared to a MAP of 107 (140/90 mm Hg). (*Adapted from* Bakris [33].)

EXPERIMENTAL TRIALS WITH ACE INHIBITORS

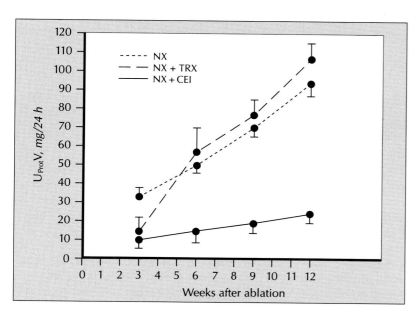

FIGURE 10-22. Anderson *et al.* [12] performed five-sixths nephrectomy in Munich-Wistar rats. This procedure results in the development of hypertension and glomerulosclerosis over a period of weeks. After nephrectomy in their study, different groups of animals were treated with either no therapy (NX), standard antihypertensive therapy (NX + TRX: hydrochlorothiazide, hydralazine, reserpine), or enalapril (NX + CEI). Sequential determinations of urinary albumin excretion ($U_{Prot}V$) over the ensuing 12 weeks demonstrated that the animals receiving enalapril had a marked diminution in albuminuria. There was a significant reduction in glomerular capillary pressure and attenuation of the development of glomerulosclerosis. Both groups had similar reductions in systemic blood pressure. Unless glomerular capillary hypertension is corrected, control of systemic blood pressure is insufficient to prevent progressive renal injury in rats with reduced renal mass. (*Adapted from* Anderson *et al.* [12].)

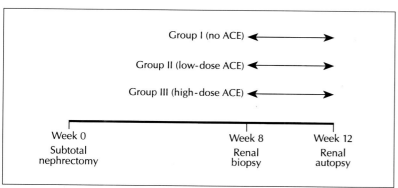

FIGURE 10-23. An experimental study was designed to assess the effectiveness of angiotensin-converting enzyme (ACE) inhibition in preventing progression after injury has occurred [34]. Rats were subjected to one-sixth and five-sixths nephrectomy and were observed over the following 8 weeks, during which time they developed hypertension and progressive glomerulosclerosis. Eight weeks after nephrectomy, a renal biopsy was performed to document the degree of glomerulosclerosis in their remaining kidneys. The animals were subdivided into three groups. One group received no therapy, and the other two groups were treated with either low or high doses of the ACE inhibitor enalapril. After 4 weeks of therapy, the animals were sacrificed and renal histology was examined. Similar reductions in both systemic and glomerular capillary pressures occurred with both low- and high-dose ACE inhibition during therapy in groups II and III. (*Adapted from* Ikoma *et al.* [34].)

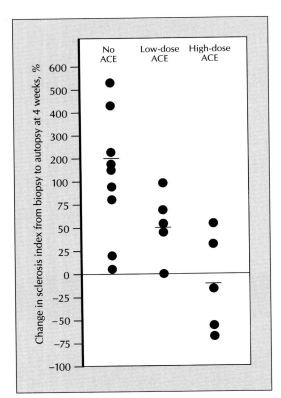

FIGURE 10-24. Ikoma *et al.* [34] evaluated the change in glomerulosclerosis from the time of biopsy to the time of autopsy 4 weeks later in three groups of rats subjected to one-sixth and five-sixths nephrectomy. In the animals receiving no therapy, there was a 200% increase in the degree of glomerulosclerosis, whereas in the low-dose angiotensin-converting enzyme (ACE) inhibitor group there was only a 50% increase in glomerulosclerosis, a fourfold reduction compared with those receiving no treatment. Remarkably, in the high-dose ACE inhibitor group, despite no greater reduction in systemic or glomerular capillary pressures, there was almost a complete attenuation of progressive glomerulosclerotic injury. Indeed, in some animals there was the suggestion that some glomerulosclerosis could be reversed. ACE inhibitors may have nonhemodynamic effects that could be important in limiting glomerulosclerotic injury. (*Adapted from* Ikoma *et al.* [34].)

HUMAN CLINICAL TRIALS

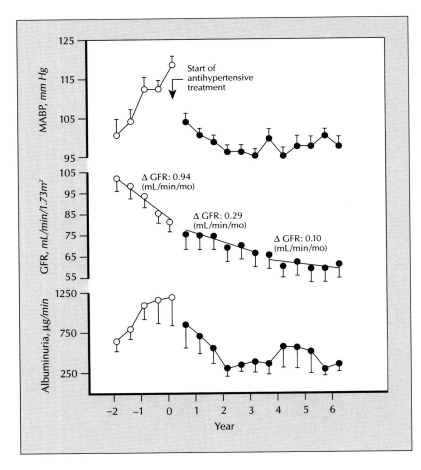

FIGURE 10-25. Although experimental studies in animals have demonstrated the beneficial influences of angiotensin-converting enzyme inhibitors and calcium channel blockers in delaying the progression of renal disease, clinical trials in humans with either primary or secondary causes of hypertension are needed to delineate differences in therapies with regard to the rate of progression of renal disease. Parving *et al.* [35] demonstrated that untreated hypertensive patients with insulin-dependent diabetes had a much higher rate of deterioration of renal function prior to the start of antihypertensive therapy (*closed circles*). When these patients received traditional therapy (diuretics and β-blockers) there was a marked attenuation of albuminuria and a slowing in the rate of loss of glomerular filtration rate (GFR: mL/min/mo) over a 6-year follow-up period. *Open circles* indicate before therapy. MABP—mean arterial blood pressure.

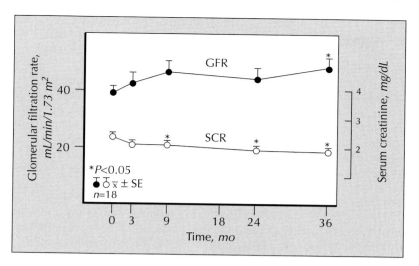

FIGURE 10-26. Pettinger *et al.* [36] demonstrated a long-term improvement in renal function after achieving strict blood pressure control with a variety of antihypertensive agents in patients with hypertensive nephrosclerosis. Seventy-nine patients were enrolled in a prospective randomized trial and renal function was assessed using radioisotopic clearance techniques. To be eligible, patients had to have a serum creatinine (SCR) of 1.6 to 7 mg/dL, or a glomerular filtration rate (GFR) less than 70 mL/min/1.73 m^2, and no known secondary causes of renal disease. Twenty-two subjects completed 36 months of treatment. The study design involved a 2- to 4-month initial period of aggressive diastolic blood pressure control (< 80 mm Hg) followed by control of diastolic blood pressure at less than 90 mm Hg. The stability of SCR and the gradual improvement in GFR over the 36-month follow-up period can be seen. (*Adapted from* Pettinger *et al.* [36].)

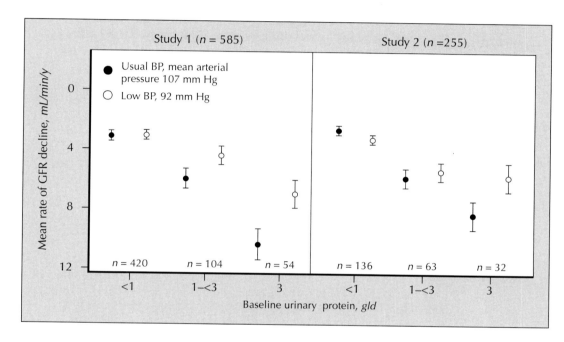

FIGURE 10-27. Influence of proteinuria and blood pressure (BP) level achieved on progression of renal disease. The decline in glomerular filtration rate (GFR) according to baseline urinary protein excretion and level of BP obtained is depicted for patients having a variety of kidney diseases who participated in the Modification of Diet in Renal Disease Study. In Study 1, the baseline GFR was 25 to 55 mL/min/1.73 m^2, and in Study 2 it was 13 to 24 mL/min/1.73 m^2. A higher level of baseline urinary protein excretion was associated with a more rapid deterioration of GFR and a larger difference in mean rate of decline in the GFR between the two BP treatment groups. Thus, proteinuric renal disease (> 1 g daily) requires more vigorous BP reduction. The number at the bottom of each panel indicates the total number of patients having follow-up GFR measurements in the two BP groups combined. (*Adapted from* Klahr *et al.* [37].)

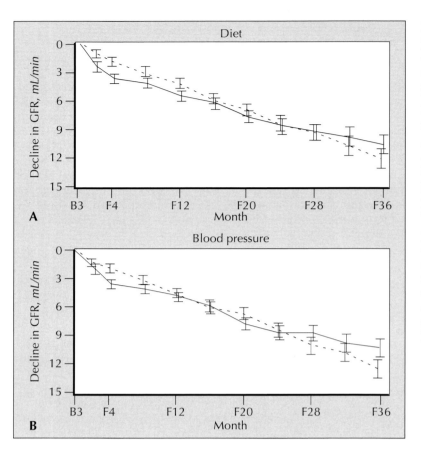

FIGURE 10-28. The effects of dietary protein restriction and blood pressure (BP) control on the progression of renal disease were evaluated in 585 patients with varying forms of kidney disease and a glomerular filtration rate (GFR) between 25 and 55 mL/min/1.73 m^2 over a mean of 2.2 years of follow-up in the Modification of Diet in Renal Disease Study. **A** and **B,** The projected mean decline in GFR did not differ significantly between the low protein diet of 0.58 g daily (*solid line*) and the usual protein diet of 1.3 g daily (*dashed line*), or the low BP group (mean arterial pressure, 92 mm Hg; *solid line*) or usual BP group (mean arterial pressure, 107 mm Hg; *dashed line*). The steeper initial decline in the GFR for both low protein diet and low BP likely reflects hemodynamic changes as opposed to progression of renal disease. The less steep slope in the GFR during later follow-up for both low protein diet and low BP is indicative of the small beneficial effect of these separate interventions on the rate of progression of renal disease. However, the interpretation of these results should not be misconstrued to suggest that reduction of dietary protein and BP offer only minor benefit. Significant confounding variables, such as race, type of renal disease, level of pretreatment proteinuria, and level of BP achieved can obscure the results. B—baseline; F—follow-up visit. (*Adapted from* Klahr *et al.* [37].)

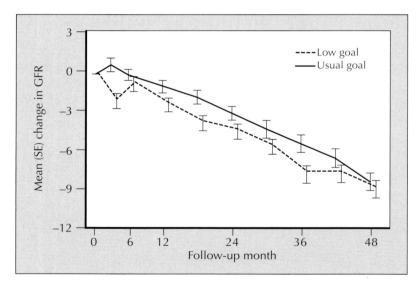

FIGURE 10-29.
The African American Study of Kidney Disease (AASK) was a randomized × 3 factorial design trial in African-Americans with hypertensive renal disease (GFR 20–65 mL/min/1.73m^2) to compare two levels of mean arterial blood pressure control (102 to 107 mm Hg [*n* = 554], or 92 mm Hg or less [*n* = 540]) and effect of initial treatment with either a beta blocker (*n* = 441), ACE inhibitor (*n* = 436) or dihydropyridine calcium channel blocker (*n* = 217) on a main outcome measure of the rate of change in glomerular filtration rate (GFR) (GFR slope) [38].

Achieved blood pressure was 127/77 mm Hg in the lower group and 140/85 mm Hg in the usual group. The mean GFR slope from baseline through 4 years did not differ significantly between the lower group and the usual group. None of the different drug group comparisons showed consistent significant differences in the GFR slope. However, the ACE inhibitor (ramipril) group manifested risk reduction in the clinical composite outcome (reduction of GFR by more than 50% or more than 25 mL/min/1.73m^2 from baseline, ESRD, or death) compared to the beta blocker (metoprolol, 22% RR; *P* = 0.04) and the calcium channel blocker (amlodipine, 38% RR; *P* = 0.004). There was no difference in clinical composite outcome based on blood pressure goal in 4 years. Numbers of patients with GFRs at years 0, 1, 2, 3, and 4 were 1094, 953, 837, 731 and 469, respectively.

The authors concluded that in this study there was no additional benefit of lower blood pressure goal in slowing the progression of hypertensive nephrosclerosis in African Americans. These data need to be interpreted carefully due to the relatively short (5 years) duration of follow-up and the lack of diabetes or significant proteinuria in the patients. Longer follow-up may show the benefit of lower blood pressure not only for the kidneys, but also for preventing cardiovascular events in African Americans with early renal insufficiency due to hypertensive nephrosclerosis.

EFFECTS OF ANTIHYPERTENSIVE DRUGS ON NONDIABETIC RENAL DISEASE

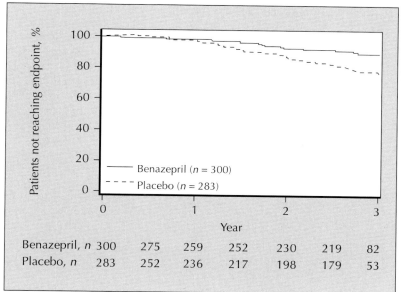

Benazepril, n: 300 275 259 252 230 219 82
Placebo, n: 283 252 236 217 198 179 53

FIGURE 10-30. Effect of angiotensin-converting enzyme inhibitors and other antihypertensive medications on progression of diabetic and nondiabetic kidney disease. A prospective, double-blind, randomized trial involving 49 European hospitals compared the effect of benazepril versus placebo, in addition to other antihypertensive therapy, on the progression rate of renal disease in patients with varying types of renal disease (glomerulopathies, $n = 192$; polycystic kidney disease, $n = 64$; diabetes, $n = 21$; and miscellaneous or unknown, $n = 104$). Most patients had significant renal impairment (creatinine clearance: 46 to 60 mL/min, $n = 227$; 30 to 45 mL/min, $n = 356$). The primary endpoint was a doubling of the baseline serum creatinine concentration or the need for dialysis. Median duration of treatment was 3.0 years for the benazepril group and 2.9 years for the placebo group. As shown, renal survival was significantly better in the benazepril group ($P < 0.001$, using Kaplan-Meier estimates). Only 31 patients in the benazepril group versus 57 in the placebo group reached the endpoint. (*Adapted from* Maschio *et al.* [39].)

OVERALL RISK REDUCTION WITH BENAZEPRIL

BASELINE FACTOR	UNADJUSTED, %	ADJUSTED FOR DIASTOLIC BP, %*	ADJUSTED FOR CHANGES IN URINARY PROTEIN EXCRETION, %
Creatinine clearance	53 (27–70)	38 (3–6)	39 (5–61)
> 45 mL/min	71 (21–90)	66 (6–88)	65 (4–87)
≤ 45 mL/min	46 (12–67)	26 (-23–55)	27 (-21–56)
Gender			
Male	56 (28–73)	42 (4–65)	40 (2–64)
Female	40 (-59–77)	22 (-107–71)	35 (-69–75)
Normal BP	58 (-72–89)	37 (-153–84)	30 (-187–83)
Treated hypertension			
Diastolic BP ≤ 90 mm Hg	51 (13–73)	42 (-4–68)	37 (-13–65)
Diastolic BP > 90 mm Hg	50 (-8–76)	32 (-47–68)	42 (-24–73)
24-H urinary protein excretion			
≤ 1 g	31 (-67–71)	3 (-137–60)	26 (-79–69)
> 1 to < 3 g	53 (-14–81)	45 (-35–77)	44 (-36–77)
≥ 3 g	66 (34–82)	56 (15–78)	52 (5–76)

*95% confidence interval.

FIGURE 10-31. Overall risk reduction of progressive renal insufficiency in the benazepril group based on pretreatment prognostic factors, with and without adjustment for changes in diastolic blood pressure (BP) and proteinuria. The risk reduction was greatest for males, patients with baseline urinary protein excretion greater than 1 g daily, and renal dysfunction due to glomerulopathies, diabetes, or miscellaneous or unknown causes. Diastolic BP reduction was 3.5 to 5.0 mm Hg in the benazepril group and increased by 0.2 to 1.5 mm Hg in the placebo group. Urine protein excretion after 3 years of treatment decreased by 29% (from 1.8 ± 2.6 g daily) in the benazepril group, whereas it increased in the placebo group by 9% (from 1.8 ± 2.2 g daily). (*Adapted from* Maschio *et al.* [39] .)

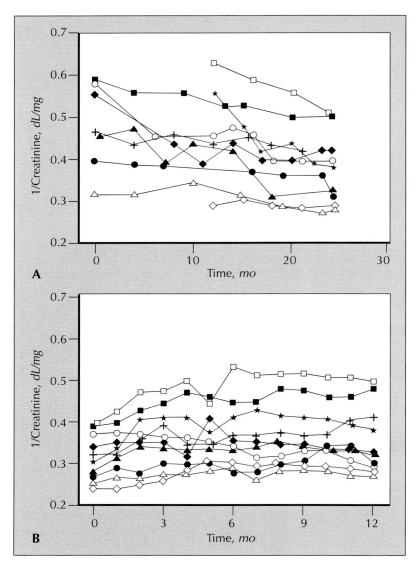

FIGURE 10-32. Ruilope *et al.* [40] studied the influence of the angiotensin-converting enzyme inhibitor captopril in patients with chronic renal failure of diverse etiology (mean baseline inulin clearance 28.2 ± 3 mL/min/1.73 m^2). Ten patients whose hypertension was controlled with triple-drug therapy (propranolol, hydralazine, furosemide) were treated for a period of 12 to 24 months (**A**) prior to transfer to therapy with captopril (**B**). Each symbol represents a different patient, all of whom continued captopril therapy for 1 year. Inulin clearance, used to measure renal function, demonstrated stability over the 1 year of captopril treatment. In contradistinction to the triple therapy, captopril therapy stabilized renal function consistently. (*Adapted from* Ruilope *et al.* [40].)

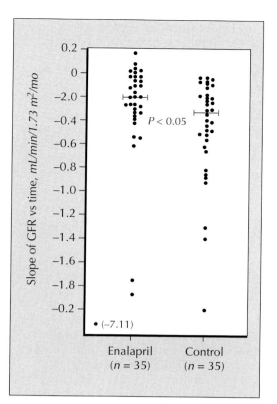

FIGURE 10-33. Kamper *et al.* [41] studied the effect of enalapril on the progression of chronic renal failure in patients whose baseline median glomerular filtration rate (GFR) was 15 mL/min/1.73 m². Patients were randomized in an open study either to traditional treatment with diuretics, β-blockers, and vasodilators, or with enalapril. Patients with both diabetic and nondiabetic renal disease were included. Blood pressure was reduced similarly by both treatments. Over the 24-month follow-up, the enalapril-treated group had a slower rate of renal function loss compared with the control group. (*Adapted from* Kamper *et al.* [41].)

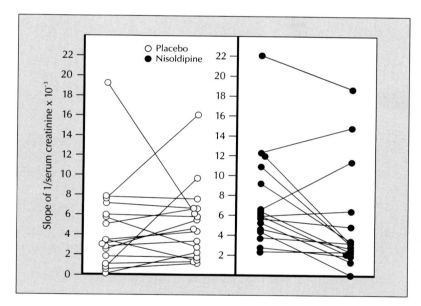

FIGURE 10-34. In a prospective, randomized, placebo-controlled trial, Eliahou *et al.* [42] studied the effect of the calcium channel blocker nisoldipine when added to a standard antihypertensive regimen in 34 patients (17 in each arm) with progressive renal failure. Diet was unrestricted, yet the mean protein intake was similar in the two groups. Blood pressure reduction was similair between groups, who received either nisoldipine or traditional antihpertensive therapy (diuretics and sympatholytics). The nisoldipine-treated group had a significant decrease in progression compared with the conventionally treated group. The authors speculated that the beneficial effect of nisoldipine may have been mediated by the ability of his calcium channel blocker to prevent calcium deposition within the kidney. The small number of subjects, short period of follow-up, other medications, and the use of creatinine clearance as the endpoint limit interpretation of this study and all of the studies published before 1994. (*Adapted from* Eliahou *et al.* [42].)

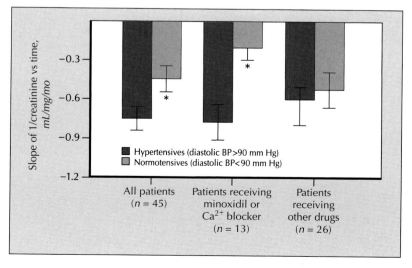

FIGURE 10-35. Brazy and Fitzwilliam [43] examined factors that might influence the rate of decline in renal function in hypertensive patients with chronic renal insufficiency. Using a multiple regression analysis, they noted that increasing age, increasing level of diastolic blood pressure (BP), and type of antihypertensive treatment used had a significant effect, whereas the patient's race and cause of renal disease did not. The authors noted that some antihypertensive medications lowered BP without affecting the slope significantly, whereas others, such as minoxidil or calcium channel blockers, when added to other medications, significantly lowered BP and the slope of reciprocal creatinine. The authors concluded that specific medications may have a favorable effect on the progression of chronic renal disease by mechanisms in addition to a reduction of BP. *T bars* represent mean ± standard error of slope from reciprocal creatinine versus time for individual patients when they were hypertensive and when they were normotensive. *Asterisks* indicate values that are significantly different by paired *t*-test. (*Adapted from* Brazy and Fitzwilliam [43].)

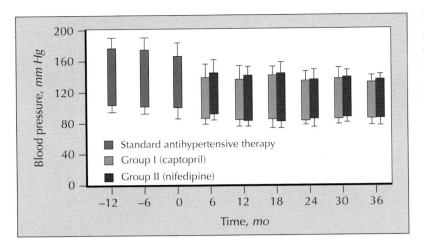

FIGURE 10-36. Zucchelli *et al.* [44] compared the effects of an angiotensin-converting enzyme inhibitor (captopril) and a calcium channel blocker (nifedipine) on both hypertension and the progression of nondiabetic renal insufficiency in a long-term study. A 4-year, multicenter, prospective, randomized trial was conducted in 142 hypertensive patients with established chronic renal failure. The subjects received standard antihypertensive treatment and a low-protein diet for 1 year prior to entering randomization to either slow-release nifedipine or captopril for a 3-year study period. Blood pressure control was significantly better after randomization than during the year of standard antihypertensive therapy. (*Adapted from* Zucchelli *et al.* [44].)

PROGRESSION OF RENAL INSUFFICIENCY

		STANDARD ANTIHYPERTENSIVE THERAPY	CAPTOPRIL THERAPY	NIFEDIPINE THERAPY
$1/S_{Cr}$, dL/mg/mo	Mean	-0.0062	0.00326*	0.00343*
	SD	± 0.0038	± 0.00340	± 0.00390
C_{Cr}, mL/min/mo	Mean	-0.46	-0.22*	-0.24*
	SD	± 0.45	± 0.38	± 0.40

* *P* < 0.001 vs standard therapy.

FIGURE 10-37. The mean slope of reciprocal serum creatinine ($1/S_{Cr}$) versus time and the mean rate of decline of creatinine clearance (C_{Cr}) during the captopril and nifedipine therapy were significantly less than with the standard antihypertensive therapy. The patients treated with captopril for 3 years did very much better than the nifedipine-treated group, but this was not a prespecified study endpoint.

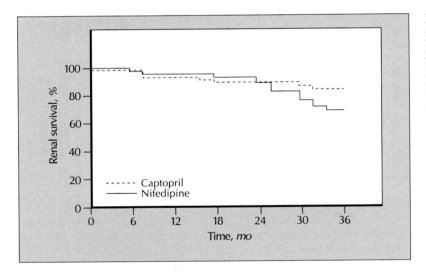

FIGURE 10-38. The renal survival curve of the captopril and nifedipine-treated groups [44]. There were no significant differences in the reduction of urinary albumin excretion. The authors concluded that better control of hypertension after randomization reduced the progression of renal insufficiency and that there were no significant differences between the angiotensin-converting enzyme (ACE) inhibitor and the calcium channel blocker. They believed their data to be consistent with the hypothesis that both ACE inhibitors and calcium channel blockers may have renoprotective effects. The results of this study differed slightly from the Bakris *et al.* [45] and Slataper *et al.* [46] studies in that the patients had nondiabetic renal disease and there was no influence of either therapy on albuminuria. (*Adapted from* Zucchelli *et al.* [44].)

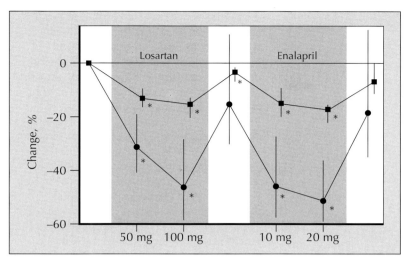

FIGURE 10-39. A randomized prospective study comparing the antihypertensive and antiproteinuric effects of an angiotensin

type 1 receptor block (losartan) versus an angiotensin-converting enzyme (ACE) inhibitor (enalapril) or placebo consisted of seven periods each lasting 1 month. All patients receive placebo, 50 mg losartan, 100 mg losartan, placebo, 10 mg enalapril, 20 mg enalapril, and placebo, respectively. Eleven nondiabetic patients with hypertension and creatinine clearance greater than 60 mL/min and proteinuria exceeding 2 g/d were included in the study. Before enrollment, all antihypertensive medications, including diuretics, were withdrawn for at least 4 weeks. At the end of each study period, proteinuria, blood pressure, and renal function were determined. The angiotensin type 1 receptor blocker (losartan) induced changes in blood pressure, renal hemodynamics, and proteinuria similar to that seen with the ACE inhibitor (enalapril). These observations support the idea that the antiproteinuric effect of an ACE inhibitor as well as its renal hemodynamic effects is related to the ability of the drug to interfere with the renin-angiotensin system as opposed to the bradykinin-related effects of the drug (*$P < 0.05$ from baseline). (*Adapted from* Gansevoort *et al.* [47].)

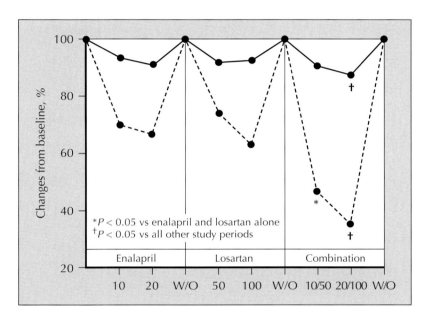

FIGURE 10-40. The effect of enalapril and losartan on ambulatory blood pressure measurements. Ten patients with normal blood pressure (118.5/75.9 mm Hg), normal renal function (creatinine clearance 109.6 mL/min/1.73 m^2), and IgA nephropathy with clinical proteinuria (1.6 ± 0.3 g/24 h) were studied to determine whether the combination of enalapril (10 or 20 mg/d) or losartan (50 or 100 mg/d) would be more effective in reducing proteinuria than the drugs administered separately. A randomized crossover clinical trial design was used. There was a dose-dependent antiproteinuric effect of the combination therapy. The study demonstrated a close correlation between blood pressure reduction and proteinuria reduction. This study also showed that lower blood pressure, even below recommended levels of 130/85 or 125/75 mm Hg, may be necessary to further reduce proteinuria in patients with kidney disease. *Dotted lines*, baseline urinary protein excretion; *solid lines*, mean ambulatory arterial blood pressure. W/O—without. (*Adapted from* Russo *et al.* [48].)

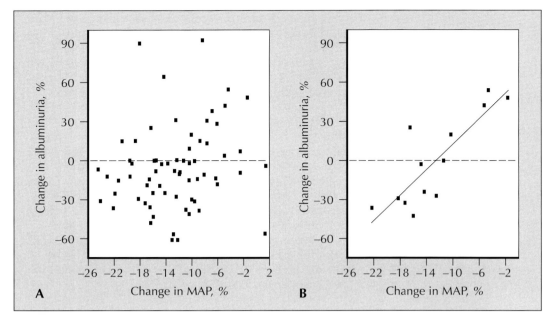

FIGURE 10-41. In clinical trials involving the use of calcium channel blockers as antihypertensive agents, an interesting paradox is evident. Dihydropyridine calcium channel blockers may increase urinary protein excretion despite lowering systemic blood pressure. In an effort to clarify this issue, Kloke *et al.* [49] combined a large series of clinical studies, conducted with various dihydropyridine calcium channel blockers, to evaluate the correlation between changes in blood pressure and changes in proteinuria. Only a very weak correlation exists between the decrease in blood pressure and the decrease in proteinuria, **A**. This may be related to the fact that measurements of blood pressure and proteinuria were not performed simultaneously. In addition, there is substantial variability in measurements of blood pressure throughout the course of the day. If one only considers the data from studies in which urine was collected over a timed interval during the day that closely approximates the time of blood pressure measurements, a significant correlation is observed, **B**. What this figure suggests is that when blood pressure is only moderately reduced, proteinuria increases, whereas a greater reduction in blood pressure is needed to produce a decrease in proteinuria. These observations parallel that which is seen in experimental studies in animals. The rationale behind this observation is that dihydropyridine calcium channel blockers preferentially dilate the afferent glomerular arteriole and, therefore, reduction in glomerular capillary pressure and proteinuria more closely depend on achieving better overall systemic blood pressure reduction. *Open symbols*— studies of patients with albuminuria < 500 mg/24h; *closed symbols*—studies of patients with albuminuria > 500 mg/24h. MAP—mean arterial pressure. (*Adapted from* Kloke *et al.* [49].)

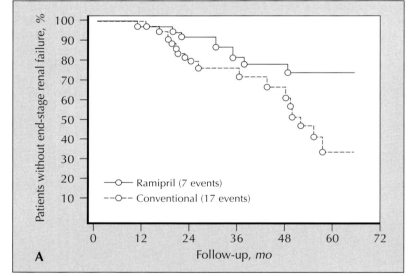

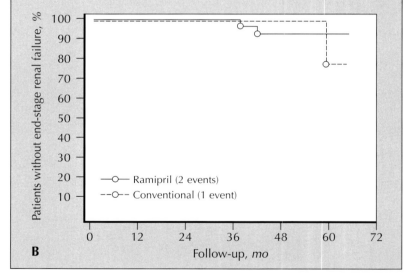

FIGURE 10-42. In stratum one of the Ramipril Efficacy in Nephropathy Trial, 186 nondiabetic patients with urinary protein < 3 g/d were randomized to receive either the angiotensin-converting enzyme (ACE) inhibitor (ramipril) or conventional antihypertensive therapy plus placebo with a target diastolic blood pressure < 90 mm Hg. The primary endpoints of the study were change in glomerular filtration rate (GFR) and time to end-stage renal failure or overt proteinuria > 3 g/24 h. Medium follow-up was 31 months. Ninety-nine patients were randomized to ramipril and 87 to conventional therapy. Baseline GFR was 49.5 mL/min/1.73 m² in the ramipril group and 43.4 mL/min/1.73 m² in the conventional group, with mean 24-hour and urinary protein excretion of 1.7 g in each group. Pretreatment blood pressure was 142/88.6 mm Hg in the ramipril group and 144.9/89.8 mm Hg in the conventional group. Decline in GFR/mo was not significantly different between the ramipril (-0.26 mL/min/mo) and control group (-0.29 mL/min/mo). Progression to renal failure was significantly less common in the ramipril group (99 vs 18/87). Progression to overt nephropathy was also less common (15/99 vs 27/87). Patients with a baseline GFR of 45 mL/min or less and proteinuria of 1.5 g/24 h or more had more rapid progression of disease and gained the most benefit from the ramipril treatment. The figure depicts the Kaplan-Meier estimation of renal survival among the patients on ramipril or conventional treatment in the subgroups based on GFR ≤ 45 mL/min/1.73 m² (**A**) and ≥ 45 mL/min/1.73 m² (**B**). Relative risk (95% confidence interval) in **A**=2.49 (1.03–6.02), P=0.036, and in **B**=1.00 (0.09–1.11), P=0.99. ACE inhibitors convey an important renal survival advantage in patients with more renal impairment and proteinuria than conventional therapy when blood pressure is reduced to 140/50 mm Hg. (*Adapted from* Ruggenenti *et al.* [50].)

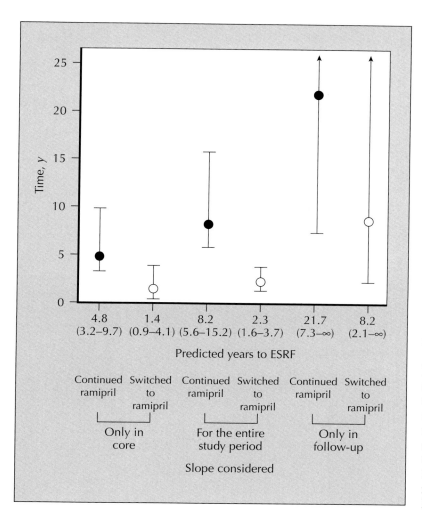

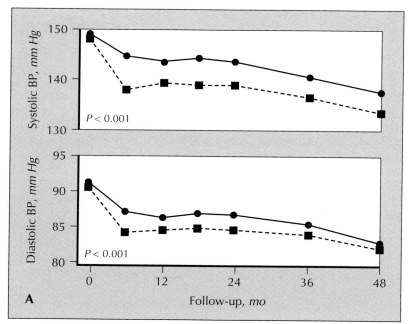

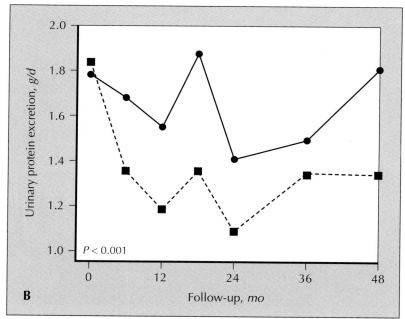

FIGURE 10-43. The Ramipril Efficacy in Nephropathy core study. More than 36 months of continued angiotensin-converting enzyme (ACE) therapy with ramipril decreased substantially the risk of end-stage renal disease and the risk of ≥ 3 g/24 h urinary protein excretion in patients with nondiabetic nephropathy compared with other antihypertensive therapy. In a follow-up study, the investigators evaluated time-dependent changes in glomerular filtration rate (GFR) in those patients who were switched from conventional therapy to ramipril therapy, as well as those patients who originally were on ramipril therapy and were maintained on it during the follow-up study. The analysis included 150 patients with nondiabetic nephropathy who were either continued on ramipril (*n* = 74) or switched to ramipril (*n* = 76). Ramipril dosages were 1.25 mg qd to 5 mg qd, and conventional therapy was added to achieve a diastolic blood pressure of < 90 mm Hg. Mean GFR at the time of randomization was 40.5 mL/min/1.73 m^2 in the ramipril group versus 38.5 mL/min/1.73 m^2 in the group that switched to ramipril. Urinary protein excretion was 5.6 g/d (ramipril) versus 4.9 g/d (switched to ramipril). The overall follow-up was 28±18 months after randomization. The figure depicts predicted time to end-stage renal disease (GFR = 10 mL/min/1.73 m^2) in the 43 patients continued on ramipril (*n* = 26), and those switched to ramipril (*n* = 17), who had at least three GFR measurements (including baseline) during the core study and at least three GFR measurements during the follow-up study. Time to end-stage renal disease is predicted on the basis of the last GFR, and mean and 95% confidence intervals of GFR, measured during both core and follow-up study periods, together and separately. Longer duration ACE inhibitor therapy appears to provide an advantage over traditional therapy in preserving kidney function in proteinuric (> 5 g/d) patients with nondiabetic nephropathy. ESRF—end-stage renal failure. (*Adapted from* Ruggenenti *et al.* [50].)

FIGURE 10-44. An individual patient meta-analysis of 1860 patients in 11 randomized controlled trials compared the efficacy of antihypertensive regimens including angiotensin-converting enzyme (ACE) inhibitors to the efficacy of regimens without ACE inhibitors in delaying progression of nondiabetic renal disease. Mean duration of follow-up was 2.2 years. As shown in the figure, patients in the ACE inhibitor group had a greater mean decrease in blood pressure (-4.5/-2.3 mm Hg) (**A**) and proteinuria (-460 mg/d) (**B**) compared with the non-ACE inhibitor group. Even after adjustment for baseline variables and changes in blood pressure and proteinuria during follow-up, the ACE inhibitor group had greater renal survival (*continued*)

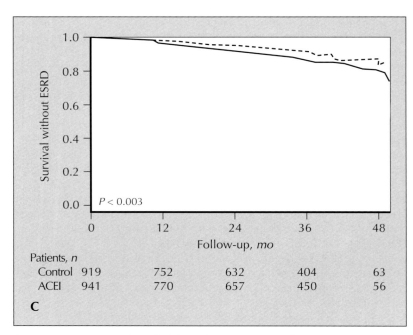

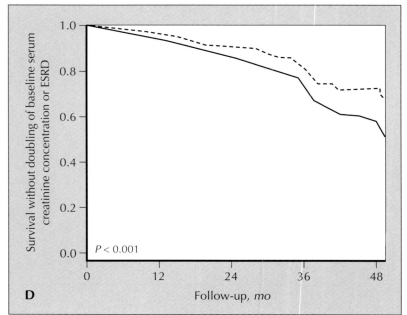

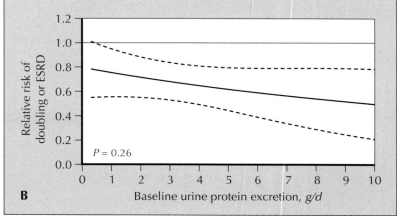

FIGURE 10-44. (*continued*) (**C**) and reduced risk for doubling of creatinine or end-stage renal disease (**D**) [13].

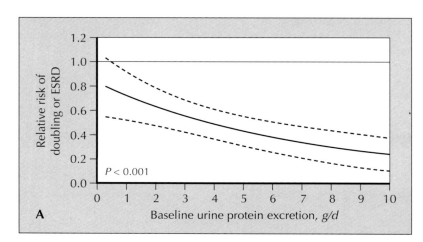

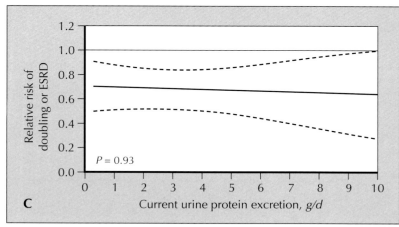

FIGURE 10-45. The 1860 patients from the individual patient meta-analysis described in Figure 10-44 had their clinical courses evaluated to assess the relationship between changes in urine protein excretion (1.9 g/d at baseline [mean]) during follow-up and the effect of angiotensin-converting enzyme (ACE) inhibitor on time to doubling of baseline serum creatinine values or onset of end-stage renal disease (ESRD). In all three panels, the vertical axis indicator indicates relative risk for ESRD. The horizontal axis is either baseline or current level of urine protein excretion. *Solid* and *dotted lines* indicate point estimates and 95% CIs for the relative risks, respectively. **A,** Note that the beneficial effect of the ACE inhibitor is greater at higher levels of baseline protein excretion. In panel **B,** which controls for change in protein excretion, note that the beneficial effect of ACE inhibitors remains significant, and is not related to level of baseline proteinuria. In panel **C,** which controls for current urine protein excretion, the beneficial effect of ACE inhibitors remains significant, but does not vary with current urine protein excretion. These data indicate that the greater beneficial effect of ACE inhibitors on progression of renal disease in patients with higher baseline proteinuria reflects their greater antiproteinuric effects in these patients. However, the level of proteinuria attained after treatment is begun is a better predictor of the risk of progression of renal disease [14].

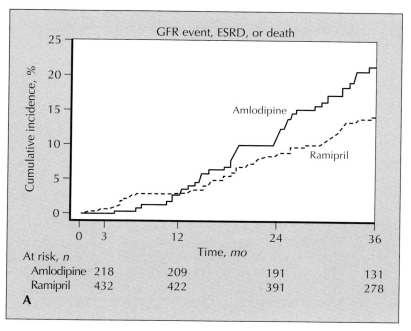

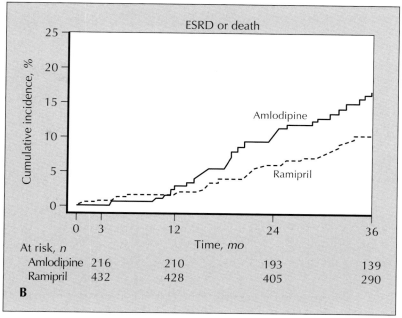

FIGURE 10-46. In the African-American Study of Kidney Disease (AASK), 1094 black patients with hypertensive renal disease (glomerular filtration rate [GFR] 20 to 65 mL/min/1.73 m²) were randomly assigned to receive an amlodipine-, atenolol-, or ramipril-based antihypertensive regimen. After 3 years of follow-up, the ramipril-based regimen retarded renal disease progress more compared with the amlodipine-based regimen, so the amlodipine arm was stopped. In this figure, the adjusted risk reduction for ramipril versus amlodipine for GFR event (50% reduction or decrease of 25 mL/min/1.73 m²), end-stage renal disease (ESRD), or death was 38% (95% CI, 13% to 56%; $P = 0.005$) (**A**), and for ESRD or death was 41% (95% CI, 14 to 60; $P = 0.007$) (**B**). This is the first study to demonstrate the advantage of ACE inhibition on a renal endpoint in black patients compared with other forms of antihypertensive therapy, and was most noticeable in patients with a urine protein/urine creatinine ratio greater than 0.22 (300 mg/d) [51].

EFFECTS OF DRUGS ON DIABETIC RENAL RESPONSE

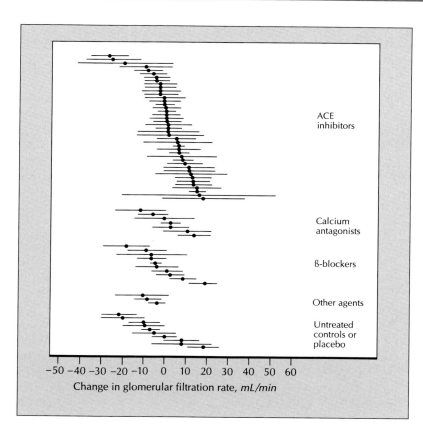

Figure 10-47. Kasiske *et al.* [52] reported a meta-analysis of 100 studies on the relative effect of different antihypertensive agents on proteinuria and renal function in hypertensive patients with diabetes. The meta-analysis confirmed that angiotensin-converting enzyme (ACE) inhibitors decrease proteinuria and preserve glomerular filtration rate in patients with diabetes, independent of changes in systemic blood pressure. In contrast, other antihypertensive agents had no effect on glomerular filtration rate, once the beneficial effects of mean arterial pressure reduction were taken into account. Thus, mean arterial pressure reduction from ACE inhibitor therapy caused a significantly greater improvement in glomerular filtration rate than did a comparable pressure reduction from other agents. The relative increase in glomerular filtration rate after ACE inhibition was not significantly different in patients treated for short or prolonged periods of time. The authors further noted that the effects of ACE inhibitors on renal function were not limited to patients with type 1 or 2 diabetes, patients with hypertension, or patients with early or more advanced diabetic nephropathy. (*Adapted from* Kasiske *et al.* [52].)

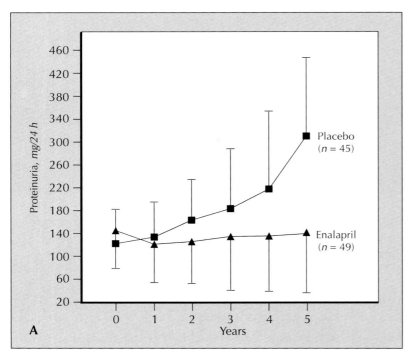

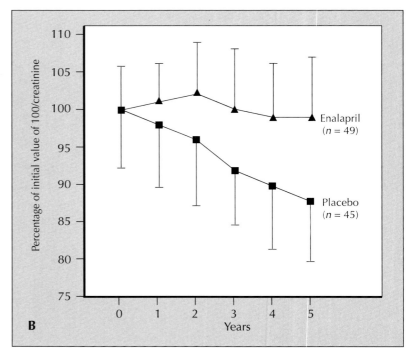

A

B

FIGURE 10-48. A total of 94 normotensive type 2 diabetic patients with microalbuminuria and normal renal function were randomized to receive 10 mg of enalapril daily or placebo. Any increase in blood pressure (BP) was treated with long-acting nifedipine. Each patient was followed-up for 5 years. The mean BP was stable in the enalapril group (initial mean, 99 ± 2.1 mm Hg; fifth-year mean, 100 ± 3.2 mm Hg) but increased in the placebo group from an initial mean of 97 ± 3.2 to 102 ± 34 mm Hg after 5 years ($P = 0.08$). **A,** Less proteinuria occurred in the enalapril group compared with placebo after the second year ($P < 0.05$ after 2 years; $P < 0.01$ after 3 years; $P < 0.005$ after 4 and 5 years). **B,** Reciprocal creatinine (100/creatinine) levels expressed as a percentage of initial value during the 5 years of follow-up demonstrate the benefit of enalapril therapy versus placebo. The mean rate of decline of reciprocal creatinine differed between the two groups ($P < 0.05$ for the second and third years; $P < 0.02$ for the fourth and fifth years). These results support the concept that early intervention with angiotensin-converting enzyme inhibitors in patients with type 2 diabetes can reduce urinary albumin loss and stabilize renal function. In this clinical trial, the enalapril therapy prevented a blood pressure increase, which likely explains not only the reduction in proteinuria but also the better preservation of renal function. Thus, it is hard to discern whether the beneficial effect of the drug is related to prevention of increasing blood pressure or a specific nonhemodynamic benefit. (*Adapted from* Ravid *et al.* [53].)

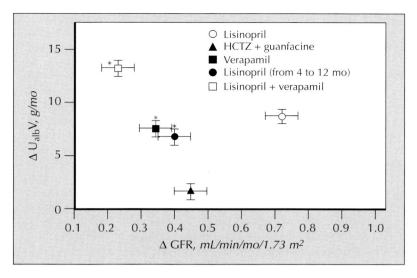

FIGURE 10-49. Bakris *et al.* [45] studied the relationship between the rate of decline of albuminuria and the rate of decline in renal function in patients with hypertension, type 2 diabetes mellitus, and mild renal insufficiency (mean creatinine clearance, 74 ± 2 mL/min and mean proteinuria, 5.9 ± 0.3 g/24 h). Patients were randomized to one of four treatment groups: group one (*n* = 8) received lisinopril, group two (*n* = 8) verapamil-SR, group three (*n* = 8) lisinopril and verapamil-SR, and group four (*n* = 6) hydrochlorothiazide (HCTZ) and guanfacine. All patients received these medications for a period of 1 year. Similar blood pressure reductions, which were titrated to reduce diastolic blood pressure to less than 90 mm Hg, occurred in each group. Note the relationship between the rate of change of glomerular filtration rate (GFR) and albuminuria for the treatment period. Note that the slower rate of decline in GFR the greater the reduction in urinary albumin excretion. *Asterisks* indicate statistical significance (*P* < 0.005) of a slower rate of decline in GFR and greater reduction in urinary albumin excretion compared with the group treated with HCTZ and guanfacine.

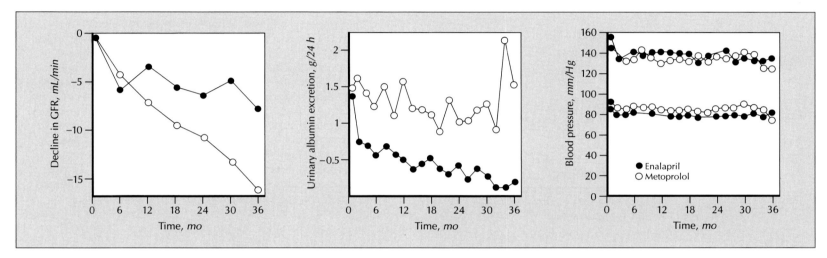

FIGURE 10-50. A prospective, randomized, open-label trial was conducted in Sweden to compare enalapril and metoprolol (both therapies usually combined with furosemide) to determine whether angiotensin-converting enzyme inhibition reduced the rate of decline in kidney function more than did blood pressure reduction with other antihypertensive treatment [54]. Forty patients with insulin-dependent diabetes were treated with either enalapril (*n* = 20; mean glomerular filtration rate [GFR], 46 mL/min/1.73 m²; mean arterial pressure [MAP], 114 mm Hg; mean proteinuria, 2.0 g/24 h) or metoprolol (*n* = 20; mean GFR, 48 mL/min/1.73 m²; MAP, 109 mm Hg; mean proteinuria, 2.0 g/24 h) plus furosemide as needed for blood pressure and volume control. As depicted, the decline in GFR was minimized (-2.0 mL/min/y) with enalapril compared with metoprolol (-5.6 mL/min/y) over a mean 2.2-year follow-up. Urinary albumin excretion decreased with enalapril. No significant changes were noted with blood pressure control between therapies. The authors concluded that treatment with enalapril can reduce the rate of decline in kidney function in patients with diabetic nephropathy more than equally effective antihypertensive treatment with metoprolol. (*Adapted from* Bjorck *et al.* [54].)

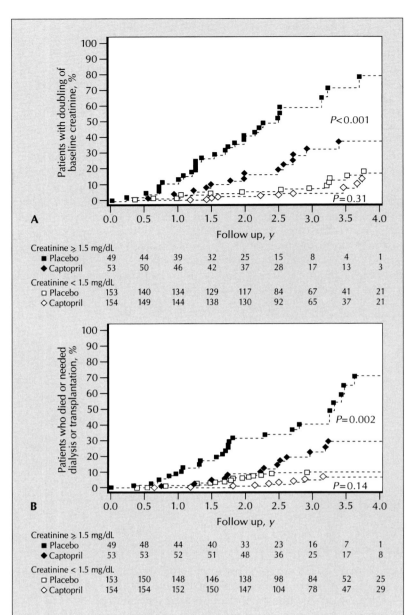

FIGURE 10-51. A pivotal study conducted by the Collaborative Study Group to assess the influence of an angiotensin-converting enzyme (ACE) inhibitor (captopril) on the progression of diabetic renal disease [55] determined whether captopril has kidney-protecting properties independent of its effect on blood pressure. A randomized, controlled trial conducted over 3 years compared captopril with placebo in patients with type 1 diabetes whose urinary protein excretion was 500 mg/d or more and whose serum creatinine concentration was 2.5 mg/dL or less. Two hundred seven patients received captopril (entry blood pressure, $137 \pm 19/85 \pm 11$ mm Hg) and 202 placebo (entry blood pressure, $140 \pm 20/86 \pm 12$ mm Hg). Blood pressure goals were defined to achieve control (systolic/diastolic 140/90 mm Hg or less) during a median follow-up of 3 years with either captopril or placebo in conjunction with antihypertensives (except ACE inhibitors or calcium channel blockers). The primary endpoint was a doubling of baseline serum creatinine concentration. Overall, serum creatinine concentrations doubled in 25 patients in the captopril group compared with 43 patients in the placebo group ($P = 0.007$). The cumulative incidence of events in patients in each group is depicted according to baseline serum creatinine concentration. A total of 102 patients had a baseline serum creatinine of 1.5 mg/dL or more, and 307 had a baseline serum creatinine concentration below 1.5 mg/dL. **A,** The cumulative percentage of patients in each subgroup who had a doubling of the serum creatinine concentration to at least 2 mg/dL. **B,** The cumulative percentage of patients in each subgroup who died or required dialysis or renal transplantation. The numbers under each graph are the numbers of patients in each subgroup at risk for the event at baseline after each 6-month period. The associated reductions in risk of a doubling of serum creatinine concentration were 48% in the captopril group as a whole, 76% in the subgroup with a baseline serum creatinine concentration of 2 mg/dL, 55% in the subgroup with a concentration of 1.5 mg/dL, and 17% in the subgroup with a concentration of 1 mg/dL. Captopril protects against the deterioration of renal function in patients with type 1 diabetes and early evidence of renal dysfunction and is more effective than is blood pressure control alone. (*Adapted from* Lewis *et al.* [55].)

UNITED KINGDOM PROSPECTIVE DIABETES STUDY RENAL DISEASE RESULTS

Proportion of patients progressing to a urinary albumin concentration ≥ 50 mg/L*
 Captopril 31% (48/153)
 Atenolol 26% (38/146) } *P = .31

Proportion of patients progressing to a clinical proteinuria > 300 mg/L†
 Captopril 5% (7/153)
 Atenolol 10% (14/146) } †P = .09

No difference in serum creatinine or in proportion of patients who had a twofold increase in creatinine over a 9-year period

FIGURE 10-52. The United Kingdom Prospective Diabetes Study was a randomized controlled trial comparing an angiotensin-converting enzyme (ACE) inhibitor (captopril, 50 mg po bid) with a β-blocker (atenolol 50 to 100 mg qd) in patients with type 2 diabetes, aiming for a blood pressure < 180/105 mm Hg (less tight) or < 150/85 mm Hg (tight). Of 11,048 patients with hypertension (mean age 56 y, mean blood pressure 160/94 mm Hg), 758 patients were allocated to tight control of blood pressure as mentioned earlier. Four hundred received captopril, and 358 received atenolol, plus additional medications to facilitate blood pressure control. Captopril and atenolol were equally effective in reducing blood pressure to a mean of 144/83 mm Hg and 143/81 mm Hg, respectively. A similar proportion of patients taking captopril (27%) and atenolol (31%) required three or more antihypertensive medications in order to achieve goal blood pressure. Both medications were equally effective in reducing the risk of macrovascular and microvascular endpoints. The renal disease results demonstrated that the proportion of patients progressing to a urinary albumin concentration ≥ 50 μg/mL were similar in both groups (captopril 31%, atenolol 26%, P = 0.31). The proportion of patients progressing to clinical proteinuria ≥ 300 μg/mL tended to be fewer in the captopril group (5%) versus the atenolol group (10%), where P = 0.09. There was no overall difference between primary therapies in serum creatinine level or those patients who had a twofold increase in creatinine over the 9-year period of follow-up. Consequently, blood pressure lowering with captopril or atenolol was similarly effective in reducing the incidence of diabetic complications of the kidney. This study provided no evidence that either drug has any specific beneficial or deleterious effect, suggesting that blood pressure reduction in itself may be more important than the treatment used. (*Adapted from* UK Prospective Diabetes Study Group [56].)

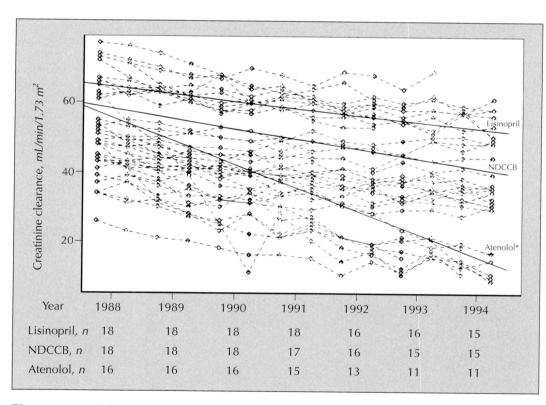

Year	1988	1989	1990	1991	1992	1993	1994
Lisinopril, n	18	18	18	18	16	16	15
NDCCB, n	18	18	18	17	16	15	15
Atenolol, n	16	16	16	15	13	11	11

Figure 10-53. Bakris *et al.* [57] prospectively randomized 52 patients having nephropathy associated with non–insulin-dependent diabetes mellitus to treatment with lisinopril (n = 18), diltiazem or verapamil (n = 18), or atenolol (n = 16), plus additional medication (furosemide, α-blocker, or hydralazine to reduce blood pressure [BP] to less than 140/90 mm Hg), in order to compare the impact of these therapies with the progression rate of renal disease. Baseline values for BP (155–161/97–99 mm Hg), 24-hour urine protein excretion (2.7 to 4.5 g), and serum creatinine level (141 to 168 mmol/L) were similar for all three groups. There were no significant differences in mean arterial pressure reduction among the groups. However, the mean rate of decline in creatinine clearance over a period of 6 years was greatest in the atenolol group (-3.48 mL/min/y/1.73 m², P < 0.0001) compared with the other two groups. There was no difference in the creatinine clearance slopes for the lisinopril or non-dihydropyridine calcium channel blocker (NDCCB) groups (P = 0.36). Proteinuria was reduced to a significant and similar extent only in the lisinopril or NDCCB groups and correlated with slowing of renal disease progression. *Asterisk* denotes P < 0.01 compared with other two slopes. (*Adapted from* Bakris *et al.* [57].)

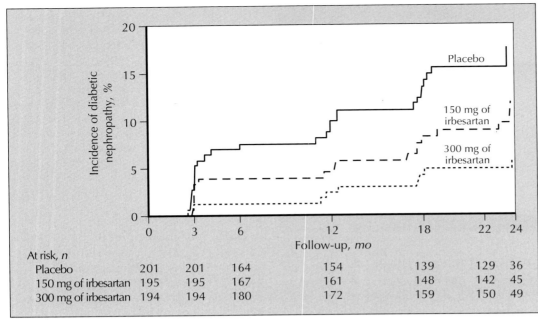

At risk, n

Placebo	201	201	164	154	139	129	36
150 mg of irbesartan	195	195	167	161	148	142	45
300 mg of irbesartan	194	194	180	172	159	150	49

FIGURE 10-54. A total of 590 patients with hypertension (153/90 mm Hg), type 2 diabetes, microalbuminuria (56 μg/min), and normal renal function (serum creatinine 1.1 mg/dL) were randomly assigned to placebo plus conventional therapy, irbesartan 150 mg plus

conventional therapy, or irbesartan 300 mg plus conventional therapy to see if there was an advantage of a specific antihypertensive regimen in preventing progression to clinical proteinuria (300 μg/min) over a 2-year period. The average follow-up blood pressure during the course of the study was approximately 143/83 mm Hg for the three groups. In this figure, one can appreciate the incidence of diabetic nephropathy based on the three therapies. Ten of 94 patients in the 300-mg irbesartan group (5.2%) and 19 of the 195 patients in the 150-mg irbesartan group (9.7%) reached clinical proteinuria, as compared with 30 of 201 patients in the placebo group: 14.9% (hazard ratios, 0.30; 95% CI, 0.14 to 0.61; $P < 0.001$) and 0.61% (95% CI, 0.34 to 1.09; $P = 0.08$), respectively. The angiotensin II receptor blocker irbesartan retards the progression to clinical proteinuria in hypertensive patients with type 2 diabetes and microalbuminuria independent of blood pressure [58].

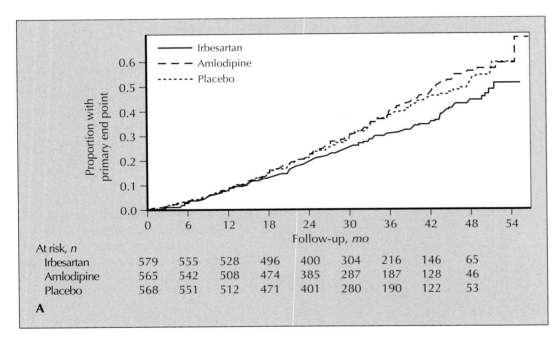

At risk, n

Irbesartan	579	555	528	496	400	304	216	146	65
Amlodipine	565	542	508	474	385	287	187	128	46
Placebo	568	551	512	471	401	280	190	122	53

A

FIGURE 10-55. A total of 1715 patients with hypertension (159/87 mm Hg), type 2 diabetes, renal disease (serum creatinine 1.7 mg/dL), and clinical proteinuria (2.9 g/24 h) were randomly assigned to placebo, amlodipine, or irbesartan plus conventional non–angiotension-converting enzyme inhibitor antihypertensive therapy to evaluate the differential effects of the regimens on progression to the composite endpoint of doubling of serum creatinine, end-stage renal disease, or death. **A,** After 2.6 years of follow-up, there was a statistically significant advantage of irbesartan-based (mean dose, 269 mg) therapy reaching the composite endpoint compared to amlodipine-based (mean dose, 8.9 mg) or placebo-based antihypertensive regimens despite all three groups reaching similar levels of blood pressure achievement (141/77 mm Hg).
(Continued on next page)

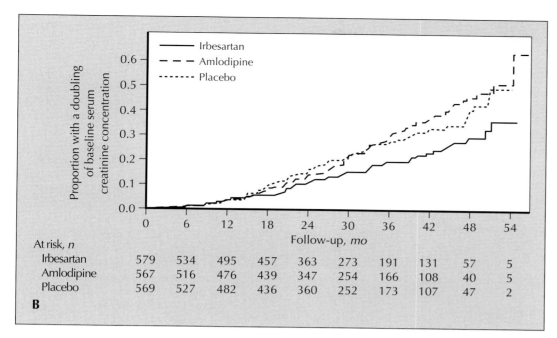

B

At risk, n										
Irbesartan	579	534	495	457	363	273	191	131	57	5
Amlodipine	567	516	476	439	347	254	166	108	40	5
Placebo	569	527	482	436	360	252	173	107	47	2

FIGURE 10-55. *(Continued)* **B,** Treatment with the angiotensin II receptor blocker (irbesartan)-based antihypertensive regimen was associated with a 20% lower risk for reaching the composite endpoint compared to the placebo-based regimen (*P* = 0.02) and 23% lower than an amlodipine-based regimen (*P* = 0.006). This study established the benefit of an angiotensin II receptor blocker as being renoprotective independent of blood pressure reduction in hypertensive type 2 diabetics with early clinical renal disease [15].

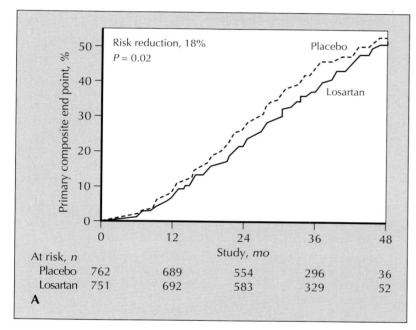

A

At risk, n					
Placebo	762	689	554	296	36
Losartan	751	692	583	329	52

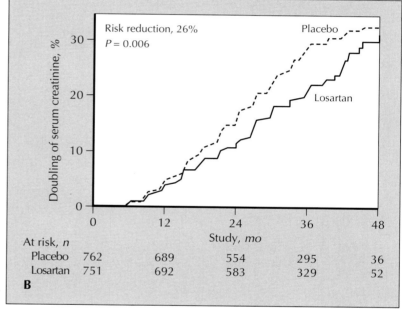

B

At risk, n					
Placebo	762	689	554	295	36
Losartan	751	692	583	329	52

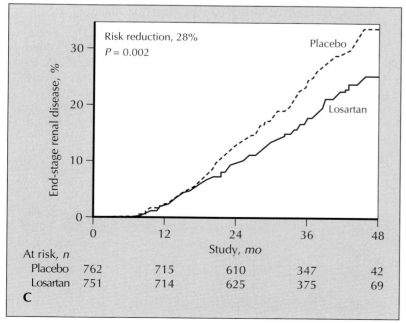

C

At risk, n					
Placebo	762	715	610	347	42
Losartan	751	714	625	375	69

FIGURE 10-56. A total of 1513 patients with hypertension (152/82 mm Hg), type 2 diabetes, renal insufficiency (creatinine 1.9 mg/dL), and proteinuria (urinary albumin/creatinine ratio, 1249) were randomly assigned in a double-blind study comparing losartan (50 to 100 mg four times daily) with placebo, in addition to conventional (non–angiotensin-converting enzyme inhibitor) antihypertensive treatment (*eg*, calcium antagonists, β-blockers, diuretics) for a mean of 3.4 years to study progression to the primary outcome of the composite endpoint of doubling of baseline serum creatinine, end-stage renal disease (ESRD), or death. Similar levels of blood pressure were achieved in both arms of the study: losartan (140/74 mm Hg) and placebo (142/74 mm Hg); *P* = 0.77. Losartan therapy led to a 35% reduction in proteinuria, whereas there was a slight increase in the placebo arm. **A,** Losartan therapy resulted in a 16% relative risk reduction for reaching the composite endpoint (*P* = 0.02) and a 25% reduction (*P* = 0.006) in the risk for doubling of baseline serum creatinine (**B**). Furthermore, patients in the losartan arm experienced a 28% reduction (*P* = 0.002) in the risk for ESRD (**C**),

Continued on next page

ANTIHYPERTENSIVE THERAPY: PROGRESSION OF RENAL INJURY
235

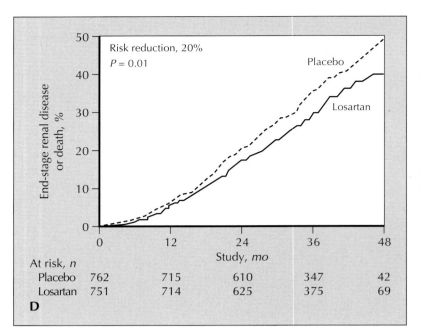

FIGURE 10-56. *(Continued)* and a 20% reduction (*P* = 0.01) in the risk of ESRD or death (**D**). This study established that the angiotensin II receptor blocker, losartan, along with conventional antihypertensive therapy, confers renal protection, independent of blood pressure reduction, in patients with type 2 diabetes and nephropathy [16].

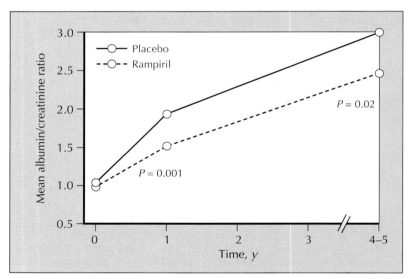

FIGURE 10-57. Heart Outcomes Prevention Evaluation (HOPE) study. In the HOPE study, 3577 patients with diabetes were included (approximately 39% of the total). These patients were individuals 55 years or older with a previous cardiovascular event, or at least one other risk factor, no clinical proteinuria, or heart failure, and who were not previously on an angiotensin-converting enzyme (ACE) inhibitor who were randomly assigned to receive ramipril 10 mg four times daily or placebo in addition to standard medically indicated therapy for hypertension or cardiovascular disease. During the course of 4.5 years of follow-up, 117 (7%) of participants on ramipril and 149 (8%) on placebo developed overt nephropathy (24% relative risk reduction; *P* = 0.027). As shown in the figure, the geometric mean urine albumin/creatinine ratio was consistently lower in all participants on ramipril with available 24-hour urine collection. These data indicate the advantage of the ACE inhibitor in preventing clinical nephropathy in a large cohort of type 2 diabetics [59].

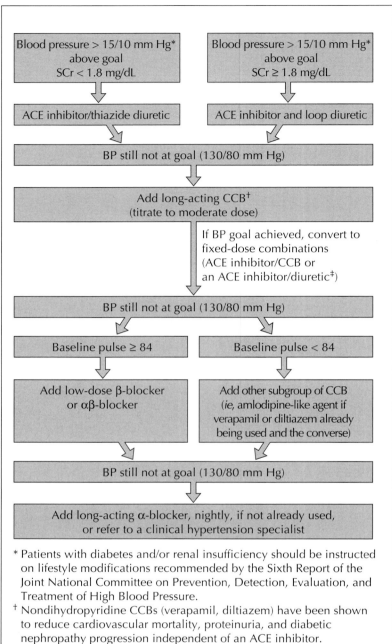

FIGURE 10-58. A recommended drug treatment algorithm for achieving blood pressure control in patients with renal insufficiency and/or diabetes by the National Kidney Foundation Hypertension and Diabetes Executive Committee Working Group. Note that an angiotensin-converting enzyme (ACE) inhibitor is recommended for all patients. To these drugs can be added diuretics, calcium antagonists, and other drugs depending on comorbid problems such as proteinuria or coronary artery disease. Note that these recommendations were drafted before the landmark trials in type 2 diabetes and nephropathy indicated an important therapeutic advantage with angiotensin II receptor blockers [60]. ACE—angiotensin-converting enzyme; BP—blood pressure; CCB—calcium channel blocker; SCr—serum creatinine.

CONSIDERATION TO SLOW PROGRESSION OF DIABETIC NEPHROPATHY WITH ANTIHYPERTENSIVE THERAPY

To reduce the risk and/or slow the progression of nephropathy, optimize blood pressure control (130/80 mm Hg)

In the treatment of albuminuria/nephropathy, both ACE inhibitors and ARBs can be used

In hypertensive and nonhypertensive type 1 diabetic patients with microalbuminuria or clinical albuminuria, ACE inhibitors are the initial agents of choice

In hypertensive type 2 diabetic patients with microalbuminuria or clinical albuminuria, ARBs are the initial agents of choice

If one class is not tolerated, the other should be substituted

Combination of ACE inhibitors and ARBs will decrease albuminuria more than use of either agent alone

Consider the use of nondihydropyridine calcium antagonists in patients unable to tolerate ACE inhibitors or ARBs

FIGURE 10-59. This table outlines the need for more intensive blood pressure control (< 130/80 mm Hg), specifically with drugs that have antihypertensive and antiproteinuric effects whose efficacy is supported by well-controlled clinical trials. Note that many patients will require multiple antihypertensive medications to achieve lower blood pressure goals. These recommendations are endorsed by the American Diabetes Association [61]. ACE—angiotensin-converting enzyme; ARBs—angiotensin II receptor blockers.

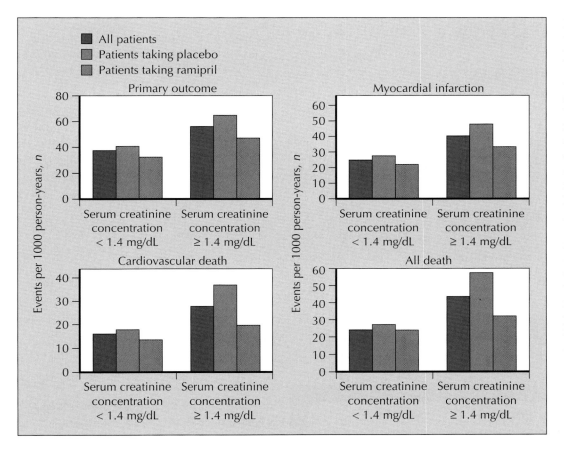

FIGURE 10-60. In analysis of the HOPE trial data, the clinical course of 980 patients with mild renal insufficiency (serum creatinine ≥ 1.4 but ≤ 2.3 mg/dL) and 8307 patients with normal renal function (serum creatinine <1.4 mg/dL) was evaluated to assess the influence of mild renal insufficiency on cardiovascular outcome and whether the angiotensin-converting enzyme inhibitor, ramipril, decreased that risk. The cumulative incidence of cardiovascular events was higher in those patients with renal insufficiency than in those without (22% vs 15.1%; $P < 0.001$) and increased with serum creatinine concentration. The effect of renal insufficiency on cardiovascular events was independent of known cardiovascular risks and treatment. As shown, ramipril therapy reduced the incidence of primary outcome (cardiovascular death, myocardial infarction, stroke) and individual endpoint, regardless of whether the patients had renal insufficiency [62].

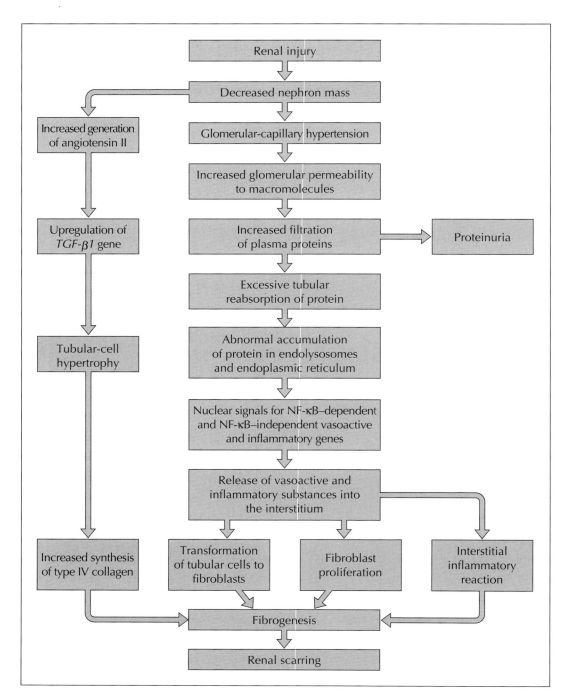

FIGURE 10-61. In patients with renal disease and proteinuria, there is clinical evidence that reducing proteinuria with drugs such as angiotensin-converting enzyme inhibitors slows the rate of loss of renal function. Elevated glomerular capillary pressure, perhaps by enlarging the radius of pores in the glomerular basement membrane, which results in a size-selective impairment of the membrane to retard transmembrane protein flux, results in increased proteinuria. Excessive reabsorption of proteins by renal tubular epithelial cells likely triggers vasoactive and inflammatory cytokine production resulting in proliferation of fibroblasts and interstitial inflammation, ultimately resulting in enhanced production of extra-cellular matrix and glomerulosclerosis. As shown here, both nuclear signals for inflammatory substance genes and the renin-angiotensin transforming growth factor-β 1 axis can be stimulated, leading to excessive renal scarring via a variety of mechanisms. These insights underscore the importance of better control of glomerular capillary pressure and reduction of proteinuria in order to protect renal function in patients with proteinuric nephropathies [63]. TGF—transforming growth factor.

CONCLUSIONS

Sufficient clinical data are evident to support the need for more intensive control of blood pressure to a systolic pressure <125 mm Hg in patients with renal disease, particularly those who have diabetes or proteinuria >1 g/24 h

Antagonism of the renin-angiotensin system more consistently provides reduction in both systemic blood pressure and glomerular capillary pressure and therefore provides a better opportunity to delay progression of renal disease

Therapies that reduce blood pressure and proteinuria appear to be beneficial in slowing progressive nephropathy

FIGURE 10-62. There are sufficient data to suggest that hypertension is an important variable in the rate of progression of all forms of renal disease. It is likely that there are many different pathways involved in the development of progressive renal injury, depending on the type of underlying disease. However, it is also likely that there is a final common pathway linking the various mechanisms, and excessive neuro-hormonal influence within the kidney may be the glue that links them together. It does appear that elevated systemic and glomerular capillary pressures are linked to glomerular proteinuria and glomerular injury, and therapy to reduce blood pressure and proteinuria appears to be beneficial in slowing progressive nephropathy. The reduction of proteinuria will likely prove to be most important in patients with diabetic renal disease.

REFERENCES

1. National Heart, Lung, and Blood Institute: *National High Blood Pressure Education Program Working Group Report: Hypertension and Chronic Renal Failure.* Rockville, MD: US Dept of Health and Human Services, National Institutes of Health; 1990. NIH publication 90-3032.

2. Multiple Risk Factor Intervention Trial (MRFIT): Risk factor changes and mortality results. *JAMA* 1982, 248:1465–1477.

3. Shulman NB, Ford CE, Hall WD, *et al.*: Prognostic value of serum creatinine and effect of treatment of hypertension on renal function. *Hypertension* 1989, 13(suppl 1):1180–1193.

4. Rostand SG, Brown G, Kirk KA, *et al.*: Renal insufficiency in treated essential hypertension. *N Engl Med* 1989, 320:684–648.

5. Tierney WM, McDonald CJ, Luft FC: Renal disease in hypertensive adults: effects of race and type II diabetes mellitus. *Am J Kidney Dis* 1989, 13:485–493.

6. Walker WG, Neaton JD, Cutler JA, *et al.*Renal function change in hypertensive members of the Multiple Risk Factor Intervention Trial: racial and treatment effects. The MRFIT Research Group. *JAMA* 1992, 268:3085–3091.

7. Navar LG, Burke TJ, Robinson RR, Clapp JR: Distal tubular feedback in the autoregulation of single nephron glomerular filtration rate. *J Clin Invest* 1974, 53:516–525.

8. Johnson RJ, Schreiner GF: Hypothesis: the role of acquired tubulointerstitial disease in the pathogenesis of salt-dependent hypertension. *Kidney Int* 1997, 52:1169–1179.

9. Brenner BM. Dworkin LD, Ichikawa I: Glomerular filtration. In *The Kidney.* Edited by Brenner BM, Rector FC. Philadelphia: WB Saunders; 1986:122–144.

10. Anderson S, Meyer TW, Rennke HG, *et al.*: Control of glomerular hypertension limits glomerular injury in rats with reduced renal mass. *J Clin Invest* 1985, 76:612–691.

11. Hostetter TH, Olson JL, Rennike HG, *et al.*: Hyperfiltration in remnant nephrons: a potentially adverse response to renal ablation. *Am J Physiol* 1981, 241:F85–F93.

12. Anderson S, Remke HG, Brenner BM: Therapeutic advantage of converting enzyme inhibitors in arresting progressive renal disease associated with systemic hypertension in the rate. *J Clin Invest* 1986, 77:1993–2000.

13. Jafar TH, Schmid CH, Landa M, *et al.*: Angiotensin-converting enzyme inhibitors and progression of non-diabetic renal disease. A meta-analysis of patient level data. *Ann Intern Med* 2001, 135:73–87.

14. Jafar TH, Stark PF, Schmid CH, *et al.*: Proteinuria as a modifiable risk factor for the progression of non-diabetic renal disease. *Kidney Int* 2001, 60:1131–1140.

15. Lewis EJ, Hunsicker LG, Clarke WR, *et al.*: Renoprotective effects of the angiotensin receptor antagonist irbesartan in patients with nephropathy due to type 2 diabetes. *N Engl J Med* 2001, 345:851–860.

16. Brenner BM, Cooper ME, deZeeuw D, *et al.*: Effects of losartan on renal and cardiovascular outcomes in patients with type 2 diabetes and nephropathy. *N Engl J Med* 2001, 345:861–869.

17. The sixth report of the Joint National Committee on Prevention, Detection, Evaluation, and Treatment of High Blood Pressure. *Arch Intern Med* 1997, 157:2413–2446.

18. Wesson LG: *Physiology of the Human Kidney.* New York: Grune and Stratton; 1969.

19. The fifth report of the Joint National Committee on Detection, Evaluation and Treatment of High Blood Pressure (JNC V). *Arch Intern Med* 1993, 153:154–183.

20. Lindeman RD, Tobin JD, Shock NW: Association between blood pressure and rate of decline of kidney function with age. *Kidney Int* 1984, 26:861–868.

21. Rosansky SJ, Hoover DR, King L, *et al.*: The association of blood pressure levels and change in renal function in hypertensive and nonhypertensive subjects. *Arch Intern Med* 1991, 151:1280–1287.

22. Brazy PC, Stead WW, Fitzwilliam JF: Progression of renal insufficiency: role of blood pressure. *Kidney Int* 1989, 35:670–674.

23. Friedman JR, Norman DC, Yoshikawa TT: Correlation of estimated renal function parameters versus 24-hour creatinine clearance in ambulatory elderly. *J Am Geriatr Soc* 1989, 37:145–149.

24. Klag MJ, Whelton PK, Randall BL, *et al.*: Blood pressure and end-stage renal disease in men. *N Engl J Med* 1996, 334:13–18.

25. National Institute of Diabetes and Digestive and Kidney Diseases. *US Renal Data System 2001 Annual Data Report: Atlas of End-Stage Renal Disease in the United States.* Bethesda, MD; National Institutes of Health; 2001.

26. Weir MR: Hypertensive nephropathy: is a more physiologic approach to blood pressure control an important concern for the presentation of renal function? *Am J Med* 1992, 93(suppl 2A):27–37.

27. Folkow B: Structural myogenic, humoral and nervous factors controlling peripheral resistance. In *Hypotensive Drugs.* Edited by Harrington M. London: Pergamon Press; 1956:163–174.

28. Lever AF: Slow pressor mechanisms in hypertension: a role for hypertrophy of resistance vessels. *J Hypertens* 1986, 4:515–524.

29. Brenner BM, Dworkin LD, Ichikawa I: Glomerular filtration. In *The Kidney.* Edited by Brenner BM, Rector FCC. Philadelphia: WB Saunders; 1986:122–144.

30. Bauer JH, Reams GP: Do calcium antagonists protect the human hypertensive kidney? *Am J Hypertens* 1989, 2:173S–178S.

31. Glassock RJ: The kidney: therapeutic implications of angiotensin-converting enzyme inhibitors. Prevention of renal disease: where do we go from here? *Am J Hypertens* 1988, 1:389S–392S.

32. Dworkin LD, Benstein JA: Impact of antihypertensive therapy on progressive kidney damage. *Am J Hypertens* 1989; 2:162S–172S.

33. Bakris GL: Maximizing cardiorenal benefits: achieve blood pressure goals. *J Clin Hypertens* 1999, 1:141–148.

34. Ikoma M, Kawamura T, Kakinuma Y, *et al.*: Cause of variable therapeutic efficiency of angiotensin converting enzyme inhibitor on glomerular lesions. *Kidney Int* 1991, 40:195–202.

35. Parving HH, Andersen AR, Smidt UM, *et al.*: Effect of antihypertensive treatment of kidney function in diabetic nephropathy. *BMJ* 1987, 294:1443–1447.

36. Pettinger WA, Lee HC, Reisch J, *et al.*: Long-term improvement in renal function after short-term strict blood pressure control in hypertensive nephrosclerosis. *Hypertension* 1989, 13:766–772.

37. Klahr S, Levey AS, Beck GJ, *et al.* for the MDRD Study Group: The effects of dietary protein restriction and blood-pressure control on the progression of chronic renal disease. *N Engl J Med* 1994, 330:877–884.

38. Wright JT, Jr, Bakris GL, Greene T, *et al.*: Effect of blood pressure lowering and antihypertensive drug class on progression of hypertensive kidney disease. *JAMA* 2002, 288 (November issue).

39. Maschio G, Alberti D, Janin G, *et al.* for the Angiotension-Converting-Enzyme Inhibition in Progressive Renal Insufficiency Study Group: Effect of the angiotensin-converting enzyme inhibitor benazepril on the progression of chronic renal insufficiency. *N Engl J Med* 1996, 334:939–945.

40. Ruilope LM, Miranda B, Morales JM, *et al.*: Converting enzyme inhibition in chronic renal failure. *Am J Kidney Dis* 1989, 13:120–126.

41. Kamper AL, Strandgaard S, Leyssac PP: Effect of enalapril on the progression of chronic renal failure: a randomized controlled trial. *Am J Hypertens* 1992, 5:423–430.

42. Eliahou HE, Cohen D, Heilberg B, *et al.*: Effect of the calcium channel blocker nisoldipine on the progression of chronic renal

failure in man. *Am J Nephrol* 1988, 8:285–290.

43. Brazy PC, Fitzwilliam JF: Progressive renal disease: role of race and antihypertensive medications. *Kidney Int* 1990, 37:1113–1119.

44. Zucchelli P, Zuccala A, Borghi M, *et al.*: Long-term comparison between captopril and nifedipine in the progression of renal insufficiency. *Kidney Int* 1992, 42:452–458.

45. Bakris GL, Barnhill BW, Sadler R: Treatment of arterial hypertension in diabetic humans: importance of therapeutic selection. *Kidney Int* 1992, 41:912–919.

46. Slataper R, Vicknair N, Sadler R, *et al.*: Comparative effects of different antihypertensive treatments on progression of diabetic renal disease. *Arch Intern Med* 1993, 153:973–980.

47. Gansevoort RT, de Zeeuw D, de Jong PE: Is the antiproteinuric effect of ACE inhibition mediated by interference in the renin-angiotensin system? *Kidney Int* 1994, 45:861–867.

48. Russo D, Minutolo R, Pisani A, *et al.*: Co-administration of losartan and enalapril exerts additive antiproteinuric effect in IgA nephropathy. *Am J Kidney Dis* 2001, 38:18–25.

49. Kloke HJ, Branten AJ, Huysmans FT, Wetzels JF: Antihypertensive treatment of patients with proteinuric renal diseases: risks or benefits of calcium channel blockers? *Kidney Int* 1998, 53:1559–1573.

50. Ruggenenti P, Perna A, Gherardi G, *et al.*: Renoprotective properties of ACE-inhibition in non-diabetic nephropathies with non-nephrotic proteinuria. *Lancet* 1999, 354:359–364.

51. Agodoa LY, Appel LJ, Bakris GL, *et al.*: Effect of ramipril vs amlodipine on renal outcomes in hypertensive nephrosclerosis: a randomized controlled trial. *JAMA* 2001, 285:2719–2728.

52. Kasiske BL, Kalel RSN, Ma JZ, *et al.*: Effect of antihypertensive therapy on the kidney in patients with diabetes: a meta-regression analysis. *Ann Intern Med* 1993, 118:129–138.

53. Ravid M, Savin H, Jutrin I, *et al.*: Long-term stabilizing effect of angiotensin-converting enzyme inhibition on plasma creatinine and on proteinuria in normotensive type II diabetic patients. *Ann Intern Med* 1993, 118:577–581.

54. Bjorck S, Mulec H, Johnsen SA, *et al.*: Renal protective effect of enalapril in diabetic nephropathy. *BMJ* 1992, 304:339–343.

55. Lewis EJ, Hunsicker LG, Bain RP, *et al.*: The effect of angiotensin-converting enzyme inhibitor on diabetic nephropathy. *N Engl J Med* 1993, 329:1456–1462.

56. UK Prospective Diabetes Study Group: Efficacy of atenolol and captopril in in reducing risk of macrovascular and microvascular complications in type 2 diabetes: UKPDS39. *BMJ* 1998, 317:713–720.

57. Bakris GL, Copley JB, Vicknair N, *et al.*: Calcium channel blockers versus other antihypertensive therapies on progression of NIDDM associated nephropathy. *Kidney Int* 1996, 50:1641–1650.

58. Parving HH, Lenhert H, Brochner-Mortensen J, *et al.*: The effect of irbesartan on the development of diabetic nephropathy in patients with type 2 diabetes. *N Engl J Med* 2001, 345:870–878.

59. Effects of ramipril on cardiovascular and microvascular outcomes in people with diabetes mellitus: results of the HOPE study and MICRO-HOPE substudy. *Lancet* 2000, 355:253–255.

60. Bakris GL, Williams M, Dworkin L, *et al.*: Preserving renal function in adults with hypertension and diabetes: a consensus approach. *Am J Kidney Dis* 2000, 36:646–661.

61. American Diabetes Association. Diabetic Nephropathy. *Diabetes Care* 2002, 25(suppl 1):585–589.

62. Mann JFE, Gerstein HC, Pogue J, *et al.*: Renal insufficiency as a predictor of cardiovascular outcomes and the impact of ramipril. The HOPE randomized trial. *Ann Intern Med* 2001, 134:629–639.

63. Remuzzi G, Bertani T: Pathophysiology of progressive nephropathies. *N Engl J Med* 1998, 339:1448–1456.

ANTIHYPERTENSIVE THERAPY: COMPLIANCE AND QUALITY OF LIFE

Richard B. Anderson and Gordon H. Williams

Health-related *quality of life* (QOL) refers to the ability of an individual to perform in a number of roles in society and to reach an acceptable level of satisfaction from functioning in these roles. A comprehensive and universal definition of QOL is difficult to achieve, probably because the precise elements for evaluating QOL vary under different circumstances and in different individuals. Furthermore, the definition of a "good" QOL may vary depending on the culture, age, gender, and personal preference of the individual.

The application of QOL techniques to the evaluation of antihypertensive therapy has received increasing emphasis for several reasons. First, it is assumed that hypertensive patients are asymptomatic. Second, many antihypertensive medications are available, and nearly all have been proven equally effective in lowering blood pressure in large, population-based studies. Third, at present there is little information to guide the physician in the selection of a particular agent for a specific patient. Fourth, all antihypertensive treatment programs have annoying, if not serious, side effects. Finally, a substantial degree of noncompliance is associated with antihypertensive therapy.

The utility of a QOL study is based not only on its ability to distinguish adequately the impact of different medications on QOL, but also on the reliability of the conclusion that there is or is no difference among agents. The clinician must carefully evaluate QOL reports for potential statistical type 2 or β errors, *ie*, the incorrect conclusion that there is no difference when one does exist. The correct interpretation of many QOL studies, therefore, is obscured because of one or more of the following problems: a substitute endpoint, too short a study period, too few subjects enrolled, inappropriate study instruments, or the absence of a positive control. Thus, in studies that report no difference among therapeutic agents, each of these five areas should be evaluated carefully.

Substantial advances have been made in the application of QOL technology to the assessment of antihypertensive therapy. Available QOL instruments can detect significant differences in patients treated with all classes of antihypertensive agents and even among drugs in the same class—a remarkable sensitivity. In addition, baseline QOL substantially affects the response of the patient to a particular drug [1]. Finally, some QOL instruments have been calibrated against life events questionnaires, thereby allowing assessment of the clinical relevance of QOL change scores. Thus the clinician now has an additional tool in deciding which drug to use in a particular hypertensive patient. In addition to efficacy and significant physical symptoms, information regarding the impact of a particular drug on the QOL of the patient is rapidly becoming available. Use of this information should improve compliance and may also have an economic impact on improved work performance and less absenteeism because of drug side effects.

BACKGROUND

COMPLIANCE

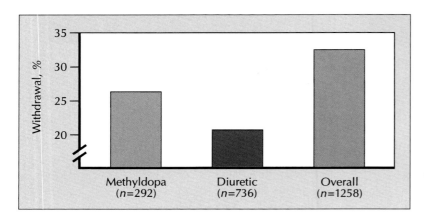

FIGURE 11-1. The Hypertension Detection and Follow-Up Program trial [2,3]. This trial was one of the largest hypertension studies ever conducted. Its goal was to compare the effects of standard and intensive stepped-care therapy on several outcome measures including death and disability. For 5 years, 3500 hypertensive patients on active treatment were followed up. Despite intensive efforts to maintain patients in the clinical trial, 33% withdrew. Nearly one fifth of the patients on diuretic therapy and more than a quarter of the patients on methyldopa had withdrawn from the study during the 5-year follow-up. (*Adapted from* The Hypertension Detection and Follow-Up Program Cooperative Group [2].)

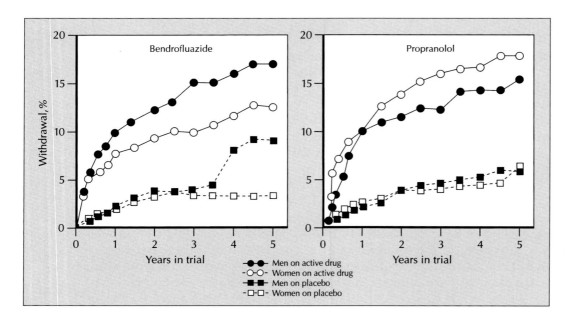

FIGURE 11-2. The Medical Research Council trial [4]. This group also provided interesting insights into the relationship between duration of treatment and dropout rates. This study enrolled over 14,000 patients; 50% received placebo, and 50% were treated with propranolol or a diuretic (bendrofluazide). Individuals treated with placebo withdrew at a rate of 3% to 5%, with the rate plateauing approximately 2 years into the study. The pattern of withdrawal in patients on active therapy was similar, with the steep part of the curve lasting for the first 18 months of therapy and a plateau occurring between 2 and 3 years. (*Adapted from* The Medical Research Council Working Party on Mild-to-Moderate Hypertension [4].)

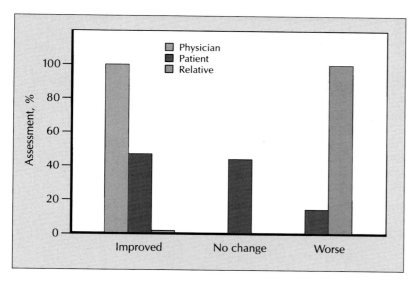

FIGURE 11-3. The problem of patient compliance may not be readily appreciated by the physician and, at least in the usual physician-patient interchange, concerns may not be expressed easily by the patient [5]. Jachuck *et al.* [6] studied 75 hypertensive patients whose blood pressures were normalized with standard therapy. A series of questions designed to determine whether the patient's general well-being was modified by normalization of his or her blood pressure was asked of the physician, the patient, and a relative of the patient. Nearly all physicians assumed the patients were improved. Only half of the patients agreed with their physicians, but only 10% assumed they were worse on therapy than off. In sharp contrast, the relatives of the patients, who had no appreciable contact with the physicians, stated almost universally that the patients were worse on therapy. Thus the discrepancy between the physician's, patients', and relatives' assessment of the utility of antihypertensive therapy may be a major factor contributing to the low compliance rate. (*Adapted from* Jachuck *et al.* [6].)

HYPERTENSION AWARENESS, TREATMENT, AND CONTROL RATES

	1971–1972, %*	1974–1975, %*	1976–1980, n (%)†	1988–1991, n (%)‡
Aware (told by physician)	51	64	73(54)	84(65)
Treated (on medication)	36	34	56(33)	73(49)
Controlled (blood pressure < 160/95 mm Hg on one-occasion measurement and reported currently taking antihypertensive medications)	16	20	34(11)	55(21)

*Data from Roberts [8].
†Data from Rowland and Roberts [9].
‡Data from NHANES III, unpublished data provided by the Centers for Disease Control and Prevention, National Center for Health Statistics.

FIGURE 11-4. Hypertension awareness, treatment, and control rates. At approximately 5-year intervals since the early 1970s the National Center for Health Statistics has evaluated the health of the US population [6]. Over a 20-year period from the early 1970s to the early 1990s, there was a substantial increase in the percentage of hypertensive patients who were aware of their disease. *Hypertensive* patients included those with a blood pressure of 160/95 mm Hg or higher on one-occasion measurement or those reported as currently taking antihypertensive medication. There has been a concomitant increase in

the percentage of hypertensives on medication. The percentage who are controlled (defined by a reduction in blood pressure < 140/90 mm Hg), however, has remained relatively flat. Thus over the past 20 years there has been a substantial increase in the general public's knowledge about hypertension but no appreciable change in its control, suggesting a substantial degree of noncompliance. *Numbers in parentheses* indicate the percentage of patients with blood pressures of 140/90 mm Hg. (*Adapted from* The Fifth Report of the Joint National Committee on Detection, Evaluation and Treatment of High Blood Pressure [7].)

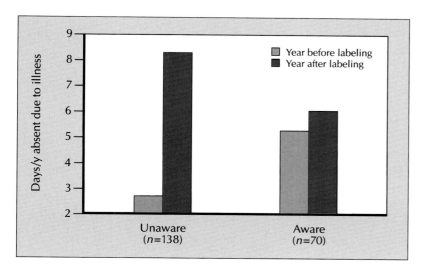

FIGURE 11-5. Effect of hypertension diagnosis on work attendance. In addition to the impact of adverse effects of drug therapy on patients' well-being, the diagnosis of hypertension per se may modify the way they behave. Absenteeism from work may be an indirect reflection of the patient's perception of his or her state of health. The rates of absenteeism before and after labeling the patient as a hypertensive are substantially different [10].

Patients were "labeled" as hypertensive on the day of a screening examination and were also asked whether they were aware that they had hypertension. In those who were unaware they had hypertension, absenteeism in the year prior to labeling was one third of that in the year after labeling. In contrast, those who knew they had hypertension showed no appreciable change in their overall absenteeism rate. Thus drug effects and the diagnosis of hypertension itself can lead to a modification in the patient's sense of well-being. (*Adapted from* Haynes *et al.* [10].)

THE FIVE DOMAINS OF QUALITY OF LIFE

Sense of well-being and life satisfaction
Physical state
Emotional state
Intellectual functioning
Work performance and social participation

FIGURE 11-6. The five domains of quality of life (QOL). Medically related QOL can be divided into five separate subsets or domains. In some studies, only one or two domains are assessed. Which domains a specific study uses is determined in part by the outcomes the investigator wishes to monitor. In general, the more complete the QOL assessment, the more reliable the conclusions. This may not be true, however, if the therapy modifies only one of the domains while the others remain relatively unaffected.

COMPONENTS OF QUALITY OF LIFE: HYPERTENSION

COMPONENT	ASSESSMENT TECHNIQUE	MEASURES
Presence of adverse reactions and physical symptoms	Clinical examination	Simple checklist of common reactions
Distress associated with symptoms	Preclinical questionnaire	Physical, sexual, somatic, cognitive
Emotional status	Preclinical questionnaire	Well-being, vitality, anxiety, depression, sleep disturbance
Life satisfaction	Preclinical questionnaire or interview	Social, personal, marital, job

FIGURE 11-7. Components of quality of life (QOL) in the setting of hypertension. For the hypertensive patient, QOL is best determined by using the same criteria as those used for healthy individuals because in most cases the patients are asymptomatic. Four components are used, each with specific assessment techniques. To assess physical symptoms, for example, usually the clinical examination is used with a simple checklist for common adverse events. An increasingly more complex approach is necessary to evaluate other components of the patient's QOL [11–16]. (*Adapted from* Williams and Testa [15].)

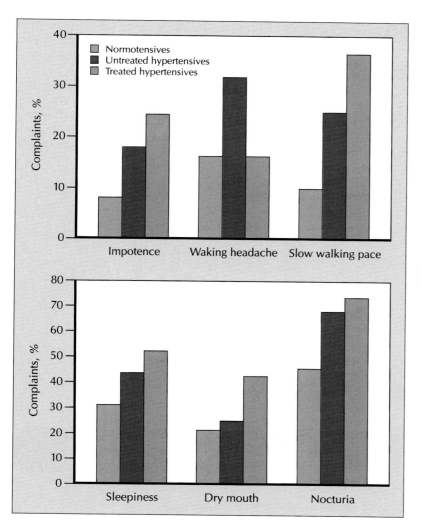

FIGURE 11-8. First-level assessment of quality of life (QOL). A study reported by Bulpitt *et al.* [17] in normotensive and hypertensive subjects provides an example of the first level of assessing QOL. In this study, several clinical questions were asked of each subject. The subjects were divided into normotensive, untreated hypertensive, and treated hypertensive groups. The importance of including a normotensive control group is readily apparent. It is generally assumed that drug treatment may be associated with an increase in impotency and nocturia. Yet from this study it is clear that hypertension alone may be accompanied by a significant frequency of these two complaints. The difference between the untreated hypertensive patients and the normotensive patients also suggests that hypertension alone may be accompanied by adverse events that could be reversed by treatment. Thus studies assessing the effect of antihypertensive therapy on QOL need to ensure that comparable reductions in blood pressure are achieved in the treatment groups in order to minimize the impact of a confounding variable. (*Adapted from* Bulpitt *et al.* [17].)

ASSESSMENT TECHNIQUES

VITALITY SUBSCALE

How much energy, pep, or vitality did you have or feel (during the past month)?
6—Very full of energy; lots of pep
5—Fairly energetic most of the time
4—My energy level varied quite a bit
3—Generally low in energy or pep
2—Very low in energy or pep most of the time
1—No energy or pep at all; I felt drained, sapped

ANXIETY SUBSCALE

Have you been anxious, worried, or upset (during the past month)?
1—Extremely so; to the point of being sick or almost sick
2—Very much so
3—Quite a bit
4—Some; enough to bother me
5—A little bit
6—Not at all

FIGURE 11-9. Sample question from the vitality subscale. Quality of life instruments are a series of questionnaires that are usually self-administered with minimal guidance from trained personnel. An alternative approach is a series of interviews by trained interviewers. The risk involved with the second approach is the introduction of an inapparent bias by the interviewer. In most cases, the questions allow for five to seven graded responses by the subject and usually ask the subject to limit his or her assessment to a certain finite period of time, *ie*, the past week or month. The responses vary from "not at all" to "extremely so" [15].

FIGURE 11-10. Sample question from the anxiety subscale. The questions are scored in such a way that desirable responses are always ranged high and undesirable responses are ranked low. Thus, depending on the nature of the question, the first response level may either be a 6 or a 1 (*see* Fig. 11-9). Questions assessing a similar dimension of quality of life are then grouped together and an average score calculated for that particular dimension. These scores are then usually normalized on a scale of 100 to 600, 1 to 10, or 1 to 100.

COMPOSITION OF QUALITY OF LIFE INDICES

	COMPOSITE INDEX		
DIMENSION	PSYCHOLOGIC WELL-BEING	PSYCHOLOGIC DISTRESS	GENERAL PERCEIVED HEALTH
Anxiety		X	
Behavioral or emotional control		X	
Depression		X	
Emotional ties	X		
General positive affect	X		
Life satisfaction	X		
Vitality			X
General health status			X
Sleep			X
Sexual functioning			
Cognitive functioning			
Work well-being			

FIGURE 11-11. The components of a quality of life (QOL) index. These components are divided into several individual dimensions. These dimensions can be grouped together to provide subscales that will provide a composite index of QOL. Each of the individual dimensions has its own specific score (*see* Figs. 11-9 and 11-10). The subindices, *eg*, psychologic well-being, general perceived health, and psychologic distress, were originally developed by the Rand Corporation [18–20] and have been adapted by a number of investigators. An overall QOL assessment would include not only the composite index but also sexual functioning, cognitive functioning, and work or social well-being [21–24]. An unresolved question is how to average the QOL subscales to produce a composite QOL index. It is unclear whether a simple mean of the scores is correct, yet weighting them may lead to erroneous conclusions if the perceptions of the patient and the investigator are not similar.

APPLICATION TO ANTIHYPERTENSIVE THERAPY

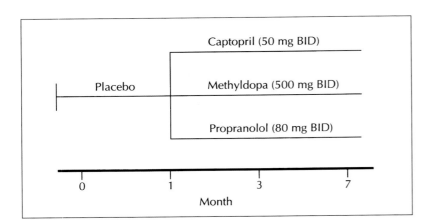

FIGURE 11-12. Results from a study on quality of life (QOL) assessment techniques. QOL assessment techniques have been used in general in cross-sectional studies of large populations to evaluate primarily medical and social issues. In 1986, Croog *et al.* [25] documented the applicability of these techniques to assess the impact of antihypertensive therapy on the QOL of patients enrolled in a clinical trial. They used a standard clinical format, enrolling over 600 subjects, and after a 4-week washout period, randomized them into three treatment groups: propranolol, methyldopa, or captopril. In each case, hydrochlorothiazide, 25 mg twice daily, was added at month 3 if blood pressure was not normalized so that the confounding effect of an elevated blood pressure per se on the patients' QOL could be avoided (*see* Fig. 11-8). This clinical trial was primarily an assessment of the utility of these techniques to measure the impact of drug therapy. Thus there was a positive (methyldopa) and a negative control (captopril). The patients completed questionnaires designed to evaluate QOL, using a format similar to that outlined in Figures 11-9, 11-10, and 11-11, at the beginning of the trial and at its completion 24 weeks later (or at the time of withdrawal). (*Adapted from* Croog *et al.* [25].)

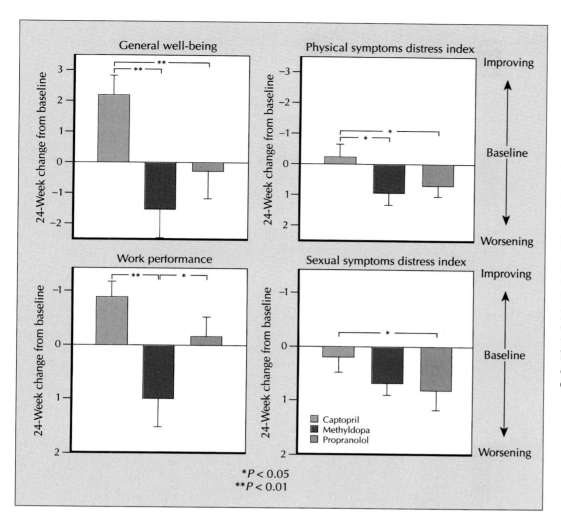

FIGURE 11-13. The overall results of the study discussed in Figure 11-12. Mean (± SEM) rates of change from baseline values for quality of life (*T bars*) are compared for each of the three treatment groups. As anticipated, for each of the indices, except sexual symptoms, methyldopa fared the worst. For most indices, propranolol had no appreciable effect except for the sexual symptoms distress index. While physical and sexual symptoms distress indices did not change while the patients were under treatment with captopril, both work performance and general well-being improved significantly. This improvement was unanticipated and suggests either that these patients had symptoms caused by their hypertension that were relieved by lowering the blood pressure with an agent that had no side effects per se, or that captopril had some unique feature to enhance general well-being and work performance independent of its antihypertensive effect. (*Adapted from* Croog *et al.* [25].)

	Therapy		
Quality	Captopril	Methyldopa	Propranolol
General well-being	■ Improved	□ Stable	□ Stable
Physical symptoms	□ Stable	■ Worse	■ Worse
Sexual dysfunction	□ Stable	■ Worse	■ Worse
Work performance	■ Improved	□ Stable	□ Stable
Sleep dysfunction	□ Stable	□ Stable	□ Stable
Cognitive function	■ Improved	■ Improved	■ Improved
Life satisfaction	□ Stable	■ Worse	■ Worse
Social participation	□ Stable	□ Stable	■ Worse

■ Improved   □ Stable   ■ Worse

FIGURE 11-14. Changes in quality of life (QOL) scales from baseline values for patients who completed Croog *et al.*'s 24-week treatment program [25]. Improvement and worsening reflect a significant (*P* < 0.05) change from baseline values. In general, the individual changes in the QOL domains paralleled the overall subscale changes. Captopril-treated patients showed either no change or an improvement, whereas patients treated with methyldopa showed a deterioration in four of the eight domains. (*Adapted from* Croog *et al.* [25].)

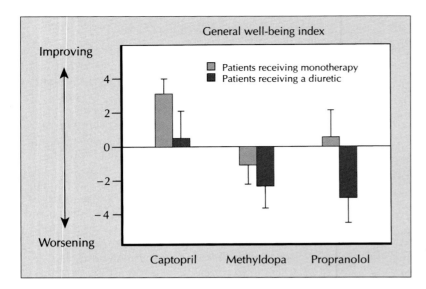

FIGURE 11-15. The effect of diuretics on general well-being. An analysis of this data set addressing the effect of diuretics was also undertaken [26]. Comparison of mean (*T bars* indicate ± SEM) changes after 24 weeks of therapy from baseline for the general well-being index is displayed with each of the three treatment groups divided into those who did and those who did not receive diuretics. Diuretics profoundly reduced quality of life (QOL) in all treatment groups, with the most dramatic effect occurring in those also treated with propranolol. Caution in interpreting these data is necessary because patients were not randomly assigned into mono- versus two-drug therapy. It is unclear whether the changes observed in the patients requiring two drugs are the result of their being part of a different population or of their having received a diuretic. However, baseline QOL indices were not different between those who did and those who did not require a diuretic. (*Adapted from* Williams *et al.* [26].)

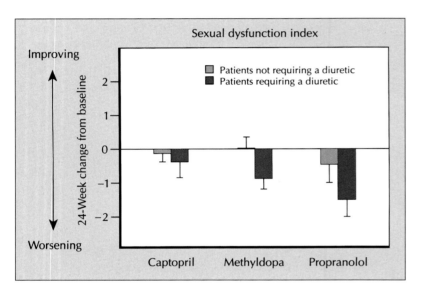

FIGURE 11-16. The effect of diuretics on sexual function. Comparison of mean (*T bars* indicate ± SEM) changes after 24 weeks of therapy from baseline for the sexual dysfunction index is displayed in patients divided into two subgroups—those on monotherapy and those also requiring a diuretic [26]. As was true for the general well-being index, diuretics also had a negative impact on this quality of life subscale beyond that produced by monotherapy. (*Adapted from* Williams *et al.* [26].)

COMMON ERRORS IN QOL STUDY DESIGN

Substitute endpoints
Inappropriate study design
Too short
Too few subjects
Inappropriate questionnaires

FIGURE 11-17. Common errors in quality of life (QOL) study design. A variety of errors are common in QOL studies [27,28]. In general these errors tend to produce a β or type 2 statistical error, *ie*, the apparent absence of a significant difference when such differences actually exist. The most common problem is an inappropriate study design. However, inappropriate questionnaires (simplified questionnaires that have not been validated) and substitute endpoints (*eg*, using a decrease in blood pressure as the primary determinant of an improvement in QOL) were also apparent in the analysis of these studies.

FIGURE 11-18. Three critical questions need to be addressed regarding the utility of quality of life (QOL) techniques in determining appropriate therapy in hypertensive patients. Limited data were available to determine the sensitivity of the QOL instruments. Most importantly, even when statistically significant differences were demonstrated among different treatment programs, their clinical relevance was unclear.

CLINICAL RELEVANCE AND SENSITIVITY

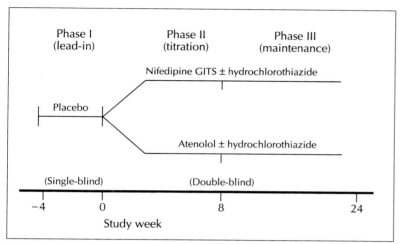

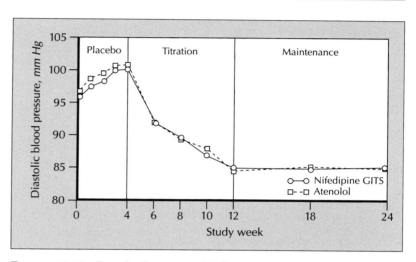

FIGURE 11-19. Nifedipine versus atenolol study. Testa *et al.* [29] reported a double-blind placebo-controlled comparison of nifedipine gastrointestinal therapeutic system (GITS) and atenolol. The authors used an approach similar to that used by Croog *et al.* [25] in that hydrochlorothiazide could be added to normalize blood pressure. The study consisted of a 4-week washout period and a 24-week treatment phase. The dose of the primary agent was titrated and hydrochlorothiazide was added (if necessary) to the highest dose. The primary goals of the study were to determine whether commonly used antihypertensive agents have a differential effect on quality of life (QOL), and the relationship of QOL changes in subjects who completed the study versus those who withdrew. Nearly 400 patients began this study; approximately one third failed to complete the entire 24-week active treatment portion. (*Adapted from* Testa *et al.* [29].)

FIGURE 11-20. Results from the nifedipine gastrointestinal therapeutic system (GITS) versus atenolol study. Both treatment programs normalized blood pressure to approximately the same extent. (*Adapted from* Testa *et al.* [29].)

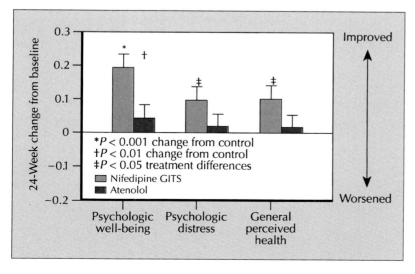

FIGURE 11-21. The change in quality of life (QOL) scores from baseline to the end of the study by Testa *et al.* [29] for three subscales depicted for those patients who completed the entire protocol. Nifedipine gastrointestinal therapeutic system (GITS) had a more positive impact on QOL scores. (*T bars* indicate mean ± SEM.) (*Adapted from* Testa *et al.* [29].)

QUALITY OF LIFE CHANGE SCORES

	TREATMENT			
	NIFEDIPINE GITS		ATENOLOL	
QOL Scale	Completed (*n* = 119)	Withdrawn (*n* = 68)	Completed (*n* = 131)	Withdrawn (*n* = 47)
Psychologic well-being	0.195 ± 0.04*	-0.117 ± 0.07	0.041 ± 0.05	-0.018 ± 0.08

* *P* < 0.001 between completers and withdrawals.

FIGURE 11-22. Quality of life (QOL) change scores. In evaluating a QOL clinical trial, careful attention must be paid to the impact of patient withdrawal from the study on the QOL indices. With some agents, the QOL of those who withdraw compared with those who remain in the study are not substantially different, whereas with other agents a substantial difference occurs. In the study by Testa *et al.* [29], in which approximately the same number of patients in each treatment group withdrew, the impact on the QOL indices was quite different between the two agents. Those patients treated with atenolol showed little difference in QOL change scores (represented by psychologic well-being; mean ± SEM) whether or not they withdrew. In contrast, individuals treated with nifedipine gastrointestinal therapeutic system (GITS) who withdrew from the study had profoundly negative QOL change scores in contrast to the positive scores of those who completed the study. (*Adapted from* Testa *et al.* [29].)

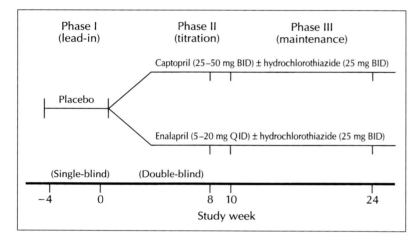

FIGURE 11-23. Further study on quality of life (QOL) change. Testa *et al.* [30] reported a second study in which the overall goals included the following: 1) to test the sensitivity of quality of life (QOL) instruments by determining whether they could measure the differential impact on QOL of two antihypertensive agents from the same class (enalapril and captopril); 2) to evaluate the impact of baseline QOL on the response to therapy; and 3) to determine the clinical relevance of any statistical differences in QOL scores. The study design was similar to that of Croog *et al.* [25] except that captopril and enalapril were used in escalating doses, with the addition of hydrochlorothiazide, if needed, to normalize blood pressure. QOL assessments were performed at the beginning and at the end of the study. Approximately 400 subjects were randomly assigned to each treatment group, with a 15% to 18% overall withdrawal rate. (*Adapted from* Testa *et al.* [30].)

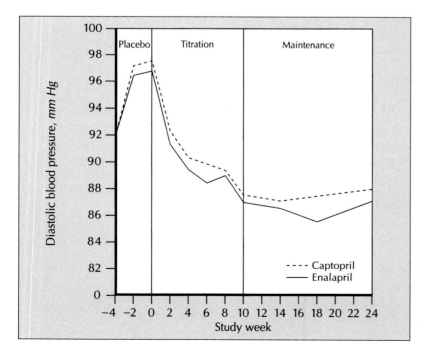

FIGURE 11-24. Blood pressure responses to therapy. Blood pressure responses to therapy were equivalent in the two treatment groups of the study described in Figure 11-23 [30]. Additionally, baseline quality of life scores were indistinguishable, suggesting that the randomization procedure produced equivalent groups.

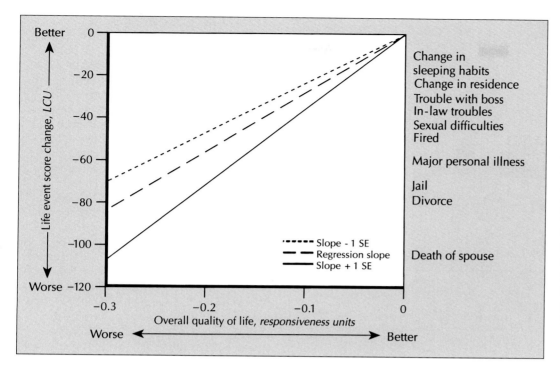

FIGURE 11-25. Clinical relevance of quality of life (QOL) change scores. One of the questions addressed in the study by Testa *et al.* [30] was the clinical relevance of QOL change scores. This was accomplished by having each subject also complete a life events questionnaire on the day he or she completed a QOL questionnaire. The life events questionnaire asks the subject whether certain events had occurred in his or her life over the previous month. The life events scores were calibrated using previously published data [31]. Overall QOL change scores in responsiveness units (modified standard deviations) are plotted against life event score changes. The life event scores varied from a -12 for a change in sleeping habits to a -100 for the death of a spouse. LCU—life change unit; SE—standard error of the mean. (*Adapted from* Testa *et al.* [30].)

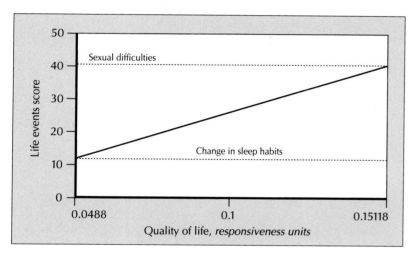

FIGURE 11-26. Minimally clinically relevant changes from Testa *et al.*'s [30] study. The upper portion of Figure 11-25 is expanded and reversed to include minimally clinically relevant changes as determined by the life events scores. Thus, these data suggest that with the quality of life (QOL) instruments used and the specific study design, clinically relevant changes in QOL responsiveness units are between 0.1 and 0.2. Changes of this magnitude are equivalent to difficulties associated with changes in sleeping habits, trouble with one's employer, or sexual difficulties. (*Adapted from* Testa *et al.* [30].)

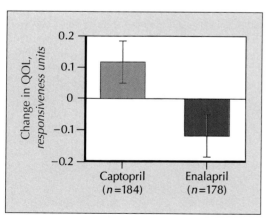

FIGURE 11-27. The overall impact of captopril versus enalapril on quality of life (QOL) is depicted as mean ± SEM (indicated by *T bars*). All subject groups are included—both those who completed and those who withdrew from the study. Changes from baseline are shown. The difference was significant ($P < 0.04$). Of equal importance, the mean difference between the two treatment groups was also clinically relevant if the changes observed with the calibration curves shown in Figures 11-25 and 11-26 are compared. (*Adapted from* Testa *et al.* [30].)

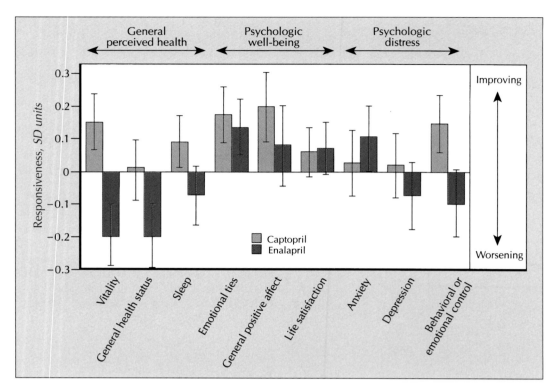

FIGURE 11-28. Comparison of the individual domains grouped together into the three major subscales (*see* Fig. 11-11). All data shown are mean ± SEM (indicated by *T bars*) for all patients in the study—both those who completed and those who withdrew. The data are displayed as changes from baseline to endpoint in standard deviation (SD) responsiveness units. Few differences were observed between the two treatment groups in psychologic well-being or psychologic distress subscales. Most of the overall differences in quality of life (QOL) occurred because of the differential effects of the two agents on general perceived health, where vitality, general health status, and sleep were significantly different ($P < 0.05$) between the two treatment groups. These data, therefore, illustrate the power of QOL technology not only to assess the overall impact of different agents on QOL but also to determine the individual components of QOL that are affected differentially by various agents. (*Adapted from* Testa *et al.* [30].)

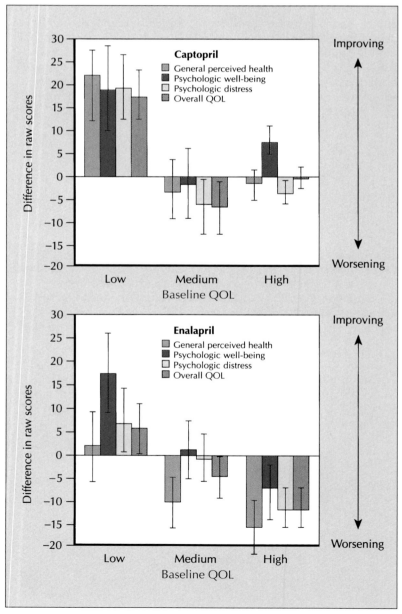

FIGURE 11-29. Baseline quality of life (QOL) of patients entering a clinical trial. It might be anticipated that the baseline QOL of patients entering a clinical trial may influence their response to therapy. For example, those individuals who begin a trial with a relatively low QOL are likely not to perceive a further reduction in QOL in response to treatment side effects, but might see an improvement in QOL caused by amelioration of disease effects. The opposite could occur in individuals with a high QOL. In this study, patients treated with enalapril showed this more typical pattern whether overall QOL or its subscales (general perceived health, psychologic well-being, and psychologic distress) were observed. In contrast, patients treated with captopril had a different response pattern. Those individuals with a low baseline QOL had an overall significant increase in QOL, whereas those in the middle and high groups showed no particular QOL change in response to treatment. These results strongly suggest that any evaluations of the impact of drug therapy on QOL should take into account the baseline QOL in the population being studied. While an alternate statistical inter-pretation of the enalapril data is possible (regression to the mean), such an explanation could not explain the captopril results unless the overall mean actually increased under treatment. Changes in QOL raw scale points are plotted (mean ± SEM) as *T bars*. The overall population was divided into thirds—low, medium, and high—based on entry QOL. The actual baseline QOL scores in the two treatment groups were identical for each subgroup. (*Adapted from* Testa *et al.* [30].)

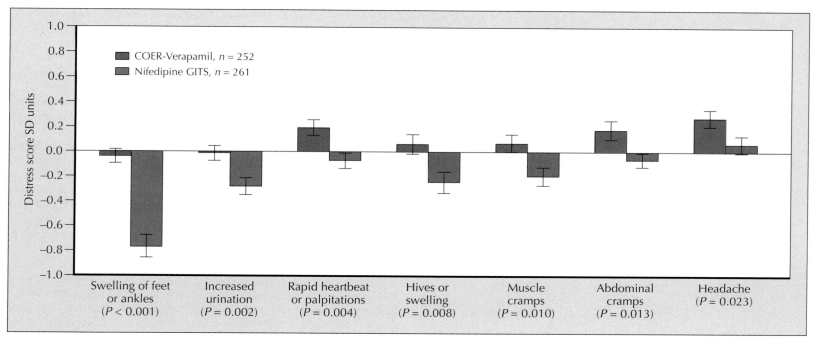

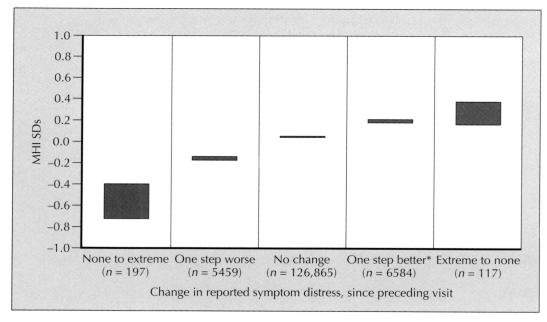

FIGURE 11-30. Assessing the impact of psychosocial instruments on drug therapy quality of life (QOL). Despite more than 20 years of using psychosocial instruments to assess the impact of drug therapy on quality of life, many physicians remain unconvinced of their utility because of the nonclinical characteristics of the generated data. Anderson [31] has bridged this gap by developing a tool that can be understood by the clinician and correlating it with the psychosocial tools commonly used by the social scientist. Anderson refined the standard symptom check by asking the subject not only whether a symptom was present, but also the degree of the distress of the symptom. To test this instrument, a standard clinical trial format was used, where two calcium channel blockers were compared: COER-verapamil and nifedipine gastrointestinal therapeutic system (GITS) after a 4-week placebo washout. The patient's symptom distress was assessed several times over a 10-week treatment period. A difference in the level of physical symptom distress was detected between treatments (P = 0.002; multivariate analysis of variance). Eight significant univariate treatment effects were noted: pedal edema, polyuria, rapid heartbeat, palpitations, hives, muscle cramps, abdominal cramps, and headaches. Interestingly, constipation-related distress increased significantly (P = 0.001) but to a similar extent with both treatments. Thus, the well-known effect of verapamil causing constipation was equally present in individuals treated with nifedipine if the distress of the symptom was considered. Importantly, the difference in symptom distress correlated with dropout rates (P = 0.066) favoring the COER-verapamil group. (*Adapted from* Anderson [31].)

FIGURE 11-31. Further correlations between psychosocial instruments and quality of life (QOL). Anderson *et al.* [32] extended their analysis to assess the correlations between the standard psychosocial quality of life indices and their newly defined symptom distress index. To obtain the broadest degree of comparability, they studied individuals with hypertension or angina. Several medicines were used to treat these individuals so that a large range in the symptom distress index or the psychosocial QOL was produced. A pool of 1003 patients was evaluated; each patient completed up to five tests, yielding over 200,000 pairs of change scores. The psychosocial QOL instrument that was primarily used was the Rand Mental Health Index (MHI). The change in the MHI score, in units of unadjusted sample standard deviation (SD) of the index, were compared with the changes in concomitantly determined changes in symptom distress. Ninety-five percent CIs for the mean changes are depicted. There was a highly consistent, albeit somewhat surprising correlation between the psychosocial index of QOL and the symptom distress index. With this study, the traditional social scientist approach to evaluating QOL has now been anchored in the terminology of the physician and biologic scientist (physical symptoms and the distress they cause). (*Adapted from* Anderson *et al.* [32].)

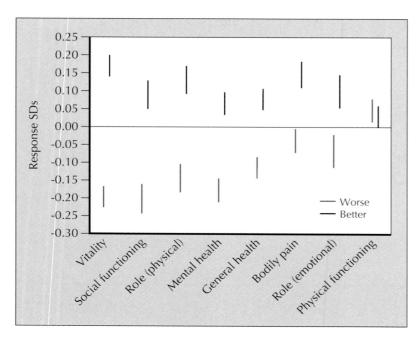

FIGURE 11-32. Mean changes (95% CIs) in SF-36 domain scores in groups of responses defined by concurrent reports of change in symptom distress. To clarify further the relationship between symptom distress and health-related quality of life (HRQOL), Hollenberg *et al.* [33] administered the SF-36 concurrently with an appropriate version of the Symptom Distress Inventory (SDI) to 241 subjects in a trial comparing amlodipine and eplerenone in the context of systolic hypertension. SF-36 is, worldwide, the most commonly adopted operational definition of HRQOL.

The investigators obtained 46,608 concurrent reports of SF-36 and symptom distress change since the preceding visit. Of these reports, 2897 reflected a worsening of symptom distress, whereas 2953 reflected improvement. The bars are 95% CIs, descriptively defined, for the associated SF-36 domain score changes in the "better" and "worse" groups of responses.

Symptom distress and SF-36 are clearly associated both strongly and positively. For all eight SF-36 domains, the domain score improved on average where it was associated with reports of symptom distress improvement. For seven domains, the mean score also typically deteriorated in association with worsening symptom distress. In magnitude, moreover, the typical SF-36 difference lies very much in the same range (one or two tenths of a raw-score standard deviation) that we observed [30] in calibrating the subscales of the Rand Mental Health Index against life events by a similar procedure.

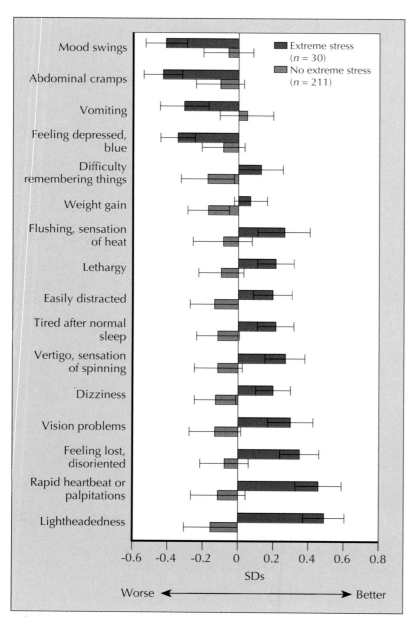

FIGURE 11-33. Symptom distress change from baseline to endpoint for patients reporting extreme stress, and for patients reporting no extreme stress (mean, ± SE).

Although the Symptom Distress Inventory shows every sign of measuring phenomena highly correlated with those addressed by SF-36, a new measure of external stress appears to bear a more complex relationship to symptom distress. At each visit in the same trial that yielded the results in Figure 11-32, each patient also completed a 12-point Life Events Stress Inventory (LESI). Secondary analysis of a descriptive, exploratory character reveals that at some point, 30 subjects reported extreme stress from external life events, whereas the remaining 211 did not. This figure contrasts four symptoms that were worse for the subjects under stress with 12 symptoms that were actually reported as better.

Tentatively, as befits exploratory analysis, one may interpret the first, negative cluster as "symptoms of stress" (the kinds of symptoms that arise when one experiences stress, whatever its origin); and the second, positive cluster as "symptoms that stress may relieve" or at least mask, by focusing the mind elsewhere and energizing the body's stress-response mechanisms. These early results require extensive replication. (*Adapted from* Anderson *et al.* [34].)

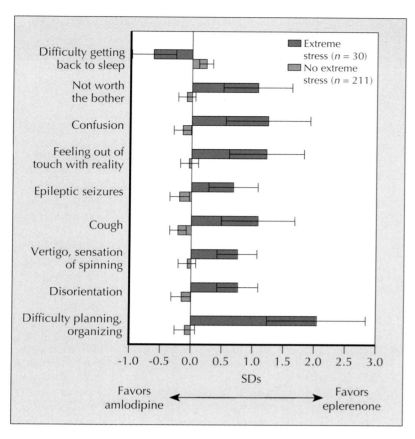

FIGURE 11-34. Symptom distress: treatment effect on change from baseline to endpoint for patients reporting extreme stress, and for patients reporting no extreme stress (mean, ± SE).

Subjects who reported extreme stress also reported, on average, a pattern of treatment effects on symptom distress nonrandomly different from that of their unstressed fellow subjects. The primary analysis of these data revealed that, relative to eplerenone, amlodipine was poorly tolerated, in that it induced a wide range of distressful symptoms. This secondary analysis suggests that this contrast holds particularly strongly for patients under external stress.

The analysis singled out one amlodipine-favoring effect (difficulty getting back to sleep), and identified a list of eight eplerenone-favoring effects on symptom distress (difficulty planning, organizing; disorientation; vertigo, sensation of spinning; cough; epileptic seizures, feeling out of touch with reality; confusion; "not worth the bother").

These stress-specific treatment effects, particularly the eplerenone-favoring ones, are very large, ranging from 0.8 to 2.1 standard deviations, a whole order of magnitude larger than 1) the average overall treatment effect, or 2) the trial's prespecified threshold of clinical significance (0.15 standard deviations).

This study marks the first time that we have looked for interactions of stress with other indicators of quality of life. When we looked, we found them. Further research will doubtless document further instances and illuminate their implications for research methodology and clinical practice. (*Adapted from* Anderson *et al.* [34].)

FUTURE DIRECTIONS

FUTURE ASSESSMENT

Standardize QOL methodology

Use QOL technology to evaluate all therapeutic agents

Expand QOL techniques to an assessment of economic impact

FIGURE 11-35. During the past decade, a number of studies clearly have established the feasibility of applying the instruments used by social scientists to evaluate quality of life (QOL) for measuring the impact of drug therapy in longitudinal studies. There are a variety of instruments and approaches that can be used to obtain this information. In some cases, erroneous conclusions may have been drawn based on inappropriate trial design or the use of inappropriate instruments. One major need in the future is to standardize the methodology by using the best techniques available as documented in specific clinical trials. With the establishment of standard methodology, it is imperative that all new therapeutic agents include an assessment of the agent's impact on the QOL of the patient, particularly in comparative trials. The power of this technology has yet to be fully exploited in assessing the economic consequences of different forms of therapy. Economic considerations are becoming increasingly important in therapeutic decision making, particularly in treating chronic diseases such as hypertension [35–38]. However, reliable and comprehensive cost data are not available. Medication costs are easily obtained but likely reflect less than 10% of the total cost of patient care. Of greater importance are the costs associated with physician, nurse, and dietitian time; laboratory tests; hospitalization because of noncompliance or poor compliance; sick days either from disease, the side effects of medications, or visits to physicians; and finally, altered work performance due to differential effects of medications on the patient's QOL. An additional hidden cost not considered in assessing the economic impact of different forms of therapy is the cost of having to switch therapy when medications are discontinued because of intolerable adverse impact on the patient's QOL. Thus, at present we have a limited ability to evaluate economic factors in clinical decision making because the readily available economic factors probably represent only a small proportion of the total economic impact of different forms of therapy.

REFERENCES

1. Grimm RH, Jr, Grandits GA, Cutler JA, et al.: Relationships of quality-of-life measures to long-term lifestyle and drug treatment in the Treatment of Mild Hypertension Study. Arch Intern Med 1997, 157:638–648.

2. Hypertension Detection and Follow-Up Program Cooperative Group: Five-year findings of the Hypertension Detection and Follow-Up Program. I: Reduction in mortality in persons with high blood pressure. JAMA 1979, 242:2562–2577.

3. Hypertension Detection and Follow-Up Program Cooperative Group: The effects of treatment on mortality in "mild" hypertension: results of the Hypertension Detection and Follow-Up Program. N Engl J Med 1982, 307:976–980.

4. Medical Research Council Working Party on Mild-to-Moderate Hypertension: Adverse reactions to bendrofluazide and propranolol for the treatment of mild hypertension. Lancet 1981, 2(8246):539–544.

5. Kitler ME: The changing face of hypertension and antihypertensive agents. Drugs Aging 1996, 8:5–11.

6. Jachuck SJ, Brierley H, Jachuck S, et al.: The effect of hypotensive drugs on the quality of life. J R Coll Gen Pract 1982, 32:103–105.

7. The Fifth Report of the Joint National Committee on Detection, Evaluation and Treatment of High Blood Pressure. Bethesda, MD: National Institutes of Health; 1993:93–1088.

8. Roberts J: Blood pressure of persons 18–74 years, United States, 1971-72. Data from the National Health Survey, Washington, DC: National Center for Health Statistics, 1975; DHEW publication no. 75-1632. (Vital and health statistics; series 11, no. 150).

9. Rowland M, Roberts J: Blood pressure levels and hypertension in persons ages 6–74 years: United States, 1976-80. Hyattsville, MD: National Center for Health Statistics, October 1982; DHHS publication no. 82-1250. (Advance data from vital and health statistics; no. 84).

10. Haynes RB, Sackett DL, Taylor DW, et al.: Increased absenteeism from work after detection and labeling of hypertensive patients. N Engl J Med 1978, 299:741–744.

11. Williams GH: Quality of life and its impact on hypertensive patients. Am J Med 1987, 82:98–105.

12. Spilker B, ed: Quality of Life Assessments in Clinical Trials. New York: Raven Press; 1990.

13. Fava GA, Magnani B: Quality of life: a review of contemporary confusion. Med Sci Res 1988, 16:1051–1054.

14. Hollenberg NK, Testa M, Williams GH: Quality of life as a therapeutic end-point. Drug Safety 1991, 6:83–93.

15. Williams GH, Testa MA: Quality of life: an important consideration in antihypertensive therapy. In Management of Hypertension: A Multifactorial Approach. Edited by Hollenberg NK. Boston: Scientific Therapeutics Information, Inc.; 1987:79–100.

16. Levine S, Croog SH: What constitutes quality of life? A conceptualization of the dimensions of life quality in healthy populations and patients with cardiovascular disease. In Assessment of Quality of Life in Clinical Trials of Cardiovascular Therapies. Edited by Wenger NK, Mattson ME, Furberg CD, et al. New York: LeJacq; 1984:46–58.

17. Bulpitt CJ, Dollery CT, Carne S: Change in symptoms of hypertensive patients after referral to hospital clinic. Br Heart J 1976; 38:121–128.

18. Ware JE, Jr, Johnston SA, Davies-Avery A, et al.: Conceptualization and Measurement of Health for Adults in the Health Insurance Study. Vol III: Mental Health. Santa Monica: Rand Corporation; 1979.

19. Brook RH, Ware JE, Jr, Davies-Avery A, et al.: Conceptualization and Measurement of Health for Adults in the Health Insurance Study. Vol VIII: Overview. Santa Monica: Rand Corporation; 1979.

20. Ware JE Jr, Johnston SA, Davies-Avery A, et al.: Conceptualization and Measurement of Health for Adults in the Health Insurance Study. Vol I: Model of Health and Methodology. Santa Monica: Rand Corporation; 1980.

21. Hogan MJ, Wallin JD, Baer RM: Antihypertensive therapy and male sexual dysfunction. Psychosomatics 1980, 21:234–237.

22. House JS: Work Stress and Social Support. Reading, MA: Addison-Wesley; 1981.

23. Croog SH, Levine S: Life After a Heart Attack: Social and Psychological Factors Eight Years Later. New York: Human Sciences Press; 1982.

24. Campbell A, Converse PE, Rodgers WL: The Quality of American Life. New York: Russell Sage Foundation; 1976.

25. Croog SH, Levine S, Testa MA, et al.: The effects of antihypertensive therapy on the quality of life. N Engl J Med 1986, 314:1657–1664.

26. Williams GH, Croog SH, Levine S, et al: Impact of antihypertensive therapy on quality of life: effect of hydrochlorothiazide. J Hypertens 1987, 5:S29–S35.

27. Beto JA, Bansal VK: Quality of life in treatment of hypertension: a meta-analysis of clinical trials. Am J Hypertens 1992, 5:125–133.

28. Guyatt GH, Van Zanten SJPV, Feeny DH, et al.: Measuring quality of life in clinical trials: a taxonomy and review. Can Med Assoc J 1989, 140:1441–1448.

29. Testa MA, Hollenberg NK, Andersen RB, et al.: Assessment of quality of life by patient and spouse during antihypertensive therapy with atenolol and nifedipine gastrointestinal therapeutic system. Am J Hypertens 1991, 4:363–373.

30. Testa MA, Anderson RA, Nackley JF, et al.: Quality of life and antihypertensive therapy in men: a comparison of captopril with enalapril. N Engl J Med 1993, 328:907–913.

31. Anderson RB: What does it mean? Anchoring psychosocial quality of life score changes with reference to concurrent changes in reported symptom distress. Drug Inf J 1999, 33:445–453.

32. Anderson RB, Hollenberg NK, Williams GH: Physical Symptoms Distress Index: a sensitive tool to evaluate the impact of pharmacological agents on quality of life. Arch Intern Med 1999, 159:693–700.

33. Hollenberg NK, Williams GH, Anderson RB: Symptoms and the distress they cause: comparison of an aldosterone antagonist and a calcium channel blocking agent in patients with systolic hypertension. Arch Intern Med 2002, in press.

34. Anderson RB, Hollenberg NK, Williams GH: Stress arising from external events: implications for assessment of drug effects. Drug Inf J 2002.

35. Weir MR, Prisant LM, Papademetriou V, et al.: Antihypertensive therapy and quality of life. Influence of blood pressure reduction, adverse events, and prior antihypertensive therapy. Am J Hypertens 1996, 9:854–859.

36. Holmes TH, Rahe RH: The Social Readjustment Rating Scale. J Psychsom Res 1967, 11:213–218.

37. Wilson TW, Chockalingam A, Quest DW: Pharmacoeconomics of hypertension control: basic principles of economic evaluation. J Hum Hypertens 1996, 10(suppl 2):19–22.

38. Menard J: Cost-effectiveness of hypertension treatment. Clin Exp Hypertens 1996, 18:399–413.

SPECIAL SITUATIONS IN THE MANAGEMENT OF HYPERTENSION

William J. Elliott and Henry R. Black

The modern physician is charged with integrating the art and science of medicine by extrapolating the results of physiologic studies and clinical trials to individual patients. Indeed, it could be argued that every clinical encounter is a "special situation" that deserves "special consideration." Nonetheless, there are clearly circumstances in which the usual rubrics used in diagnosis and treatment must be modified. This is particularly true when the patient falls into the extremes in terms of demographic groups (*eg*, childhood or old age), when blood pressure (BP) is particularly high (*eg*, hypertensive emergencies), or when BP measurement is accomplished using techniques other than the indirect sphygmomanometric determinations in the physician's office. This chapter attempts to address some of these special situations.

Hypertension involving extremes of age may require special attention not only because of the different pathophysiology of the hypertensive state in childhood and old age, but also because treatment decisions differ among these groups and from those in the more common middle-aged hypertensive individual.

Pregnancy is another important example because during pregnancy there are two patients involved—the mother and the fetus. Obstetricians often choose drug therapy for hypertension in pregnancy. Drug selection in this setting is predicated on the past history of success in treating these women, perhaps influenced by medicolegal concerns, and the resultant difficulty in evaluating new approaches to therapy. During pregnancy, angiotensin-converting enzyme (ACE) inhibitors or angiotensin II receptor blockers (ARBs) are contraindicated due to the risk of fetal malformations. Diuretics should be used only if the patient had been taking them before becoming pregnant or if no other drug is effective in reducing BP. Other antihypertensive agents would probably work but have not been tested. Many pediatricians are reluctant to begin antihypertensive drug therapy in children because no clinical trials have shown that such therapy is beneficial, and some antihypertensive drugs are poorly tolerated by otherwise active children.

The elderly are at greater absolute risk for the adverse clinical sequelae of hypertension, have an increased likelihood of target organ damage, and have a higher probability that other cardiac risk factors are present. Many studies now indicate that significant reductions in stroke, myocardial infarction, and death in elderly patients treated for only a few years (on average) can be achieved using effective antihypertensive drug therapy. There is no longer any question that hypertension in older patients should be treated.

The magnitude of BP elevation is also a special situation that clearly influences prognosis and therapy. Patients with very high BP accompanied by signs or symptoms of acute target organ damage are said to have "hypertensive emergencies." Patients with these syndromes should be treated in the hospital with short-acting, rapidly titratable, and usually parenteral drugs. Therapy leads to a very dramatic improvement in short- and long-term outcome compared with historical controls. Recent clinical trials from the United States, Europe, and China have shown that drug therapy for the most common form of hypertension in elderly patients, isolated systolic hypertension, can successfully and safely reduce BP and, more importantly, prevent stroke and cardiovascular endpoints. Several ongoing clinical trials comparing newer and older agents may prove the benefits of treatment in younger individuals, as well as those patients with less profound elevations in blood pressure.

Another demographic feature, race, has been cited frequently as affecting blood pressure and therapy. Blacks have a higher frequency of hypertensive sequelae, especially stroke and renal insufficiency, and often acquire hypertension at earlier ages than do whites. Some investigators have attributed this difference to specific pathophysiologic features of hypertension in blacks, but these hypotheses may apply more to groups than to specific individuals. Recent research has indicated that, in large groups, diuretics and calcium antagonists appear to achieve BP control more frequently in blacks than do β-blockers or ACE inhibitors (used alone), but blacks still benefit from β-blockers (after myocardial infarction) and from ACE inhibitors (when renal impairment is present). Whether small differences in BP observed in large populations of blacks are important for individual patients is still controversial.

Although most patients with hypertension have no identifiable cause for elevated BP, it can sometimes be attributed to concomitant drug therapy. This special situation also has therapeutic implications. Cocaine, erythropoietin, and cyclosporine all cause elevations in BP; however, when the offending agent cannot be stopped (*eg*, in transplant patients treated with cyclosporine), some antihypertensive therapies have been found generally to be more effective than others.

Although essentially all data used for prognosis and therapy of hypertension are derived from office-based measurements of BP using indirect sphygmomanometry, there is interest (and perhaps some virtue) in measurement of BP outside this setting. Many patients are now using home devices to monitor their BP and therapy. In addition, some patients are being asked to wear BP monitors during their daily activities; this practice has led to entirely new classifications of hypertension, *eg*, "white coat" hypertension, which is present only in the doctor's office. We now have adequate data on normotensive persons that will allow us to decide which BP measurements outside the office are abnormal, but much more work is necessary to use these measurements as guides to prognosis and therapy.

HYPERTENSION IN PREGNANCY

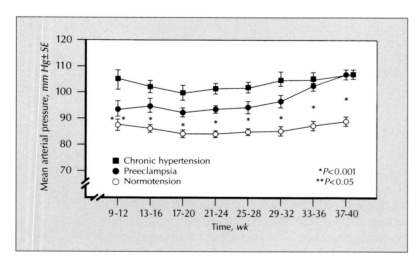

FIGURE 12-1. Because both the mother and the fetus are involved, hypertension in pregnancy has several important implications. This figure illustrates the changes in mean arterial pressure during pregnancy for control patients (*n* = 710), chronically hypertensive women (*n* = 37), and those with preeclampsia (*n* = 46) [1]. Note that blood pressure normally *decreases* during the first trimester and generally remains low until delivery nears. It is currently impossible to predict with certainty which women will develop the higher levels of blood pressure seen in preeclampsia before the last trimester, despite the significantly higher baseline blood pressure on retrospective analysis. There is too much overlap [2].

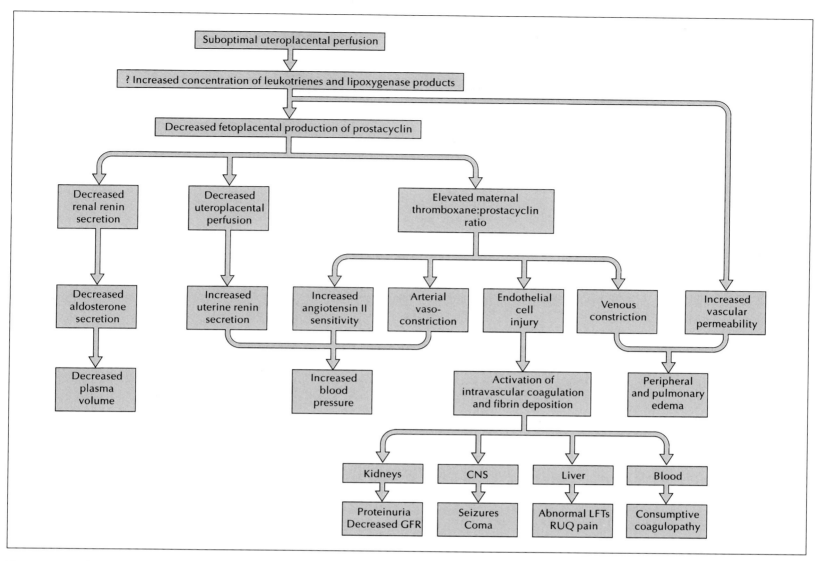

FIGURE 12-2. Scheme proposed to explain some of the patho-physiologic factors thought to be operative in preeclampsia and their consequences [3]. Note that hypertension is but one feature of this complex illness. CNS—central nervous system; GFR—glomerular filtration rate; LFTs—liver function tests; RUQ—right upper quadrant.

HYPERTENSIVE DISORDERS OF PREGNANCY

Chronic hypertension

  BP ≥ 140/90 mm Hg before the 20th week of gestation

Preeclampsia

  Elevated BP (≥ 140/90 mm Hg) in a patient who was normotensive before 20 weeks
    of gestation, accompanied by

  Urinary excretion of ≥ 0.3 g of protein in a 24-h collection

Other features that increase the certainty of the diagnosis of preeclampsia

  BP ≥ 160/110 mm Hg

  Proteinuria ≥ 2.0 g/24 h that appears initially during pregnancy and regresses postpartum

  Newly-elevated serum creatinine concentration (> 1.2 mg/dL)

  Platelet count < 100,000/mm^3 and/or evidence of microangiopathic hemolytic anemia

  Elevated hepatic enzymes (ALT or AST)

Preeclampsia superimposed upon chronic hypertension (which carries a worse prognosis
    than either condition alone) **is more likely with one or more of the following:**

  New onset proteinuria (≥ 0.3 g/24 h)

  Hypertension and proteinuria before 20 weeks of gestation

  Sudden increase in proteinuria

  Sudden increase in BP, despite previous good control

  Thrombocytopenia (platelets < 100,000 mm^3)

  Increase in ALT or AST to abnormal levels

Eclampsia

Occurrence of seizures that cannot be attributed to other causes in a
    patient with preeclampsia

Gestational hypertension

  Transient hypertension of pregnancy (if preeclampsia is not present at time of delivery
    and BP returns to normal by 12 weeks postpartum)

  Chronic hypertension (if the elevated BP seen during pregnancy persists longer than
    12 weeks postpartum)

FIGURE 12-3. Classification of hypertensive disorders of pregnancy. Knowledge of blood pressure (BP) before the 20th week of pregnancy is necessary to identify chronic hypertension. Although edema is commonly found in preeclampsia, its presence is no longer required for the diagnosis [4]. ALT—alanine aminotransferase; AST—aspartate aminotransferase; DBP—diastolic blood pressure.

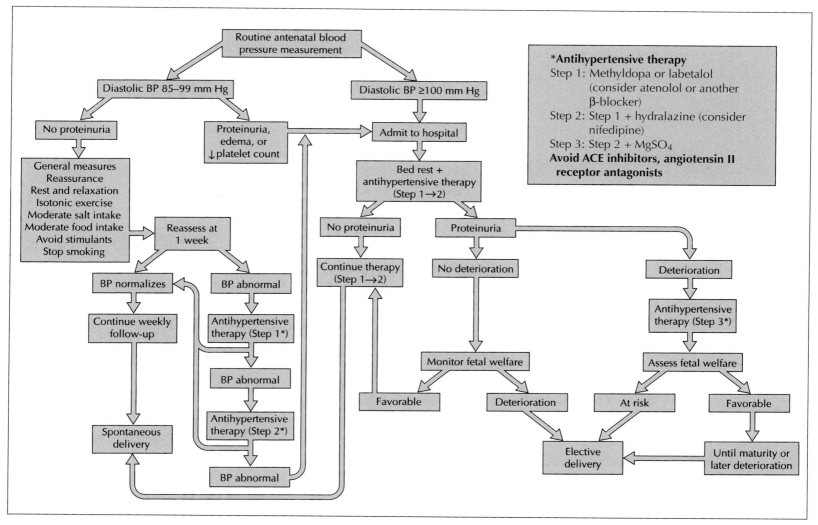

FIGURE 12-4. A conservative approach for management of hypertension in pregnancy. Angiotensin-converting enzyme (ACE) inhibitors and angiotensin II receptor antagonists are contraindicated in pregnancy and in women trying to become pregnant. ACE inhibitors can cause adverse effects on uterine blood flow and lethal acute renal failure in neonates of women treated with them in the last trimester [5]; similar effects are expected with angiotensin II receptor antagonists. BP—blood pressure. (*Adapted from* the Working Group on High Blood Pressure in Pregnancy [4] and Lubbe [6].)

DRUG THERAPY FOR HYPERTENSION IN PREGNANCY

Recommended	Methyldopa—initial drug of choice against which all other antihypertensive agents must be tested; used for the longest time in the treatment of hypertension in pregnancy, so it has the best long-term follow-up data supporting its lack of toxicity; also lowers the number of midtrimester abortions in hypertensive women compared with placebo
	Hydralazine—used extensively, usually with methyldopa, and considered safe for mother and fetus by most obstetricians
	β-blockers (typically atenolol or labetalol)—used with caution and concern about growth retardation, fetal bradycardia, and the ability of the fetus to withstand hypoxic stress
	Nifedipine—teratogenic in rats (at 30× the recommended dose in humans); sometimes acutely used in preterm labor, but without FDA approval
Not recommended	Diuretics—cause volume depletion, which has been associated with poor fetal outcomes
Contraindicated	ACE inhibitors or angiotensin II receptor antagonists—associated with lethal acute renal failure in neonates of women treated in the third trimester

FIGURE 12-5. Drug therapy for hypertension in pregnancy, according to the Working Group on High Blood Pressure in Pregnancy [4]. Angiotensin-converting enzyme (ACE) inhibitors and angiotensin II receptor antagonists are contraindicated, and both dietary sodium restriction and the use of diuretics are controversial and not recommended unless such agents were necessary in the pregravid state. FDA—Food and Drug Administration.

Author, date	Treatment	Control		Weight	Odds ratio (95% CI)
Low-risk* women (US)					
CPEP, 1997	158/2163	168/2173		74.0	0.94 (0.77–1.16)
Low-risk women (outside US)					
Belizan, 1991	15/579	23/588		8.9	0.66 (0.35–1.26)
Crowther, 1999	10/227	23/229		6.6	0.44 (0.21–0.90)
Punwar, 1996	2/97	11/93		1.6	0.17 (0.04–0.77)
Villar, 1987	1/25	3/27		0.7	0.36 (0.04–3.24)
Villar, 1990	0/90	3/88		<0.1	0.14 (0.01–2.67)
Subtotal	28/1018	63/1025		17.9	0.37 (0.24–0.72)
High-risk women (outside US)					
Jaramillo, 1990	0/22	8/34		<0.1	0.09 (0.01–1.48)
Jaramillo, 1997	4/125	21/135		3.2	0.21 (0.07–0.58)
Niromanesh, 2001	1/15	7/15		0.7	0.14 (0.02–1.02)
Sanchez-Ramos, 1994	4/29	15/34		2.5	0.31 (0.01–2.67)
Jaramillo, 1989	2/55	12/51		1.6	0.15 (0.04–0.77)
Subtotal	11/224	63/225		8.1	0.14 (0.08–0.31)
Overall total	**189/3427**	**294/3467**		**100.0**	**0.65 (0.56–0.84)**

0.1 0.5   1   5 10

Calcium supplementation better   Control better

Odds ratio (calcium/control)

*Low-risk women have < 15% incidence of preeclampsia in the placebo group

FIGURE 12-6. Relative risk estimates for the difference in incidence of preeclampsia for calcium supplementation vs placebo. Results are shown from a National Institutes of Health-sponsored, randomized, multicenter clinical trial done in the United States among 4589 nulliparas at low risk (< 15% incidence in the placebo group) [7], multiple small clinical trials outside the United States in low-risk women, and multiple small clinical trials outside the United States in high-risk women (≥ 15% incidence in the placebo group). Previous meta-analyses of these trials showed large degrees of inhomogeneity across studies [8], which may be avoided by grouping the studies as shown. Possible reasons for the inhomogeneity include differences in baseline consumption of calcium, recruitment of primarily low-risk women in the United States clinical trial, or the proper role of meta-analysis, which is a research tool useful in designing better trials, rather than the definitive method by which to answer important clinical questions [9].

EFFICACY OF ANTIPLATELET AGENTS VS PLACEBO IN PREVENTING PREECLAMPSIA

	INCIDENCE		
OUTCOME	ANTIPLATELET AGENTS	PLACEBO	RELATIVE RISK (95% CI)
Pregnancy-induced hypertension	795/8464 (9.4%)	810/8450 (9.6%)	0.96 (0.88–1.05)
Proteinuric preeclampsia	951/13,991 (6.8%)	1110/13,973 (7.9%)	0.85 (0.79–0.93)
Preterm delivery	1772/13,473 (13.1%)	1928/13,534 (14.2%)	0.92 (0.87–0.97)
Fetal, neonatal, or infant death	361/14,325 (2.5%)	407/14,353 (2.8%)	0.88 (0.77–1.01)
Small for gestational age	668/9439 (7.1%)	701/9448 (7.4%)	0.94 (0.85–1.04)

FIGURE 12-7. Summary of the efficacy of anti-platelet agents (primarily aspirin) vs placebo to prevent preeclampsia and its complications [10]. Early studies enrolling a relatively small number of patients showed significant benefits, but subsequent and much larger studies did not confirm the initial results. Although there was little evidence of harm, most practicing obstetricians agree with the recommendation of the Working Group on Hypertension in Pregnancy [4] and do not routinely recommend low-dose aspirin (≈ 60 mg/d) for women with a high risk of eclampsia and preeclampsia. CI—confidence interval.

CHILDHOOD

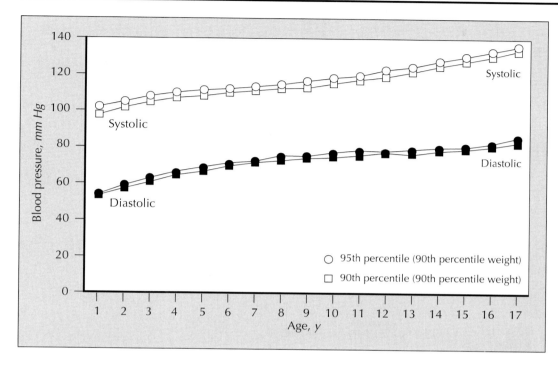

FIGURE 12-8. Age-specific values for systolic (*upper lines*) and diastolic (*lower lines*) blood pressure (BP) in boys [11]. A separate but similar graph exists for girls. Boys with BP higher than the 90th percentile (*squares*) should be monitored closely. Three measurements above the 95th percentile (*circles*) constitute significant hypertension and may require treatment (lifestyle modifications or pharmacologic treatment). The values given are for children at or below the 90th percentile for height (using standard growth charts); typically there are only a few mm Hg separating children with median and high levels of BP. On average, children with BP levels between the 90th and 95th percentiles are allowed approximately 4 mm Hg higher BPs before hypertension is suspected. Many authorities now recommend yearly BP determinations for children, with the values plotted on a graph similar to this; when a child begins to cross lines (as in growth charts), more interest in managing BP becomes appropriate.

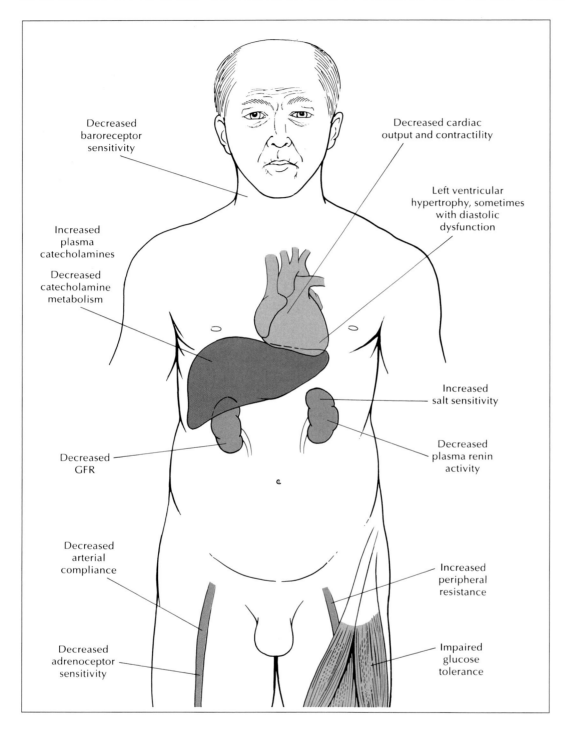

FIGURE 12-9. Some of the pathophysiologic features of hypertension in the elderly. Although some features are common in many elderly patients with elevated blood pressure, it is unusual for all of these features to be present in any one patient. GFR—glomerular filtration rate.

Decreased baroreceptor sensitivity

Decreased cardiac output and contractility

Left ventricular hypertrophy, sometimes with diastolic dysfunction

Increased plasma catecholamines

Decreased catecholamine metabolism

Increased salt sensitivity

Decreased GFR

Decreased plasma renin activity

Decreased arterial compliance

Increased peripheral resistance

Decreased adrenoceptor sensitivity

Impaired glucose tolerance

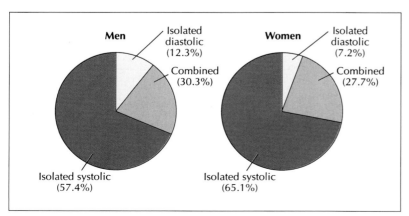

Men

Isolated diastolic (12.3%)

Combined (30.3%)

Isolated systolic (57.4%)

Women

Isolated diastolic (7.2%)

Combined (27.7%)

Isolated systolic (65.1%)

FIGURE 12-10. Gender-specific prevalence of types of hypertension in elderly (65 to 89 years old) residents of Framingham, MA [12]. At the beginning of this study, systolic blood pressure of 160 mm Hg or higher was considered abnormal, as was diastolic blood pressure of 95 mm Hg or higher; these definitions are no longer current. The smallest fraction denotes individuals with isolated diastolic hypertension. In each gender, isolated systolic hypertension is by far the most common form of elevated blood pressure. For 55- or 65-year-old residents of Framingham, MA, the lifetime risk of developing hypertension is about 90% [13].

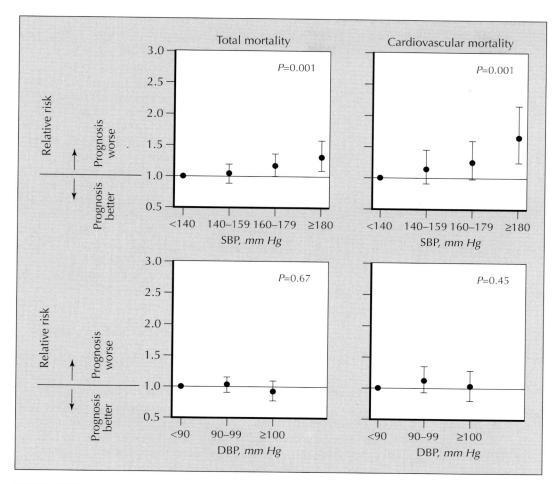

FIGURE 12-11. Ten-year total, *left*, and cardiovascular, *right*, mortality, according to the average systolic blood pressures (SBP) and diastolic blood pressures (DBP) obtained during six visits to general practitioners during the first year of follow-up among 3858 Italian patients (over age 65) with hypertension [14]. These and many other data suggest that systolic blood pressure is a much better predictor of future adverse events in the elderly than the diastolic measurement; undertreatment of systolic hypertension from 1983 to 1993 may have been part of the explanation for this observation [15].

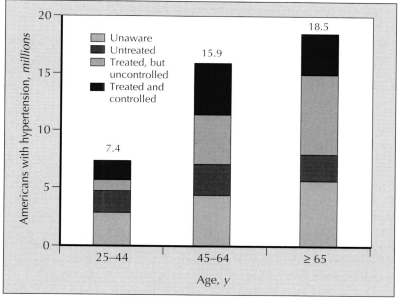

FIGURE 12-12. Numbers (in millions) of persons with various categories of hypertension, aged 25 and older, in the noninstitutionalized, civilian population in the United States, according to the National Health and Nutrition Examination Survey (NHANES) III (1988–1994). These data suggest that treated, but uncontrolled, hypertension is most common among those over 65 years of age; approximately 88% of these patients have uncontrolled systolic (≥ 140 mm Hg) but controlled diastolic blood pressures (< 90 mm Hg) [16].

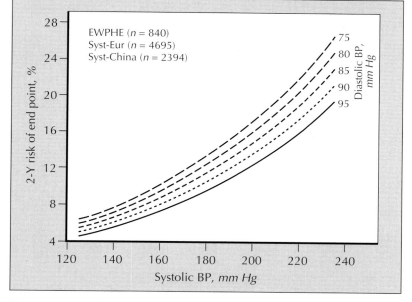

FIGURE 12-13. Schematized results of a meta-analysis of individual patient data from three studies (EWPHE [European Working Party on Hypertension in the Elderly], Syst-Eur [Systolic Hypertension in Europe], and Syst-China [Systolic Hypertension in China]). These results show the 2-year risk of cardiovascular events according to systolic pressure at fixed levels of diastolic pressure, after adjusting statistically for drug treatment, gender, age, previous cardiovascular events, and smoking [17]. Note that overall risk increases as diastolic pressure decreases. For older people, pulse pressure was the best predictor of mortality in the population-based Established Populations for Epidemiologic Studies of the Elderly (drawn from three communities in the United States) [18]. A similarly statistically significant 12% increase in 1-year mortality among 37,069 patients on hemodialysis in the United States was seen with each 10-mm Hg increase in pulse pressure, measured post-dialysis [19].

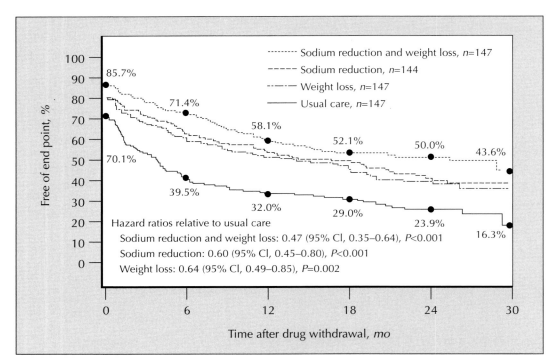

FIGURE 12-14. Results of the Trials of Nutrition in the Elderly (TONE) study. The group randomized to both weight reduction and sodium restriction had fewer than half as many patients returning to antihypertensive medication or having clinical events during the 15 to 36 months of follow-up, compared with individuals given usual care [20]. Although this study provides strong evidence that antihypertensive medication *can* be withdrawn from older patients with hypertension *if* they are provided with expert advice about nutrition and exercise, the cost of nutritionists, exercise physiologists, and quarterly visits for blood pressure monitoring is likely to be greater than simply keeping most people on their effective medication.

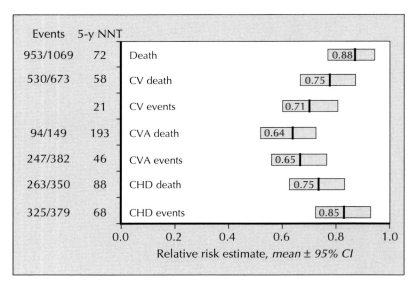

FIGURE 12-15. Results of meta-analyses of placebo-controlled hypertension trials in the elderly, according to types of clinical event, showing both the percent reduction in events [21] and the number needed to treat (NNT) for 5 years to avoid an event [22]. Unlike the situation in younger patients, the treatment groups (using diuretics and β-blocking agents) received nearly all of the expected beneficial reductions in fatal and nonfatal cerebrovascular accident (CVA) and coronary artery disease (CAD) events. Noncardiovascular deaths were not increased significantly by effective antihypertensive therapy. These conclusions have been extended to patients with hypertension over age 80 years, based on a meta-analysis of 1670 participants in seven clinical trials [23]. CHD—coronary heart disease; CI—confidence interval; CV—cardiovascular.

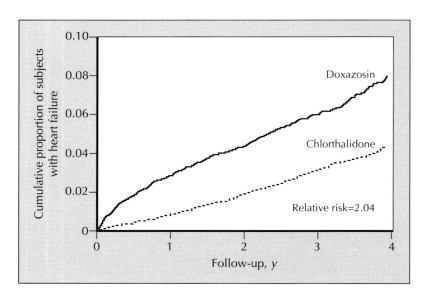

FIGURE 12-16. Results of two of four arms of the Antihypertensive and Lipid Lowering [treatment to prevent] Heart Attack Trial (ALLHAT), comparing the incidence of heart failure among hypertensive patients randomized to chlorthalidone (*n* = 15,268) or doxazosin (*n* = 9067) [24]. The doxazosin arm of this clinical trial was terminated early due to a very low probability that the α-blocker would show superiority over the diuretic in preventing the primary endpoint, fatal or nonfatal myocardial infarction. Although the chlorthalidone group had, on average, a 3.3-mm Hg lower systolic blood pressure throughout follow-up, this study suggests that an α-blocker should not be prescribed as initial therapy for hypertension. The results of the other two arms of ALLHAT (in which subjects were randomized to either amlodipine or lisinopril) are expected to guide public policy regarding the best initial drug choice for otherwise uncomplicated hypertension. P < 0.001.

HYPERTENSIVE EMERGENCIES

DEFINITIONS OF HYPERTENSIVE EMERGENCIES AND URGENCIES

HYPERTENSIVE EMERGENCY

Severe elevation in blood pressure with signs or symptoms of acute, severe target organ damage, which must be reduced *within minutes* (typically using parenteral therapy)

HYPERTENSIVE URGENCY

Severe elevation in blood pressure with mild or no acute target organ damage, which must be reduced *within hours* (typically with oral therapy)

FIGURE 12-17. Definitions of hypertensive emergencies and hypertensive urgencies [25]. Note that the older terms *accelerated hypertension* and *malignant hypertension* have been eliminated (with the exception of the terminology used by hospital administrators, as mandated by the Federal Diagnosis-Related Groups Handbook). Severe hypertension without acute target organ damage is never an emergency and does not require parenteral therapy.

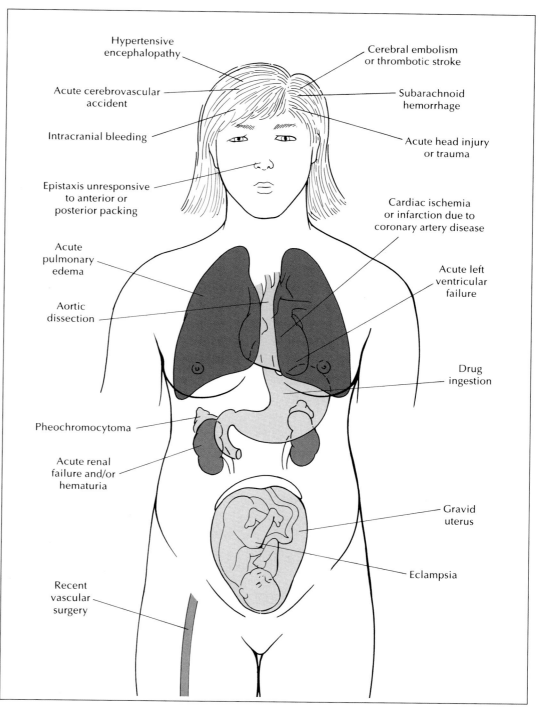

FIGURE 12-18. Common clinical conditions that are often considered hypertensive emergencies. Severe *acute* target organ damage is the major distinguishing factor between emergencies and urgencies.

DRUGS FOR HYPERTENSIVE EMERGENCIES

CONDITION	DRUG OF CHOICE	CONTRAINDICATED
Hypertensive encephalopathy	Nitroprusside*	Methyldopa
CNS catastrophes	Nitroprusside*	Methyldopa
Subarachnoid hemorrhage	Nimodipine	
Aortic dissection	β-Blocker + nitroprusside*	Hydralazine, diazoxide
Eclampsia	Hydralazine	Nitroprusside, trimethaphan
Heart failure	Nitroprusside*, nitroglycerin	Labetalol
Cardiac ischemia or angina	Nitroglycerin	Hydralazine
Catecholamine-related emergencies	Phentolamine	
Clonidine withdrawal	Clonidine	
Postoperative hypertension	Nitroprusside*	
Post-CABG hypertension	Nitroglycerin	

*Instead of nitroprusside, some clinicians prefer either intravenous nicardipine or fenoldopam (especially in the setting of renal impairment) because of the lack of potentially toxic metabolites.

FIGURE 12-19. Drug treatment options for various hypertensive emergencies [25]. The table also lists those drugs that are contraindicated in certain conditions. CABG—coronary artery bypass graft; CNS—central nervous system.

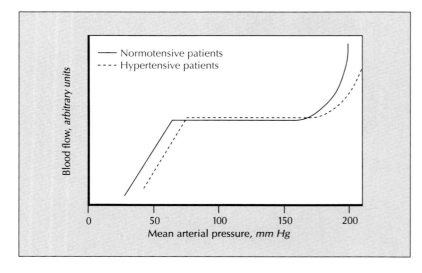

FIGURE 12-20. The blood pressure–blood flow curve for normotensive and hypertensive patients. The figure demonstrates why severely hypertensive patients often have deleterious reductions in organ perfusion when blood pressure is normalized too quickly after they present with a hypertensive emergency [26]. In this situation, autoregulatory capacity is exceeded and blood flow falls below that necessary to sustain normal organ function, even though the blood pressure is reduced into a range that would be considered acceptable for normotensive patients. This shift to the right of the blood pressure–blood flow curve in hypertensive patients also explains why chronically hypertensive patients seldom have hypertensive encephalopathy (as they autoregulate their cerebral blood flow to compensate), whereas individuals who experience sudden increases in blood pressure (*eg*, women with eclampsia or youngsters with rapidly progressing glomerulonephritis) can develop encephalopathy with lower blood pressure and a much shorter duration of hypertension.

FIGURE 12-21. Improvement in 1-year survival rates for patients in various countries presenting with hypertensive emergencies or "malignant hypertension" [27]. The incremental jump in survival around 1951 was caused in large part by the introduction of effective antihypertensive medications. These agents have been continuously refined, resulting in enhanced survival; now, most series show a greater than 90% survival rate at 1 year after diagnosis.

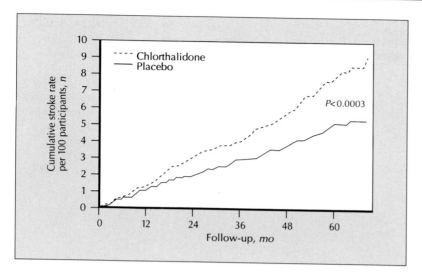

FIGURE 12-22. The occurrence of fatal and nonfatal strokes (the primary outcome measure) during the Systolic Hypertension in the Elderly Program [28]. In these elderly patients, compared with placebo, low-dose chlorthalidone therapy statistically was associated with a 36% decreased risk of stroke after an average of 4.5 years of therapy.

SECONDARY ENDPOINT REDUCTIONS IN THE SHEP TRIAL

ENDPOINT	TREATED	PLACEBO	REDUCTION, % (95% CI)	P VALUE
Nonfatal MI or CAD death	104	141	27 (6–43)	< 0.05
CVA, nonfatal MI, or CAD death	199	289	33 (20–44)	< 0.01
Any coronary event*	140	184	25 (6–40)	< 0.05
Any cardiovascular event†	289	414	32 (21–42)	< 0.01

*Coronary events included MI, sudden or rapid cardiac death, aortocoronary bypass surgery, or coronary angioplasty.

†Cardiovascular events included coronary event or stroke, transient ischemic attack, intracranial aneurysm, or carotid endarterectomy.

FIGURE 12-23. Reductions in other (secondary) endpoints during the Systolic Hypertension in the Elderly Program (SHEP) [28]. Reductions in all endpoints were statistically significant and clearly show that the benefits of low-dose thiazide diuretic therapy in patients with only the systolic form of hypertension extend far beyond reduction of fatal and nonfatal strokes. CAD—coronary artery disease; CI—confidence interval; CVA—cerebrovascular accident; MI—myocardial infarction.

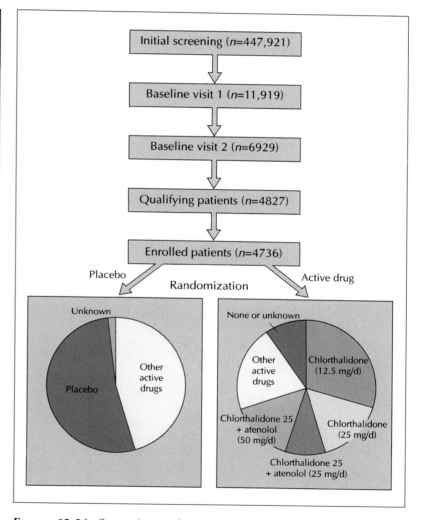

FIGURE 12-24. Screening and study design algorithm of the Systolic Hypertension in the Elderly Program [28]. Patients with normal diastolic blood pressure were enrolled to determine whether antihypertensive drug therapy could reduce systolic blood pressure and fatal and nonfatal stroke rates. The pie charts represent the fractions of patients taking a specific therapy at the conclusion of the trial.

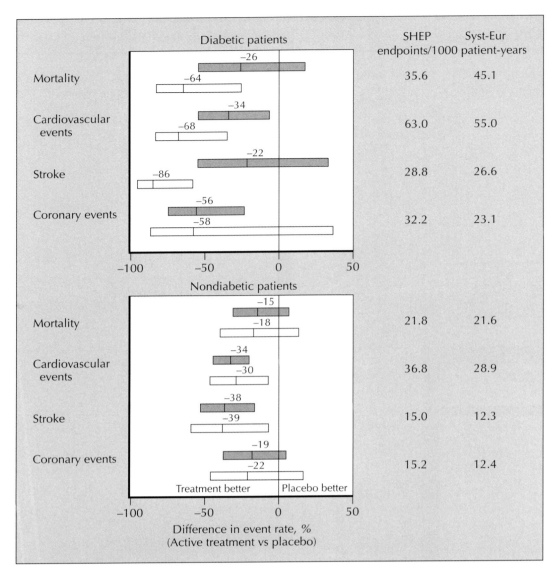

	SHEP	Syst-Eur
	endpoints/1000 patient-years	

FIGURE 12-25. Comparison of the efficacy of two treatment regimens for "isolated systolic hypertension" in older diabetic patients: a diuretic-based regimen (used in SHEP [*dark bars*, Systolic Hypertension in the Elderly Program]) and a calcium antagonist-based treatment (Syst-EUR [*light bars*, Systolic Hypertension in Europe]) [29]. The authors attributed the apparent improvement to the initial drug treatment, but differences between studies (American vs European patients, early termination vs scheduled termination, and percentage of patients taking the placebo at the end of the study) may be partially responsible.

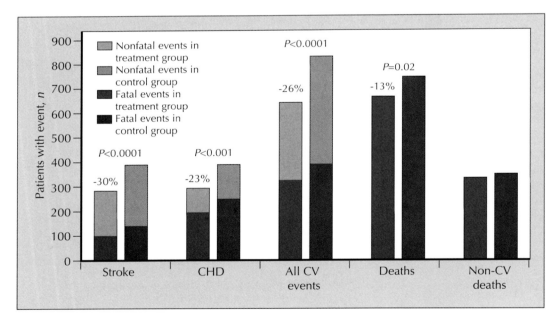

FIGURE 12-26. Results of a meta-analysis of eight clinical trials involving 15,693 patients with "isolated systolic hypertension." The average initial blood pressure in these patients was 174/83 mm Hg, and was reduced by an average of 10.4/4.1 mm Hg in patients who received antihypertensive drug therapy [30]. This reduction was associated with a significant reduction in fatal and nonfatal stroke (30%), fatal and nonfatal coronary heart disease (CHD) (23%), fatal and nonfatal cardiovascular (CV) events (26%), and all-cause mortality (13%).

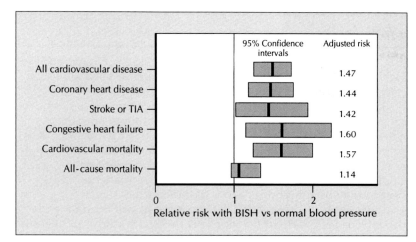

FIGURE 12-27. Adjusted risk estimates with 95% confidence intervals of adverse clinical outcomes in patients with what was formerly called borderline isolated systolic hypertension (BISH; *n* = 351; systolic blood pressure between 140 and 159 mm Hg) compared with patients having normal blood pressure (*n* = 2416) as noted in the Framingham Heart Study [31]. Since the Fifth Joint National Committee on the Detection, Evaluation, and Treatment of High Blood Pressure summary, the patients with higher blood pressures are diagnosed with stage 1 systolic hypertension. Except for all-cause mortality, the risk (adjusted for gender, age, cholesterol, obesity, cigarettes, and diabetes) for each cardio-vascular event usually associated with hypertension was statistically significant for those patients with only borderline elevated systolic pressure. TIA—transient ischemic attack.

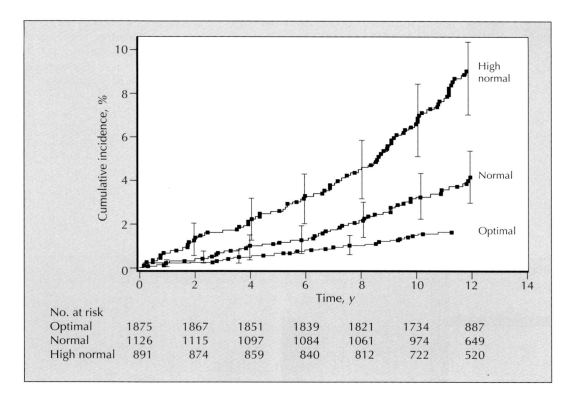

FIGURE 12-28. Incidence of cardiovascular events in 3892 women enrolled in the Framingham Heart Study, according to the Joint National Committee (JNC)-VI classification of blood pressure (BP) [32]. "Optimal" blood pressure (BP) includes systolic BP < 120 mm Hg and diastolic BP < 80 mm Hg. "Normal" BP includes systolic BP between 120–129 mm Hg and diastolic BP between 80–84 mm Hg. "High-normal" BP includes systolic BP between 130–139 mm Hg and diastolic BP between 85–89 mm Hg. Similar results were seen for the 2967 men in this cohort. Vertical bars indicate 95% confidence limits.

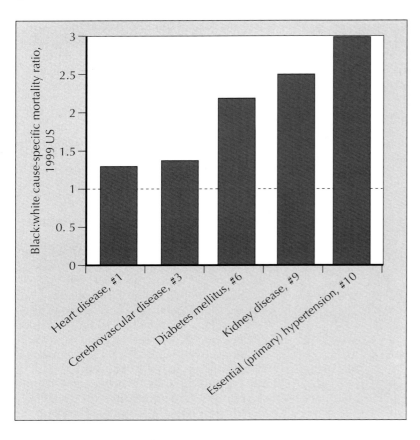

FIGURE 12-29. Ratios of black:white differences in mortality, as estimated in the Report of the Center for Health Statistics for 1999 death certificates [33]. The national ranking of the disease listed as the cause of death on the death certificate is shown after the name of the disease. In 1999, for the first time since the mid-1960s, primary hypertension and hypertension-related renal disease re-entered the top 15 causes of death in the United States. Comparisons of data from 1999 with previous years are confounded by different versions of the International Classifications of Disease (ICD). Comparisons of 1998 data with those from 1979 (both of which use ICD-9 codes) show an overall reduction in the number of Americans dying from heart disease (-27.2%) and stroke (-35.2%). However, the clinical sequelae of hypertension continue to be more common among blacks. In 1998, blacks had a 50% higher rate of age-adjusted mortality from heart disease and an 80% higher rate of stroke. The nearly threefold elevated incidence of end-stage renal disease in blacks (compared with whites) has been attributed to both higher blood pressure and lower socioeconomic status [34].

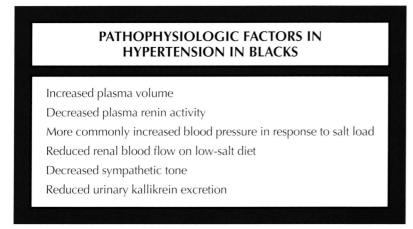

PATHOPHYSIOLOGIC FACTORS IN HYPERTENSION IN BLACKS

Increased plasma volume

Decreased plasma renin activity

More commonly increased blood pressure in response to salt load

Reduced renal blood flow on low-salt diet

Decreased sympathetic tone

Reduced urinary kallikrein excretion

FIGURE 12-30. Some factors thought to play a prominent role in the pathophysiology of hypertension in blacks. It is unlikely that all of these factors are found in all black patients; individual patients vary in their responses, which may not fit the paradigm.

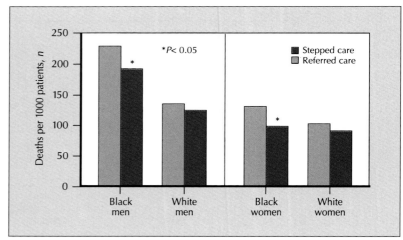

FIGURE 12-31. Death rates in black and white men and women during 8.3 years of follow-up in the Hypertension Detection and Follow-up Program [35]. Intensively treated (stepped care) black men showed a significant 16.6% reduction in death (compared with referred care); such therapy in white men reduced death rates only by a nonsignificant 7.8%. Black women enjoyed a significant 24.1% reduction in mortality, compared with a nonsignificant 11.5% reduction in white women. This follow-up period included a 2-year interval after the completion of the trial. Two earlier analyses (at 5 and 6.7 years) showed somewhat less impressive differences between the two races. The authors nonetheless attributed the reduction in death highlighted here to the more effective regimens in the intensively treated group.

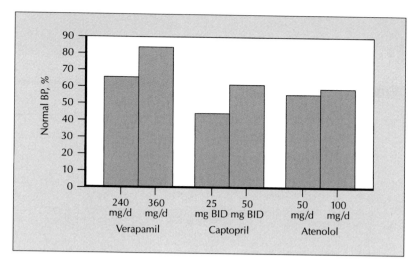

FIGURE 12-32. Differences in response to three antihypertensive medications in blacks [36]. The most generally effective class of medications for lowering blood pressure in this ethnic group, diuretics, was used as a second step for all treated patients who did not reach goal blood pressure (BP) with the β-blocker (atenolol), angiotensin-converting enzyme inhibitor (captopril), or calcium antagonist (verapamil). The response to the higher dose of atenolol used in these patients was somewhat blunted compared with the higher dose of the other two drugs. BID—twice a day.

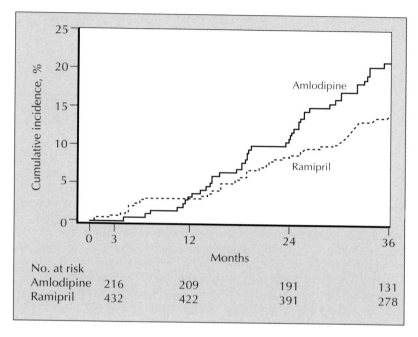

FIGURE 12-33. Results of the main secondary outcome measure of the ramipril and amlodipine arms of the African American Study of Kidney Disease and Hypertension (AASK) [37]. The primary endpoint, the rate of change in glomerular filtration rate between 3 months and 3 years of treatment, was also 36% slower in the ramipril group (P = 0.002). The figure shows a 38% reduction in the composite endpoint: glomerular event (decline by either 50% or by 25 mL/min per 1.73 m^2/y), end-stage renal disease, or death (P = 0.005). The amlodipine arm of this clinical trial was prematurely terminated because of these results. These data indicate that angiotensin-converting enzyme inhibitors have major long-term beneficial effects in blacks with nondiabetic renal disease and hypertension, despite what some perceive as a reduced short-term efficacy in lowering blood pressure (as monotherapy) and a somewhat higher incidence of both angioedema and cough.

CYCLOSPORINE

CONDITIONS IN WHICH CYCLOSPORINE ELEVATES BLOOD PRESSURE

TRANSPLANTATION

Renal

Cardiac

Hepatic

Bone marrow

Cardiopulmonary

OCULAR DISORDERS

Uveitis

"Birdshot" retinochoroidopathy

OTHER POTENTIAL "AUTOIMMUNE" DISEASES

Psoriasis

Other dermatologic conditions

Systemic lupus erythematosus

Insulin-dependent diabetes mellitus (of recent onset)

Chronic inflammatory demyelinating polyradiculoneuropathy

Rheumatoid arthritis

FIGURE 12-34. Some conditions in which cyclosporine has been found (in clinical trials or in controlled case reports) to elevate blood pressure. The wide variety of these conditions, each with a unique pathophysiology, suggests that cyclosporine is the common substance that predisposes patients with these illnesses to hypertension.

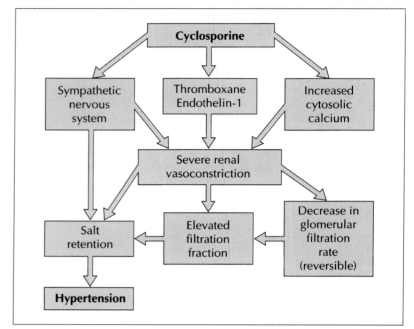

FIGURE 12-35. Suggested mechanisms for the hypertensive effect of cyclosporine [38]. Additional hypertensive effects are thought to result from direct nephrotoxicity of cyclosporine (particularly in patients with chronic renal impairment), a change in local eicosanoid or endothelin production (which may be involved in renal vasoconstriction), or thrombotic microangiopathy (which sometimes responds to withdrawal of cyclosporine, if recognized early enough). Effects of cyclosporine on the sympathetic nervous system have been noted but are controversial, particularly because hypertension often appears before a transplanted organ is re-innervated.

TREATMENT OPTIONS FOR CYCLOSPORINE-RELATED HYPERTENSION

Diuretics (most centers use loop diuretics as first-line therapy)

Calcium antagonists (note that diltiazem, verapamil, and nicardipine may interfere with excretion of cyclosporine; this has been used advantageously to decrease cyclosporine dosing requirements)

ACE inhibitors (generally felt to work best with concomitant diuretic therapy, and to be much less effective when given alone)

Labetalol

Centrally acting α_2-agonists (eg, clonidine)

ω3 Fatty acid dietary supplements

FIGURE 12-36. Treatment of cyclosporine-related hypertension [38,39]. No randomized, long-term head-to-head comparison of any two drug classes has yet been reported. Experience at most centers suggests that two drugs are frequently necessary to normalize cyclosporine-associated hypertension. ACE—angiotensin-converting enzyme.

ERYTHROPOIETIN

POSSIBLE MECHANISMS FOR THE HYPERTENSIVE EFFECT OF ERYTHROPOIETIN

Rise of hematocrit and erythrocyte mass

Changes in production or sensitivity to endogenous vasopressors

Alterations in vascular smooth muscle ionic milieu

Dysregulation of production or responsiveness to endogenous vasodilatory factors

Direct vasopressor action of erythropoietin

Arterial remodeling through stimulation of vascular cell growth

FIGURE 12-37. Possible mechanisms by which erythropoietin increases blood pressure [40]. The relative importance of the contribution of each of the suggested mechanisms has not yet been delineated.

TREATMENT OPTIONS FOR ERYTHROPOIETIN-RELATED HYPERTENSION

Diuretics (generally considered first-line therapy because of antagonist effects on erythropoietin's effect to increase circulating blood volume)

Vasodilators (*eg*, hydralazine)

Calcium antagonists

ACE inhibitors

Centrally acting α_2-agonists (*eg*, clonidine)

FIGURE 12-38. Treatment of erythropoietin-related hypertension. As mentioned earlier, no randomized, long-term head-to-head comparison of any two drug classes has yet been reported. ACE—angiotensin-converting enzyme.

COCAINE

POSSIBLE MECHANISMS FOR THE HYPERTENSIVE EFFECT OF COCAINE

Increased release of catecholamines (especially norepinephrine) from nerves, brain, or adrenals

Inhibition of neuronal uptake of catecholamines (especially norepinephrine) at nearly all neuromuscular junctions (including those involved in regulating arteriolar tone)

Increased cardiac output

Increased predilection for vasospasm in cerebral and coronary arteries and arterioles

Inhibition of peripheral vasodilatory effect of local nitric oxide production

FIGURE 12-39. Possible mechanisms by which cocaine increases blood pressure [41]. Most authorities agree that acute α-receptor blockade (*eg*, with intravenous phentolamine) is the treatment of choice for cocaine-induced hypertension, perhaps followed by β-blockade if cardiac dysrhythmia is also a feature of the temporary excess of catecholamines.

SPECIALIZED METHODS OF BLOOD PRESSURE MEASUREMENT

HOME BLOOD PRESSURE MEASUREMENT

METHODS OF AVAILABLE OUT-OF-OFFICE BLOOD PRESSURE MEASUREMENT

Anaeroid sphygmomanometry ("the dial")
  Using cuff around upper arm
  Using stethoscope
  Using oscillometry
Digital sphygmomanometry ("digital" readout)
  Using cuff around upper arm
  Using cuff around finger
  Using cuff around wrist

FIGURE 12-40. Commonly available methods of measuring blood pressure by patients in settings other than in the physician's office. Many authorities recommend caution when interpreting data from monitors worn around the finger, because these pressures often correlate poorly with traditional measurements. Patients who use any of these devices (and prefer their own readings) should be reminded that the vast majority of data accumulated in clinical trials of hypertension have been based on measurements taken in the offices of health care professionals.

METHODS OF BP MEASUREMENT AVAILABLE TO THE OUTPATIENT: ADVANTAGES AND DISADVANTAGES

ATTRIBUTE	ANAEROID WITH STETHOSCOPE	OSCILLOMETRIC WITH STETHOSCOPE	OSCILLOMETRIC WITH DIGITAL READOUT
Coordination necessary	Yes	Yes	Less so
Affected by presbyacusis	Yes	Yes	No
Affected by presbyopia	Yes	Less so	Less so
Widely available	Yes	Less so	Increasingly
Inexpensive	Yes	Less so	Increasingly
Good quality results	Yes, with effort	Yes, with effort	Yes
Increases patients' interest in managing BP	Yes	Yes	Yes
Battery-powered	No	Yes	Yes
Affected by impaired grip strength	Yes	No	No
Utility validated in prospective studies	No	No	No

FIGURE 12-41. Advantages and disadvantages of the types of machines commonly used to measure blood pressure (BP). It is recommended that anaeroid and digital devices be calibrated against a mercury column (using a Y-connector) to ensure the accuracy of such devices [42].

BLOOD PRESSURE CUFF CHARACTERISTICS

NAME	TYPICAL BLADDER SIZE (W X L), cm	APPROXIMATE ARM CIRCUMFERENCE, cm
Newborn	2.5–4 X 5–9	< 12
Infant	4–6 X 11.5–18	13–20
Child	7.5–9 X 17–19	20–24
Normal adult	11.5–13 X 22–26	24–32
Large adult	14–15 X 30.5–35	32.5–41
Thigh	18–19 X 36–38	> 41

FIGURE 12-42. Names, bladder sizes, and approximate arm circumferences for each of the six types of blood pressure cuffs that should be used in routine indirect measurement of blood pressure by the Korotkoff method. The appearance of rhythmic sound (Korotkoff I) as systolic and the disappearance of such sounds (Korotkoff V) as diastolic should be used. Muffling of sounds (Korotkoff IV) is no longer recommended as the diastolic pressure in pregnancy [4] or in children or adolescents [11]. The bladder cuff should be at least 80% of the circumference of the arm [43].

AUTOMATIC AMBULATORY BLOOD PRESSURE MODELS

DIRECT

Oxford intra-arterial method

INDIRECT

Oscillometric
  Spacelabs (many models; Redmond, WA)
  Takeda (Lincolnshire, IL)
  Del Mar Avionics (Irvine, CA)
R-wave gated microphonic
  Accutracker (used in space flights; Suntech, Raleigh, NC)
Finger cuff methods
  Portapres (TNO BMI, Belgium)
  Finapres (TNO BMI, Belgium)

FIGURE 12-43. Methods used in the measurement of blood pressure (BP) with ambulatory monitors. The direct intra-arterial measurement of BP is not commonly used in the United States, although several European centers have a great deal of experience in the utility and safety of this method.

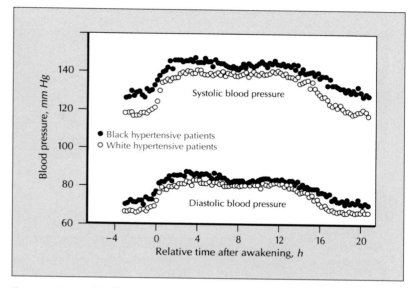

FIGURE 12-44. Differences in blood pressures (BPs) during a day-long period in 275 black and 246 white untreated hypertensive patients. Two important points are that 1) there is a large diurnal variation in the average BP in both groups and 2) the nocturnal decrease in BP is less in blacks than whites [44].

AMBULATORY BLOOD PRESSURE MEASUREMENTS IN 4577 NORMOTENSIVE SUBJECTS

PERIOD	24-h AVERAGE	DAYTIME	NIGHTTIME
	BLOOD PRESSURE, mm Hg		
90th Percentile	129/79	136/85	120/72
95th Percentile	133/82	140/88	125/76
97.5th Percentile	136/84	143/91	128/78

FIGURE 12-45. The 90th, 95th, and 97.5th percentile thresholds for ambulatory blood pressure (BP) in 4577 normotensive patients for 24 hours, daytime, and nighttime [45]. As yet, there are no results from large prospective, randomized trials using ambulatory BP monitoring for therapeutic decision-making, so what constitutes a "normal" pressure by this method is not known. Furthermore, it is likely that today no patient with an "abnormal" BP by ambulatory BP measurement will go untreated, so it is unlikely that we will ever have data to answer the question of "What is the relative risk of this level of BP by ambulatory BP measurement, if left untreated?"

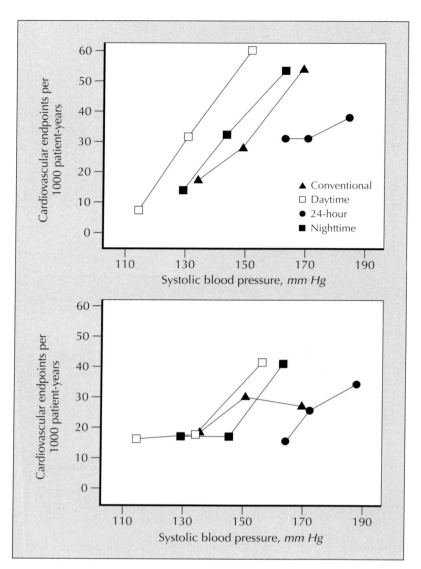

FIGURE 12-46. Comparison of four types of blood pressure measurements as predictors of cardiovascular endpoints in the Systolic Hypertension in Europe trial [46]. Among patients randomized to placebo, *upper panel*, conventional office blood pressure measurements were poor predictors of future risk and nighttime measurements were the best. In the actively treated group, *lower panel*, systolic blood pressure, regardless of how it was measured, was not a useful predictor of future risk, presumably because of the effective treatment. The authors suggest that a conventional office systolic blood pressure measurement of 160 mm Hg carries the same risk for future cardiovascular events as a 24-hour average at 142 mm Hg, a daytime average of 145 mm Hg, or a nighttime average of 132 mm Hg.

NHBPEP INDICATIONS FOR ABPM

Borderline hypertension without target organ damage

? Drug resistance

Episodic hypertension

Hypotensive symptoms on medications

"Office" or "white coat" hypertension

Blood pressure changes at night with angina or pulmonary congestion

Autonomic dysfunction

Carotid sinus syncope, pacemaker syndromes

FIGURE 12-47. Indications for ambulatory blood pressure monitoring (ABPM) according to the National High Blood Pressure Education Program (NHBPEP) [47]. These are remarkably similar to more recent recommendations from the British Hypertension Society [48]. The use of ABPM in the United States is expected to increase, in response to a Center for Medicare and Medicaid Services decision issued in 2001 to allow Medicare reimbursement for the procedure for suspected "white coat hypertension" [49]. Several cost-effectiveness calculations have indicated that if 20% of patients having ABPM are diagnosed with "white coat hypertension" and do not require intensification of their costly antihypertensive drug regimen, the health care system will actually save money.

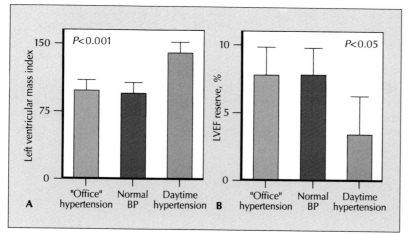

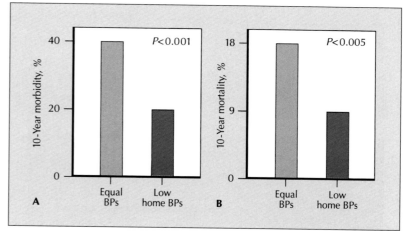

FIGURE 12-48. Relation between "office" (or "white coat") hypertension and left ventricular mass (**A**) and left ventricular reserve (**B**): exercise compared with rest ejection fraction [50]. Note that patients with office hypertension have left ventricular masses and cardiac reserve about the same as normotensive patients but different from those with sustained (or "daytime") hypertension. Although these patients were carefully selected, these observations suggest that office hypertension is sufficiently sporadic that it does not influence left ventricular mass or cardiac reserve. *T-bars* indicate SEM. BP—blood pressure; LVEF—left ventricular ejection fraction.

FIGURE 12-49. Long-term morbidity (**A**) and mortality (**B**) data in patients who monitored their blood pressures (BPs; *n* = 1076) at home [51]. *Equal BPs* indicate patients in whom BP taken in the office was equal to BP taken at home. *Low home BPs* indicate patients in whom the home BP was consistently lower than pressure measured in the office. Patients with lower home readings clearly do better than individuals with elevated pressures at home and in the office, but whether the patients with lower readings at home do as well as individuals with normal pressures in both locations has not been demonstrated.

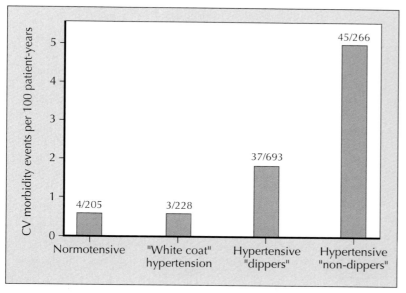

FIGURE 12-50. Rates of hypertension-related adverse outcomes observed in 1187 hypertensive patients and 206 normotensive volunteers undergoing ambulatory blood pressure (BP) monitoring (ABPM) [52]. Although the number of adverse events in each group was small, the average length of follow-up was only 3.2 years. Multivariate adjustments led to significance of ABPM data only in women. These data suggest that "white coat" hypertensive patients have a risk of adverse events about equal to normotensive patients, and that nocturnal "dippers," in whom BP drops at night, have a better prognosis than do "non-dippers." CV—cardiovascular.

ADVANTAGES AND DISADVANTAGES OF AMBULATORY BLOOD PRESSURE MONITORING

ADVANTAGES

Can take many BP measurements during 24-h period

Measures diurnal variation (BPs during sleep)

Measures BP during daily activities

Can identify "white coat" hypertension

No "alerting response"

No placebo effect

Apparent better correlation with target organ damage than other methods of BP measurement

DISADVANTAGES

Cost

Limited availability of equipment

Disruption of daily activities from noise or discomfort (*eg,* sleep quality, flaccid arm during measurement)

Lack of "normal" data and treatment guidelines

Paucity of long-term prospective studies demonstrating utility compared with traditional (and much less expensive) BP measurements

FIGURE 12-51. Advantages and disadvantages of ambulatory blood pressure (BP) monitoring. Because of the large number of readings and generally absent placebo effect, BP monitoring is used frequently in the evaluation of new antihypertensive therapies, particularly when the optimal dosing interval has not been well defined.

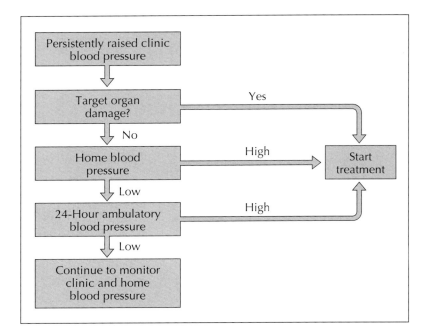

FIGURE 12-52. Algorithm for establishing diagnosis of hypertension, which incorporates office, home, and ambulatory blood pressure measurements (ABPMs), according to an Ad Hoc panel of the American Society of Hypertension [53]. Other authors suggest that, because of the potential high cost of ambulatory blood pressure monitoring in eligible Americans (which could add up to $6 billion per year to the national health care budget), ABPM should be reserved for otherwise difficult cases or used in settings in which cost is not an issue [54].

REFERENCES

1. Moutquin JM, Rainville C, Giroux L, *et al.*: A prospective study of blood pressure in pregnancy: prediction of preeclampsia. *Am J Obstet Gynecol* 1985, 151:191–196.

2. Sibai BM, Ewell M, Levine RJ, *et al.*: Risk factors associated with preeclampsia in healthy nulliparous women. The Calcium for Preeclampsia Prevention (CPEP) Study Group. *Am J Obstet Gynecol* 1997, 177:1003–1010.

3. Friedman SA: Preeclampsia: a review of the role of prostaglandins. *Obstet Gynecol* 1988, 71:122–137.

4. Report of the National High Blood Pressure Education Program Working Group on High Blood Pressure in Pregnancy. *Am J Obstet Gynecol* 2000, 183:S1–S22.

5. National High Blood Pressure Education Program Working Group on High Blood Pressure in Pregnancy. Working Group report on high blood pressure in pregnancy. *Am J Obstet Gynecol* 1990, 163:1689–1712.

6. Lubbe WF: Hypertension in pregnancy. Pathophysiology and management. *Drugs* 1984, 28:170–188.

7. Levine RJ, Hauth JC, Curet LB, *et al.*: Trial of calcium to prevent preeclampsia. *N Engl J Med* 1997, 337:69–76.

8. Atallah AN, Hofmeyr GJ, Duley L: Calcium supplementation during pregnancy for preventing hypertensive disorders and related problems. *The Cochrane Library* 2002, Issue 1. http://www.gateway2.ovid.com/ovidweb.cgi?View+Image=0007 5320-100000000-01029. Accessed March 6, 2002.

9. DerSimonian R, Levine RJ: Resolving discrepancies between a meta-analysis and a subsequent large controlled trial. *JAMA* 1999, 282:664–670.

10. Knight M, Duley L, Henderson-Smart DJ, King JF: Antiplatelet agents for preventing and treating pre-eclampsia. *The Cochrane Library* 2002, Issue 1. http://www.gateway2.ovid.com/ovidweb.cgi?View+Image=0007 5320-100000000-01104. Accessed March 5, 2002.

11. Update on the Task Force Report (1987) on High Blood Pressure in Children and Adolescents: a Working Group Report from the National High Blood Pressure Education Program. *Pediatrics* 1996, 98:649–658.

12. Wilking SV, Belanger A, Kannel WB, *et al.*: Determinants of isolated systolic hypertension. *JAMA* 1988, 260:3451–3455.

13. Vasan RS, Beiser A, Seshadri S, *et al.*: Residual lifetime risk for developing hypertension in middle-aged women and men: The Framingham Heart Study. *JAMA* 2002, 287:1003-1010.

14. Alli C, Avanzini F, Bettelli G, *et al.*: The long-term prognostic significance of repeated blood pressure measurements in the elderly: SPAA (Studio sulla Pressione Arteriosa nell'Anziano) 10-Year Follow-up. *Arch Intern Med* 1999, 159:1205-1212.

15. Elliott WJ: Which blood pressure is more important? [Editorial]. *Arch Intern Med* 1999, 159:1165-1166.

16. Hyman DJ, Pavlik VN: Characteristics of patients with uncontrolled hypertension in the United States. *N Engl J Med* 2001, 345:479-486.

17. Blacher J, Staessen JA, Girerd X, *et al.*: Pulse pressure not mean pressure determines cardiovascular risk in older hypertensive patients. *Arch Intern Med* 2000, 160:1085–1089.

18. Glynn RJ, Chae CU, Guralnik JM, *et al.*: Pulse pressure and mortality in older people. *Arch Intern Med* 2000, 160:2765–2772.

19. Klassen PS, Lowrie EG, Reddan DN, *et al.*: Association between pulse pressure and mortality in patients undergoing maintenance hemodialysis. *JAMA* 2002, 287:1548–1555.

20. Whelton PK, Appel LJ, Espeland MA, *et al.*: Sodium reduction and weight loss in the treatment of hypertension in older persons: a randomized controlled trial of nonpharmacologic interventions in the elderly (TONE). *JAMA* 1998, 279:839–846.

21. Insua JT, Sacks HS, Lau TS, *et al.*: Drug treatment of hypertension in the elderly: a meta-analysis. *Ann Intern Med* 1994, 121:355–362.

22. Mulrow CD, Cornell JA, Herrera CR, *et al.*: Hypertension in the elderly: Implications and generalizability of randomized trials. *JAMA* 1994, 272:1932–1938.

23. Gueyffier F, Bulpitt C, Boissel JP, *et al.*: Antihypertensive drugs in very old people: a subgroup meta-analysis of randomised controlled trials. *Lancet* 1999, 353:793–796.

24. Major cardiovascular events in hypertensive patients randomized to doxazosin vs. chlorthalidone: The Antihypertensive and Lipid-Lowering treatment to prevent Heart Attack Trial (ALLHAT). ALLHAT Collaborative Research Group. *JAMA* 2000, 283:1967–1975.

25. The sixth report of the Joint National Committee on Prevention, Detection, Evaluation, and Treatment of High Blood Pressure (JNC VI). *Arch Intern Med* 1997, 157:2413–2446.

26. Johansson B, Strandgaard S, Lassen NA: The hypertensive "breakthrough" of autoregulation of cerebral blood flow with forced vasodilatation, flow increase, and blood–brain barrier damage. *Circ Res* 1974, 34–35 (Suppl. I):I167–I171.

27. Elliott WJ: Malignant hypertension. In *Principles of Critical Care.* Edited by Hall JB, Schmidt GA, Wood LDH. New York: McGraw-Hill; 1992:1563–1571.

28. SHEP Cooperative Research Group: Prevention of stroke by anti-hypertensive drug treatment in older persons with isolated systolic hypertension: final results of the Systolic Hypertension in the Elderly Program. *JAMA* 1991, 265:3255–3264.

29. Toumilehto J, Rastenyte D, Birkenhäger WH, *et al.*: Effects of calcium channel blockade in older patients with diabetes and systolic hypertension. *N Engl J Med* 1999, 340:677–684.

30. Staessen JA, Gasowski J, Wang JG, *et al.*: Risks of untreated and treated isolated systolic hypertension in the elderly: meta-analysis of outcome trials. *Lancet* 2000, 355:865–872.

31. Sagie A, Larson MG, Levy D: The natural history of borderline isolated systolic hypertension. *N Engl J Med* 1993, 329:1912–1917.

32. Vasan RS, Larson MG, Leip EP, *et al.*: Impact of high-normal blood pressure on the risk of cardiovascular disease. *N Engl J Med* 2001, 345:1291–1297.

33. Hoyert DL, Arias E, Smith BL, *et al.*: In *Deaths: Final Data for 1999.* National Vital Statistics Reports, Volume 49, No. 8. Hyattsville, MD: National Center for Health Statistics; 2001.

34. Klag MJ, Whelton PK, Randall BL, *et al.*: End-stage renal disease in African-American and white men: 16 year MRFIT findings. *JAMA* 1997, 277:1293–1298.

35. Hypertension Detection and Follow-up Cooperative Group: Persistence of reduction in blood pressure and mortality of participants in the Hypertension Detection and Follow-up Program. *JAMA* 1988, 259:2113–2122.

36. Saunders E, Weir MR, Kong BW, *et al.*: A comparison of the efficacy and safety of a beta-blocker, a calcium channel blocker, and a converting enzyme inhibitor in hypertensive blacks. *Arch Intern Med* 1990, 150:1707–1713.

37. Agodoa LY, Appel L, Bakris GL, *et al.*: African American Study of Kidney Disease and Hypertension (AASK) Study Group. Effect of ramipril vs. amlodipine on renal outcomes in hypertensive nephrosclerosis: A randomized controlled trial. *JAMA* 2001, 285:2719–2728.

38. Taler SJ, Textor SC, Canzanello VJ, Schwartz L: Cyclosporin-induced hypertension: Incidence, pathogenesis, and management. *Drug Safety* 1999, 20:437–449.

39. Curtis JJ: Posttransplant hypertension. *Transplantation Proceedings* 1998, 30:2009–2011.

40. Vaziri ND: Mechanism of erythropoietin-induced hypertension. *Am J Kidney Dis* 1999, 33:821–828.

41. Williams RG, Kavanagh KM, Teo KK: Pathophysiology and treatment of cocaine toxicity: Implications for the heart and cardio-vascular system. *Can J Cardiol* 1996, 12:1295–1301.

42. Frolich ED, Grim C, Labarthe DR, *et al.*: Recommendations for Human Blood Pressure Determination by Sphygmomanometers: Report of a Special Task Force Appointed by the Steering Committee, American Heart Association. *Hypertension* 1988, 11:210A–222A.

43. Perloff D, Grim C, Flack J, *et al.*: Human blood pressure deter-mination by sphygmomanometry. *Circulation* 1993, 88:2460–2467.

44. Gretler DD, Fumo MT, Nelson KS, Murphy MB: Ethnic differences in circadian hemodynamic profile. *Am J Hypertension* 1994, 7:7–14.

45. Staessen JA, O'Brien ET, Atkins N, Amery AK: Short report: ambulatory blood pressure in normotensive compared with hypertensive subjects. *J Hypertension* 1994, 12 (Suppl. 7):S1–S12.

46. Staessen JA, Thijs L, Fagard R, *et al.*: Predicting cardiovascular risk using conventional vs. ambulatory blood pressure in older patients with systolic hypertension. *JAMA* 1999, 282:539–546.

47. National High Blood Pressure Education Program Working Group report on ambulatory blood pressure monitoring. *Arch Intern Med* 1990, 150:2270–2280.

48. O'Brien E, Coats A, Owens P, *et al.*: Use and interpretation of ambulatory blood pressure monitoring: recommendations of the British Hypertension Society. *BMJ* 2000, 320:1128–1134.

49. Tunis S, Kendall P, Londner M, Whyte J: Medicare Coverage Policy. Decisions: Ambulatory Blood Pressure Monitoring (#CAG-00067N): Decision Memorandum. Washington, DC. Health Care Financing Administration, October 17, 2001. http://www.hcfa.gov/coverage/8b3-ff2.htm. Accessed April 1, 2002.

50. White WB, Schulman P, McCabe EJ, Dey HM: Average daily blood pressure, not office blood pressure, determines cardiac function in patients with hypertension. *JAMA* 1989, 261:873–877.

51. Perloff D, Sokolow M, Cowan R: The prognostic value of ambulatory blood pressures. *JAMA* 1983, 249:2792–2798.

52. Verdecchia P, Porcellati C, Schillaci G, *et al.*: Ambulatory blood pressure. An independent predictor of prognosis in essential hypertension. *Hypertension* 1994, 24:793–801.

53. Pickering TG: Recommendations for the use of home (self) and ambulatory blood pressure monitoring. *Am J Hypertension* 1996, 9:1–11.

54. Appel LJ, Stason WB: Ambulatory blood pressure monitoring and blood pressure self-measurement in the diagnosis and management of hypertension. *Ann Intern Med* 1993; 118:867–882.

RECOMMENDATIONS OF THE ADA AND SUMMARY OF THE JNC AND WHO–ISH SPECIAL REPORTS

Norman K. Hollenberg

Hypertension is one of those fields in medicine about which there are regular reports from committees describing guidelines on evaluation and treatment. Although many physicians express mixed feelings about committee reports, the range of choices available for treatment and the magnitude of the healthcare problem makes these consensus statements a valuable source of information. In 1993, the two most widely cited consensus reports were updated. The 1993 Joint National Committee on the Detection, Evaluation, and Treatment of High Blood Pressure [1] was the fifth such meeting in the United States (JNC-V). As was the case for the previous meetings, the Committee's efforts are supported by US federal funds, and all of its members reside in the United States. The World Health Organization–International Society of Hypertension (WHO–ISH) Subcommittee [2] is selected by those two organizations and is largely European, although this committee report also reflects American and Canadian views, as well as views of two members of the Japanese Hypertension Society.

The illustrations from each report are reproduced here as they appeared in the original articles. Although there is inevitably some overlap not only between the two statements, but also with individual chapters in this volume, it seems useful to make both consensus statements available in one location. Although the similarities between the two reports are much more compelling than the differences, there are some differences. The JNC-V report provides a much more detailed set of guidelines. In such a large document, with so many illustrations, emphasis tends to be lost. In the WHO–ISH Report, principles are stressed, and special emphasis is given to associated cardiovascular risk factors that favor treatment and to the overall status of the patient with hypertension.

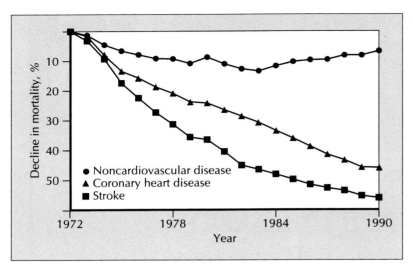

FIGURE 13-1. Decline in age-adjusted mortality for coronary heart disease, stroke, and noncardiovascular disease since 1972. A change in the natural history of any process is likely to reflect multiple factors. In the case of stroke, in which hypertension makes such a large contribution, the striking decline is likely to reflect more effective and more widespread antihypertensive therapy. The extension of treatment to the large number of individuals currently untreated presumably will reduce mortality further. There has been an identical reduction in morbidity. On the other hand, treatment of hypertension in cases of coronary heart disease with the agents used in the 1970s and 1980s probably has contributed much less to the improvement in natural history (*see* Chapter 8). The improvement in the natural history of cardiovascular events has not been matched in the area of noncardiovascular diseases. Data for 1990 are provisional. (*Data from* the National Center for Health Statistics data calculated by the National Heart, Lung, and Blood Institute.)

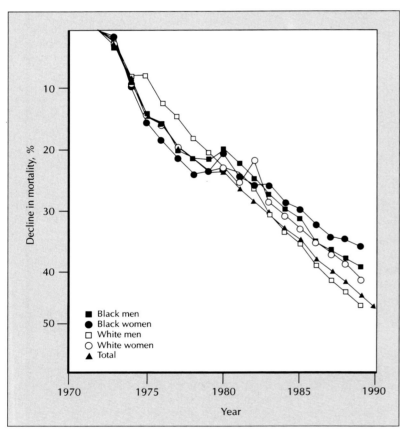

FIGURE 13-2. Decline in age-adjusted mortality for coronary heart disease by race and sex since 1972. Although both sexes and both white and black individuals have participated in the improvement, there has been less improvement in mortality in blacks. The increased incidence and severity of hypertension in blacks may well have contributed to this lag. Data for 1990 are provisional; race and sex data for 1990 were not yet available. (*Data from* the National Center for Health Statistics data calculated by the National Heart, Lung, and Blood Institute.)

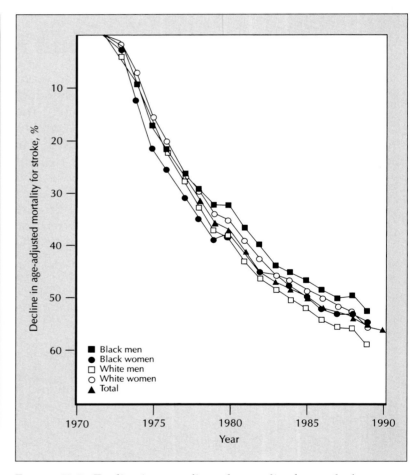

FIGURE 13-3. Decline in age-adjusted mortality for stroke by race and sex since 1972. Both sexes and both races have shown a decline in age-adjusted mortality for stroke, but black men have tended to lag somewhat. The difference in the reduction in stroke rate is smaller, and less consistent, than the race difference for coronary events. Data for 1990 are provisional; race and sex data for 1990 were not yet available. (*Data from* the National Center for Health Statistics data calculated by the National Heart, Lung, and Blood Institute.)

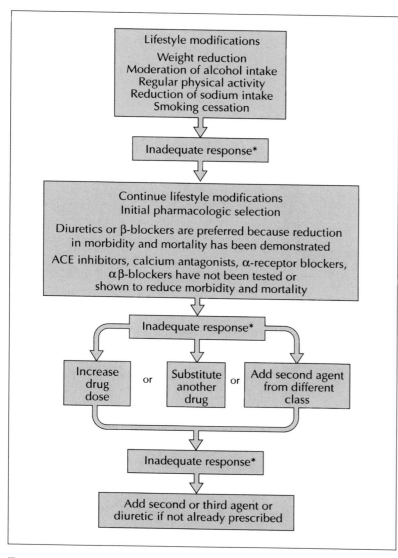

FIGURE 13-4. Treatment algorithm for hypertension. *Asterisks* indicate that response means the patient achieved goal blood pressure or is making considerable progress toward that goal. ACE—angiotensin-converting enzyme.

CLASSIFICATION OF BLOOD PRESSURE FOR ADULTS AGED 18 YEARS AND OLDER

Category	Systolic pressure, mm Hg	Diastolic pressure, mm Hg
Normal*	< 130	< 85
High normal	130–139	85–89
Hypertension†		
Stage 1 (mild)	140–159	90–99
Stage 2 (moderate)	160–179	100–109
Stage 3 (severe)	180–209	110–119
Stage 4 (very severe)	≥ 210	≥ 120

*Optimal blood pressure with respect to cardiovascular risk is < 120/80 mm Hg. However, unusually low readings should be evaluated for clinical significance.

†Based on the average of ≥ 2 readings taken at each of two or more visits after an initial screening.

FIGURE 13-5. Classification of blood pressure for adults 18 years and older not taking antihypertensive drugs and not acutely ill. When systolic and diastolic pressures fall into different categories, the higher category should be selected to classify the individual's blood pressure status. For instance, 160/92 mm Hg should be classified as stage 2, and 180/120 mm Hg should be classified as stage 4. *Isolated systolic hypertension* is defined as a systolic blood pressure of 140 mm Hg or more and a diastolic blood pressure of less than 90 mm Hg and staged appropriately (*eg*, 170/85 mm Hg is categorized as stage 2 isolated systolic hypertension). In addition to classifying stages of hypertension on the basis of average blood pressure levels, the clinician should specify the presence or absence of target-organ disease and additional risk factors. For example, a patient with diabetes and a blood pressure of 142/94 mm Hg, plus left ventricular hypertrophy, should be classified as having "stage 1 hypertension with target-organ disease (left ventricular hypertrophy) and with another major risk factor (diabetes)." This specificity is important for risk classification and management.

HYPERTENSION AWARENESS, TREATMENT, AND CONTROL RATES

	1971–1972	1974–1975	1976–1980	1988–1991
Aware, %	51	64	(54)73	(65)84
Treated, %	36	34	(33)56	(49)73
Controlled, %	16	20	(11)34	(21)55

FIGURE 13-6. Hypertension awareness, treatment, and control rates. Patients with *hypertension* are defined as those with a one-occasion measurement of 160/95 mm Hg or more or those currently taking antihypertensive medication. *Aware* indicates those told by their physicians that they are hypertensive; *treated* indicates those hypertensives taking medication. Numbers in parentheses are percentages of patients with blood pressures of 140/90 mm Hg or more. The source of data for 1971 to 1972 and 1974 to 1975: National Health and Nutrition Examination Survey I [3]; for 1976 to 1980: National Health and Nutrition Examination Survey II [4]; and for 1988 to 1991: National Health and Nutrition Examination Survey III (unpublished data provided by the Centers for Disease Control and Prevention, National Center for Health Statistics).

MANIFESTATIONS OF TARGET-ORGAN DISEASE

ORGAN SYSTEM	MANIFESTATIONS
Cardiac	Clinical, electrocardiographic, or radiologic evidence of coronary artery disease; left ventricular hypertrophy or "strain" by electrocardiography or left ventricular hypertrophy by echocardiography; left ventricular dysfunction or cardiac failure
Cerebrovascular	Transient ischemic heart attack or stroke
Peripheral vascular	Absence of 1 or more major pulses in extremities (except for dorsalis pedis) with or without intermittent claudication; aneurysm
Renal	Serum creatinine ≥130 µmol/L (1.5 mg/dL); proteinuria (1+ or greater); microalbuminuria
Retinopathy	Hemorrhages or exudates, with or without papilledema

FIGURE 13-7. Manifestations of target-organ disease.

RECOMMENDATIONS FOR FOLLOW-UP BASED ON INITIAL SET OF BLOOD PRESSURE MEASUREMENTS FOR ADULTS

INITIAL SCREENING BLOOD PRESSURE, *mm Hg*		FOLLOW-UP RECOMMENDED
SYSTOLIC	DIASTOLIC	
< 130	< 85	Recheck in 2 y
130–139	85–89	Recheck in 1 y
140–159	90–99	Confirm within 2 mo
160–179	100–109	Evaluate or refer to source of care within 1 mo
180–209	110–119	Evaluate or refer to source of care within 1 wk
≥ 210	≥ 120	Evaluate or refer to source of care immediately

FIGURE 13-8. Follow-up recommendations for adults based on initial blood pressure measurements. If the systolic and diastolic categories are different in the initial screening, recommendations for the shorter term follow-up should be followed. That is, someone with a blood pressure of 160/85 mm Hg should be evaluated or referred to the source of care within 1 month. The scheduling of follow-up should be modified by reliable information about past blood pressure measurements, other cardiovascular risk factors, or target-organ disease. For patients with systolic pressures of 130 to 139 mm Hg and diastolic pressures of 85 to 89 mm Hg, the clinician should consider providing advice about lifestyle modifications.

SITUATIONS IN WHICH AUTOMATED NONINVASIVE AMBULATORY BLOOD PRESSURE MONITORING DEVICES MAY BE USEFUL

"Office" or "white-coat" hypertension: blood pressure repeatedly elevated in office setting but repeatedly normal out of office

Evaluation of drug resistance

Evaluation of nocturnal blood pressure changes

Episodic hypertension

Hypotensive symptoms associated with antihypertensive medications or autonomic dysfunction

Carotid sinus syncope and pacemaker syndromes

FIGURE 13-9. Situations in which automated noninvasive ambulatory blood pressure monitoring devices may be useful. For carotid sinus syncope and pacemaker syndromes, electrocardiographic monitoring should also be used.

LIFESTYLE MODIFICATIONS FOR HYPERTENSION CONTROL OR OVERALL CARDIOVASCULAR RISK

Lose weight if overweight

Limit alcohol intake to ≤ 1 oz/d of ethanol (24 oz of beer, 8 oz of wine, or 2 oz of 100-proof whiskey)

Exercise (aerobic) regularly

Reduce sodium intake to < 100 mmol/d (< 2.3 g of sodium or approximately < 6 g of sodium chloride)

Maintain adequate dietary potassium, calcium, and magnesium intake

Stop smoking and reduce dietary saturated fat and cholesterol intake for overall cardiovascular health; reducing fat intake also helps reduce caloric intake—important for control of weight and type II diabetes

---

FIGURE 13-10. Lifestyle modifications for hypertension control or overall cardiovascular risk.

ANTIHYPERTENSIVE AGENTS

A. DIURETICS (INITIAL ANTIHYPERTENSIVE AGENTS)

Type of drug	Usual dosage range, *total mg/d*	Frequency, *times/d*	Mechanisms	Comments
Thiazides and related agents			Decreased plasma volume and decreased extracellular fluid volume; decreased cardiac output initially, followed by decreased total peripheral resistance with normalization of cardiac output; long-term effects include slight decrease in extracellular fluid volume	Lower doses and dietary counseling should be used to avoid metabolic changes; more effective antihypertensive than loop diuretics except in patients with serum creatinine ≥ 221 μmol/L (2.5 mg/dL); hydrochlorothiazide or chlorthalidone is generally preferred; used in most clinical trials
Bendroflumethiazide	2.5–5	1		
Benzthiazide	12.5–50	1		
Chlorothiazide	125–500	2		
Chlorthalidone	12.5–50	1		
Cyclothiazide	1.0–2	1		
Hydrochlorothiazide	12.5–50	1		
Hydroflumethiazide	12.5–50	1		
Indapamide	2.5–5	1		
Methyclothiazide	2.5–5	1		
Metolazone	0.5–5	1		
Polythiazide	1.0–4	1		
Quinethazone	25.0–100	1		
Trichlormethiazide	1.0–4	2		
Loop diuretics			*See* above	Higher doses of loop diuretics may be needed for patients with renal impairment or congestive heart failure; ethacrynic acid is only alternative for patients with allergy to thiazide and sulfur-containing diuretics
Bumetanide	0.5–5	2		
Ethacrynic acid	25.0–100	2		
Furosemide	20.0–320	1 or 2		
Potassium-sparing drugs				Weak diuretics; used mainly in combination with other diuretics to avoid or reverse hypokalemia from other diuretics; avoid when serum creatinine ≥ 221 μmol/L (2.5 mg/dL); may cause hyperkalemia, and this may be exaggerated when combined with ACE inhibitors or potassium supplements
Amiloride	5–10	2 or 3	Increased potassium resorption	
Spironolactone	25–100	1 or 2	Aldosterone antagonist	
Triamterene	50–150			

FIGURE 13-11. Antihypertensive agents. **A,** Diuretics. (*continued*)

B. ADRENERGIC INHIBITORS (INITIAL ANTIHYPERTENSIVE AGENTS)

Type of drug	Usual dosage range, *total mg/d*	Frequency, *times/d*	Mechanisms	Comments
β-Blockers			Decreased cardiac output and increased total peripheral resistance; decreased plasma renin activity; atenolol, betaxolol, bisoprolol and metoprolol are cardioselective	Selective agents will also inhibit β_2-receptors in higher doses, *eg,* all may aggravate asthma
Atenolol	25–100*	1		
Betaxolol	5–40	1		
Bisoprolol	5–20	1		
Metoprolol	50–200	1 or 2		
Metoprolol (extended release)	50–200	1		
Nadolol	20–240*	1		
Propranolol	40–240	2		
Propranolol (long acting)	60–240	1		
Timolol	20–40	2		
β-Blockers with ISA			Acebutolol is cardioselective	No clear advantage for agents with ISA except in those with bradycardia who must receive a β-blocker; they produce fewer or no metabolic side effects
Acebutolol	200–1200*	2		
Carteolol	2.5–10*	1		
Penbutolol	20–80	1		
Pindolol	10–60	2		
αβ-Blocker			Same as β-blockers, plus α_1-blockade	Possibly more effective in blacks than other β-blockers; may cause postural effects; titration should be based on standing blood pressure
Labetalol	200–1200	2		
α_1-Receptor blockers			Block postsynaptic α_1-receptors and cause vasodilation	All may cause postural effects; titration should be based on standing blood pressure
Doxazosin	1.0–16	1		
Prazosin	1.0–20	2 or 3		
Terazosin	1.0–20	1		

C. ACE INHIBITORS (INITIAL ANTIHYPERTENSIVE AGENTS)

Type of drug	Usual dosage range, *total mg/d*	Frequency, *times/d*	Mechanisms	Comments
Benazepril	10.0–40*	1 or 2	Block formation of angiotensin II, promoting vasodilation and decreased aldosterone; also increased bradykinin and vasodilatory prostaglandins	Diuretic doses should be reduced or discontinued before starting ACE inhibitors whenever possible to prevent excessive hypotension; reduce dose of those drugs marked with asterisks in patients with serum creatinine ≥ 221 µmol/L (2.5 mg/dL); may cause hyperkalemia in patients with renal impairment or in those receiving potassium-sparing agents; can cause acute renal failure in patients with severe bilateral renal artery stenosis or severe stenosis in artery to solitary kidney
Captopril	12.5–150*	2		
Cilazapril	2.5–5.0	1 or 2		
Enalapril	2.5–40*	1 or 2		
Fosinopril	10.0–40	1 or 2		
Lisinopril	5.0–40	1 or 2		
Perindopril	1.0–16	1 or 2		
Quinapril	5.0–80	1 or 2		
Ramipril	1.25–20	1 or 2		
Spirapril	12.5–50	1 or 2		

FIGURE 13-11. *(continued)* **B,** Adrenergic inhibitors. **C,** Angiotensin-converting enzyme (ACE) inhibitors. **D,** Calcium antagonists. **E,** Supplemental agents. For all patients, lifestyle modification should be advised. In each case, the lower dosage of the usual dose range is preferred, and the higher dose is the maximum daily dose. Most agents require 2 to 4 weeks for complete efficacy, and more frequent dosage adjustments are not advised except for severe hypertension. *(continued)*

D. CALCIUM ANTAGONISTS (INITIAL ANTIHYPERTENSIVE AGENTS)

Type of drug	Usual dosage range, *total mg/d*	Frequency, *times/d*	Mechanisms	Comments
Diltiazem	90–360	3	Block inward movement of calcium ion across cell membranes and cause smooth-muscle relaxation	These agents also block slow channels in heart and may reduce sinus rate and produce heart block
Diltiazem (sustained release)	120–360	2		
Diltiazem (extended release)	180–360	1		
Verapamil	80–480	2		
Verapamil (long acting)	120–480	1 or 2		
Dihydropyridines				
Amlodipine	2.5–10	1		Dihydropyridines are more potent peripheral vasodilators than diltiazem and verapamil and may cause more dizziness, headache, flushing, peripheral edema, and tachycardia
Felodipine	5–20	1		
Isradipine	2.5–10	2		
Nicardipine	60–120	3		
Nifedipine	30–120	3		
Nifedipine (GITS)	30–90	1		

E. α₂-AGONISTS, ADRENERGIC ANTAGONISTS, DIRECT VASODILATORS (SUPPLEMENTAL ANTIHYPERTENSIVE AGENTS)

Type of drug	Usual dosage range, *total mg/d*	Frequency, *times/d*	Mechanisms	Comments
Centrally acting α₂-agonists				
Clonidine	0.1–1.2	2	Stimulate central α₂-receptors that inhibit efferent sympathetic activity	Clonidine patch is replaced once/wk; none of these agents should be withdrawn abruptly; avoid in patients who do not adhere to treatment
Clonidine (patch)*	0.1–0.3	1 weekly		
Guanabenz	4–64	2		
Guanfacine	1–3	1		
Methyldopa	250–2000	2		
Peripheral-acting adrenergic antagonists				
Guanadrel	10–75	2	Inhibits catecholamine release from neuronal storage sites	May cause serious orthostatic and exercise-induced hypotension
Guanethidine	10–100	1		
Rauwolfia alkaloids				
Rauwolfia serpentina	50–200	1	Depletion of tissue stores of catecholamines	
Reserpine	0.05†–0.25	1		
Direct vasodilators				
Hydralazine	50–300	2–4	Direct smooth-muscle relaxation (primarily arteriolar)	Hydralazine is subject to phenotypically determined metabolism (acetylation); for both agents, should treat concomitantly with diuretic and β-blocker due to fluid retention and reflex tachycardia
Minoxidil	2.5–80	1 or 2		

*Weekly patch is 1, 2, 3, equivalent to 0.1 to 0.3 mg/d.

†A 0.1-mg dose may be given every other day to achieve this dosage.

FIGURE 13-11. *(continued)* The dosage range may differ slightly from the recommended dosage in the *Physician's Desk Reference* or package insert. *Asterisks* indicate drugs that are excreted by the kidney and require dosage reduction in patients with renal impairment (serum creatinine ≥ 221 µmol/L [≥ 2.5 mg/dL]). ISA—intrinsic sympathomimetic activity; GITS—gastrointestinal therapeutic system.

ANTIHYPERTENSIVE DRUG THERAPY: INDIVIDUALIZATION BASED ON SPECIAL CONSIDERATIONS (GUIDELINES FOR SELECTING INITIAL THERAPY)

A. CARDIOVASCULAR

Clinical situation	Preferred	Requires special monitoring	Relatively or absolutely contraindicated
Angina pectoris	β-Blockers, calcium antagonists	—	Direct vasodilators
Bradycardia/heart block, sick sinus syndrome	—	—	β-Blockers, labetalol, verapamil, diltiazem
Cardiac failure	Diuretics, ACE inhibitors	—	β-Blockers, calcium antagonists, labetalol
Hypertrophic cardiomyopathy with severe diastolic dysfunction	β-Blockers, diltiazem, verapamil	—	Diuretics, ACE inhibitors, α_1-blockers, hydralazine, minoxidil
Hyperdynamic circulation	β-Blockers	—	Direct vasodilators
Peripheral vascular occlusive disease	—	β-Blockers	—
After myocardial infarction	Non-ISA β-blockers	—	Direct vasodilators

B. RENAL

Clinical situation	Preferred	Requires special monitoring	Relatively or absolutely contraindicated
Bilateral renal arterial disease or severe stenosis in artery to solitary kidney	—	—	ACE inhibitors
Renal insufficiency			
Early (serum creatinine, 130–221 μmol/L [1.5–2.5 mg/dL])	—	—	Potassium-sparing agents, potassium supplements
Advanced (serum creatinine, ≥221 μmol/L [≥ 2.5 mg/dL])	Loop diuretics	ACE inhibitors	Potassium-sparing agents, potassium supplements

C. OTHER

Clinical situation	Preferred	Requires special monitoring	Relatively or absolutely contraindicated
Asthma/COPD	—	—	β-Blockers, labetalol
Cyclosporine-associated hypertension	Nifedipine, labetalol	Verapamil, nicardipine, diltiazem	—
Depression	—	α_2-Agonists	Reserpine
Diabetes mellitus			
Type I (insulin-dependent)	—	β-Blockers	—
Type II	—	β-Blockers, diuretics	—
Dyslipidemia	—	Diuretics, β-blockers	—
Liver disease	—	Labetalol	Methyldopa
Vascular headache	β-Blockers	—	—
Pregnancy			
Preeclampsia	Methyldopa, hydralazine	—	Diuretics, ACE inhibitors
Chronic hypertension	Methyldopa	—	ACE inhibitors

FIGURE 13-12. A–C, Individualization of antihypertensive drug therapy based on special considerations and clinical situations. For cyclosporine-associated hypertension, verapamil, nicardipine, and diltiazem can increase serum levels of cyclosporine. ACE—angiotensin-converting enzyme; ISA—intrinsic sympathomimetic activity; COPD—chronic obstructive pulmonary disease.

SELECTED DRUG INTERACTIONS WITH ANTIHYPERTENSIVE THERAPY

A. DIURETICS

Possible situations for decreased antihypertensive effects
  Cholestyramine and colestipol decrease absorption
  NSAIDs (including aspirin and over-the-counter ibuprofen) may antagonize diuretic effectiveness
Possible situations for increased antihypertensive effects
  Combinations of thiazides (especially metolazone) with furosemide can produce profound diuresis, natriuresis, and kaliuresis in renal impairment

Effects of diuretics on other drugs
  Diuretics can raise serum lithium levels and increase toxic effects by enhancing proximal tubular resorption of lithium
  Diuretics may make it more difficult to control dyslipidemia and diabetes

B. β-BLOCKERS

Possible situations for decreased antihypertensive effects
NSAIDs may decrease effects of β-blockers
Rifampin, smoking, and phenobarbital decrease serum levels of agents primarily metabolized by liver, owing to enzyme induction
Possible situations for increased antihypertensive effects
Cimetidine may increase serum levels of β-blockers that are primarily metabolized by liver, owing to enzyme inhibition
Quinidine may increase risk of hypotension

Effects of β-blockers on other drugs
Combinations of diltiazem or verapamil with β-blockers may have additive sinoatrial and atrioventricular node depressant effects and may also promote negative inotropic effects on failing myocardium
Combination of β-blockers and reserpine may cause marked bradycardia and syncope
β-Blockers may increase serum levels of theophylline, lidocaine, and chlorpromazine, owing to reduced hepatic clearance
Nonselective β-blockers prolong insulin-induced hypoglycemia and promote rebound hypertension due to unopposed α stimulation; all β-blockers mask adrenergically mediated symptoms of hypoglycemia and have potential to aggravate diabetes
β-Blockers may make it more difficult to control dyslipidemia
Phenylpropanolamine (which can be obtained over the counter in cold and diet preparations), pseudoephedrine, ephedrine, and epinephrine can cause elevations in blood pressure, owing to unopposed α-receptor–induced vasoconstriction

C. CALCIUM ANTAGONISTS

Possible situations for decreased antihypertensive effects
  Serum levels and antihypertensive effects of calcium antagonists may be diminished by these interactions: rifampin-verapamil; carbamazepine-diltiazem and verapamil; phenobarbital and phenytoin-verapamil
Possible situations for increased antihypertensive effects
  Cimetidine may increase pharmacologic effects of all calcium antagonists, owing to inhibition of hepatic metabolizing enzymes resulting in increased serum levels
Effects of calcium antagonists on other drugs
  Digoxin and carbamazepine serum levels and toxic effects may be increased by verapamil and possibly by diltiazem
  Serum levels of prazosin, quinidine, and theophylline may be increased by verapamil
Serum levels of cyclosporine may be increased by diltiazem, nicardipine, and verapamil; cyclosporine dose may need to be decreased

D. ACE INHIBITORS

Possible situations for decreased antihypertensive effects
  NSAIDs (including aspirin and over-the-counter ibuprofen) may decrease blood pressure control
  Antacids may decrease the bioavailability of ACE inhibitors

Possible situations for increased antihypertensive effects
  Diuretics may lead to excessive hypotensive effects (hypovolemia)

Effects of ACE inhibitors on other drugs
  Hyperkalemia may occur with potassium supplements, potassium-sparing agents, and NSAIDs
  ACE inhibitors may increase serum lithium level.

FIGURE 13-13. Selected drug interactions with antihypertensive therapy, including diuretics (**A**), β-blockers (**B**), calcium antagonists (**C**), angiotensin-converting enzyme (ACE) inhibitors (**D**),

Continued on next page

E. α-BLOCKERS AND SYMPATHOLYTICS

α-BLOCKERS

Possible situations for increased antihypertensive effects

Concomitant antihypertensive drug therapy (especially diuretics) may
  increase chance of postural hypotension

SYMPATHOLYTICS

Possible situations for decreased antihypertensive effects

  Tricyclic antidepressants may decrease effects of centrally acting and peripheral
    norepinephrine depleters

  Sympathomimetics, including over-the-counter cold and diet preparations,
    amphetamines, phenothiazines, and cocaine, may interfere with
    antihypertensive effects of guanethidine and guanadrel

  Severity of clonidine withdrawal reaction can be increased by β-blockers

  Monoamine oxidase inhibitors may prevent degradation and metabolism of
    norepinephrine released by tyramine-containing foods and may cause
    hypertension; they may also cause hypertensive reactions when combined
    with reserpine or guanethidine

Effects of sympatholytics on other drugs

  Methyldopa may increase serum lithium levels

FIGURE 13-13. (*continued*) and α-blockers and sympatholytics (**E**). These lists do not include all potential drug interactions with antihypertensive drugs. NSAID—nonsteroidal anti-inflammatory drug.

ADVERSE DRUG EFFECTS

A. DIURETICS

DRUGS	SELECTED SIDE EFFECTS	PRECAUTIONS AND SPECIAL CONSIDERATIONS
Thiazides and related diuretics	Hypokalemia, hypomagnesemia, hyponatremia, hyperuricemia, hypercalcemia, hyperglycemia, hypercholesterolemia, hypertriglyceridemia, sexual dysfunction, weakness	Except for metolazone and indapamide, ineffective in renal failure (serum creatine ≥ 221 μmol/L [≥ 2.5 mg/dL]); hypokalemia increases digitalis toxic effect; may precipitate acute gout
Loop diuretics	Same as for thiazides except loop diuretics do not cause hypercalcemia	Effective in chronic renal failure
Potassium-sparing agents	Hyperkalemia	Danger of hyperkalemia in patients with renal failure, in patients treated with ACE inhibitor or with NSAIDs
Amiloride	—	—
Spironolactone	Gynecomastia, mastodynia, menstrual irregularities, diminished libido in males	—
Triamterene	—	Danger of renal calculi

FIGURE 13-14. **A** through **F**, Adverse drug effects (*see* Fig. 13-11 for a list of drugs). This listing of side effects is not all-inclusive, and clinicians are urged to refer to the package inserts for a more detailed listing. Sexual dysfunction, particularly impotence in men, has been reported with the use of all antihypertensive agents. Few data are available on the effect of antihypertensive agents on sexual function in women. Some of the metabolic side effects of diuretics and β-blockers can be minimized by appropriate dietary counseling. ACE—angiotensin-converting enzyme; CHF—congestive heart failure; COPD—chronic obstructive pulmonary disease; ISA—intrinsic sympathomimetic activity; NSAID—nonsteroidal anti-inflammatory drug. *Continued on next page*

B. ADRENERGIC INHIBITORS

DRUGS	SELECTED SIDE EFFECTS	PRECAUTIONS AND SPECIAL CONSIDERATIONS
β-Blockers	Bronchospasm, may aggravate peripheral arterial insufficiency, fatigue, insomnia, exacerbation of CHF, masking of symptoms of hypoglycemia; also, hypertriglyceridemia, decreased high-density lipoprotein cholesterol (except for drugs with ISA); reduces exercise tolerance	Should not be used in patients with asthma, COPD, CHF with systolic dysfunction, heart block (greater than 1st degree), and sick sinus syndrome; use with caution in insulin-treated diabetics and patients with peripheral vascular disease; should not be discontinued abruptly in patients with ischemic heart disease
αβ-Blocker Labetalol	Bronchospasm, may aggravate peripheral vascular insufficiency, orthostatic hypotension	Should not be used in patients with asthma, COPD, CHF, heart block (greater than 1st degree), and sick sinus syndrome; use with caution in insulin-treated diabetics and patients with peripheral vascular disease
α₁-Receptor blockers	Orthostatic hypotension, syncope, weakness, palpitations, headache	Use cautiously in older patients because of orthostatic hypotension

C. ACE INHIBITORS

SELECTED SIDE EFFECTS	PRECAUTIONS AND SPECIAL CONSIDERATIONS
Cough, rash, angioneurotic edema, hyperkalemia, dysgeusia	Hyperkalemia can develop, particularly in patients with renal insufficiency; hypotension has been observed with initiation of ACE inhibitors, especially in patients with high plasma renin activity or receiving diuretic therapy; can cause reversible, acute renal failure in patients with bilateral renal arterial stenosis or unilateral stenosis in solitary kidney and in patients with cardiac failure and with volume depletion; rarely can induce neutropenia or proteinuria; absolutely contraindicated in 2nd and 3rd trimesters of pregnancy

D. CALCIUM ANTAGONISTS

DRUGS	SELECTED SIDE EFFECTS	PRECAUTIONS AND SPECIAL CONSIDERATIONS
Dihydropyridines Amlodipine Felodipine Isradipine Nicardipine Nifedipine	Headache, dizziness, peripheral edema, tachycardia, gingival hyperplasia	Use with caution in patients with CHF; may aggravate angina and myocardial ischemia
Diltiazem Verapamil	Headache, dizziness, peripheral edema (less common than with dihydropyridines), gingival hyperplasia, constipation (especially verapamil), atrioventricular block, bradycardia	Use with caution in patients with cardiac failure; contraindicated in patients with 2nd- or 3rd-degree heart block, or sick sinus syndrome

FIGURE 13-14. (*Continued*)

E. CENTRALLY ACTING α₂-AGONISTS

DRUGS	SELECTED SIDE EFFECTS	PRECAUTIONS AND SPECIAL CONSIDERATIONS
Clonidine Guanabenz Guanfacine hydrochloride	Drowsiness, sedation, dry mouth, fatigue, orthostatic dizziness	Rebound hypertension may occur with abrupt discontinuance, particularly with previous administration of high doses or with continuation of concomitant β-blocker therapy
Clonidine patch	Same as for clonidine; localized skin reaction to patch	—
Methyldopa	—	May cause liver damage, fever, and Coombs-positive hemolytic anemia

F. PERIPHERAL-ACTING ADRENERGIC ANTAGONISTS AND DIRECT VASODILATORS

DRUGS	SELECTED SIDE EFFECTS	PRECAUTIONS AND SPECIAL CONSIDERATIONS
Peripheral-acting adrenergic antagonists		
Guanadrel sulfate Guanethidine monosulfate	Diarrhea, orthostatic and exercise hypotension	Use cautiously because of orthostatic hypotension
Rauwolfia alkaloids Reserpine	Lethargy, nasal congestion, depression	Contraindicated in patients with history of mental depression or with active peptic ulcer
Direct vasodilators	Headache, tachycardia, fluid retention	May precipitate angina pectoris in patients with coronary artery disease; generally, use with diuretic and β-blocker
Hydralazine	Positive antinuclear antibody test	Lupus syndrome may occur (rare at recommended doses)
Minoxidil	Hypertrichosis	May cause or aggravate pleural and pericardial effusions

FIGURE 13-14. (*Continued*)

CAUSES OF LACK OF RESPONSIVENESS TO THERAPY

A. NONADHERENCE TO THERAPY

Cost of medication

Instructions not clear and/or not given to patient in writing

Inadequate or no patient education

Lack of involvement of patient in treatment plan

Side effects of medication

Organic brain syndrome (*eg*, memory deficit)

Inconvenient dosing

FIGURE 13-15. Causes of lack of responsiveness to antihypertensive therapy, including nonadherence (**A**), drug-related causes (**B**), and associated conditions (**C**).

B. DRUG-RELATED CAUSES

Doses too low

Inappropriate combinations (*eg*, two centrally acting adrenergic inhibitors)

Rapid inactivation (*eg*, hydralazine)

Drug interactions

   Nonsteroidal anti-inflammatory drugs

   Oral contraceptives

   Sympathomimetics

   Antidepressants

   Adrenal steroids

   Nasal decongestants

   Licorice-containing substances (*eg*, chewing tobacco)

   Cocaine

   Cyclosporine

   Erythropoietin

C. ASSOCIATED CONDITIONS

Increasing obesity

Alcohol intake more than 1 oz/d of ethanol

Secondary hypertension

   Renal insufficiency

   Renovascular hypertension

   Pheochromocytoma

   Primary aldosteronism

Volume overload

   Inadequate diuretic therapy

   Excess sodium intake

   Fluid retention from reduction of blood pressure

   Progressive renal damage

Pseudohypertension

A. PARENTERAL VASODILATORS

DRUG	DOSE	ONSET	CAUTIONS
Sodium nitroprusside	0.25–10 µg/kg/min as IV infusion; maximal dose for 10 min only	Instantaneous	Nausea, vomiting, muscle twitching; with prolonged use may cause thiocyanate intoxication, methemoglobinemia acidosis, cyanide poisoning; bags, bottles, and delivery sets must be light resistant
Nitroglycerin	5–100 µg as IV infusion	2–5 min	Headache, tachycardia, vomiting, flushing, methemoglobinemia; requires special delivery system due to drug binding to PVC tubing
Diazoxide	50–150 mg as IV bolus, repeated, or 15–30 mg/min by IV infusion	1–2 min	Hypotension, tachycardia, aggravation of angina pectoris, nausea and vomiting, hyperglycemia with repeated injections
Hydralazine	10–20 mg as IV bolus / 10–40 mg IM	10 min / 20–30 min	Tachycardia, headache, vomiting, aggravation of angina pectoris
Enalaprilat	0.625–1.25 mg every 6 h IV	15–60 min	Renal failure in patients with bilateral renal artery stenosis, hypotension

B. PARENTERAL ADRENERGIC INHIBITORS

DRUG	DOSE	ONSET	CAUTIONS
Phentolamine	5–15 mg as IV bolus	1–2 min	Tachycardia, orthostatic hypotension
Trimethaphan camsylate	1–4 mg/min as IV infusion	1–5 min	Paresis of bowel and bladder, orthostatic hypotension, blurred vision, dry mouth
Labetalol	20–80 mg as IV bolus every 10 min; 2 mg/min as IV infusion	5–10 min	Bronchoconstriction, heart block, orthostatic hypotension
Methyldopate	250–500 mg as IV infusion every 6 h	30–60 min	Drowsiness

C. ORAL AGENTS

DRUG	DOSE	ONSET	CAUTIONS
Nifedipine (not extended release)	10–20 mg PO, repeat after 30 min	15–30 min	Rapid, uncontrolled reduction in blood pressure may precipitate circulatory collapse in patients with aortic stenosis
Captopril	25 mg PO, repeat as required	15–30 min	Hypotension, renal failure in bilateral renal artery stenosis
Clonidine	0.1–0.2 mg PO, repeated every hour as required to a total dose of 0.6 mg	30–60 min	Hypotension, drowsiness, dry mouth
Labetalol	200–400 mg PO, repeat every 2–3 h	30 min–2 h	Bronchoconstriction, heart block, orthostatic hypotension

FIGURE 13-16. A through C, Emergencies and urgencies with various drugs in the management of hypertensive crises. It is sometimes appropriate to administer a diuretic agent with any of these drugs. IM—intramuscular; IV—intravenous; PO—orally; PVC—polyvinyl chloride.

CLASSIFICATION OF HYPERTENSION IN THE YOUNG BY AGE GROUP

Age group	High normal (90–94th percentile), *mm Hg*	Significant hypertension (95th–99th percentile), *mm Hg*	Severe hypertension (>99th percentile), *mm Hg*
Newborns (SBP)			
7 d	—	96–105	≥ 106
8–30 d	—	104–109	≥ 110
Infants (≤2 y)			
SBP	104–111	112–117	≥ 118
DBP	70–73	74–81	≥ 82
Children			
3–5 y			
SBP	108–115	116–123	≥ 124
DBP	70–75	76–83	≥ 84
6–9 y			
SBP	114–121	122–129	≥ 130
DBP	74–77	78–85	≥ 86
10–12 y			
SBP	122–125	126–133	≥ 134
DBP	78–81	82–89	≥ 90
13–15 y			
SBP	130–135	136–143	≥ 144
DBP	80–85	86–91	≥ 92
Adolescents (16–18 y)			
SBP	136–141	142–149	≥ 150
DBP	84–91	92–97	≥ 98

FIGURE 13-17. Classification of hypertension in the young by age group. Adult classifications differ. DBP—diastolic blood pressure; SBP—systolic blood pressure. (*Adapted from* the Report of the Task Force on Blood Pressure Control in Children [5].)

EFFECTS OF THERAPY IN OLDER HYPERTENSIVE PATIENTS

	Australian [6]	EWPHE [7]	Coope and Warrender [8]	STOP-Hypertension [9]	MRC [10]	SHEP [11]	HDFP [12]*
Patients, *n*	582	840	884	1627	4396	4736	2374
Age range, *y*	60–69	>60	60–79	70–84	65–74	60–≥80	60–69
Mean BP at entry, *mm Hg*	165/101	182/101	197/100	195/102	185/91	170/77	170/101
Relative risk of event (treated vs control)							
Stroke	0.67	0.64	0.58[†]	0.53[†]	0.75[†]	0.67[†]	0.56[†]
CAD	0.82	0.80	1.03	0.87[‡]	0.81	0.73[†]	0.85[†]
CHF	—	0.78	0.68	0.49[†]	—	0.45[†]	—
All CVD	0.69	0.71[†]	0.76[†]	0.60[†]	0.83[†]	0.68[†]	0.84[†]

*Includes data calculated by the Hypertension Detection and Follow-up Program (HDFP) Coordinating Center.
[†]Statistically significant.
[‡]Myocardial infarction only; sudden deaths decreased from 13 to 4.

FIGURE 13-18. Effects of therapy in older hypertensive patients. BP—blood pressure; CAD—coronary artery disease; CHF—congestive heart failure; CVD—cardiovascular disease; EWPHE—European Working Party on High Blood Pressure in the Elderly; MRC—Medical Research Council; SHEP—Systolic Hypertension in the Elderly; STOP-Hypertension—Swedish Trial in Old Patients with Hypertension.

CARDIOVASCULAR RISK FACTORS FAVORING TREATMENT

Age*

Gender*

Family history of premature
  cardiovascular disease*

Raised systolic blood pressure

Raised diastolic blood pressure

Smoking

Raised total and LDL cholesterol

Reduced HDL cholesterol

Left ventricular hypertrophy

Previous cardiovascular events*

Previous cerebrovascular events*

Diabetes

Renal disease

Microalbuminuria

Obesity

Sedentary lifestyle

FIGURE 13-19. Cardiovascular risk factors favoring treatment. Factors marked with *asterisks* are not modifiable. HDL—high-density lipoprotein; LDL—low-density lipoprotein.

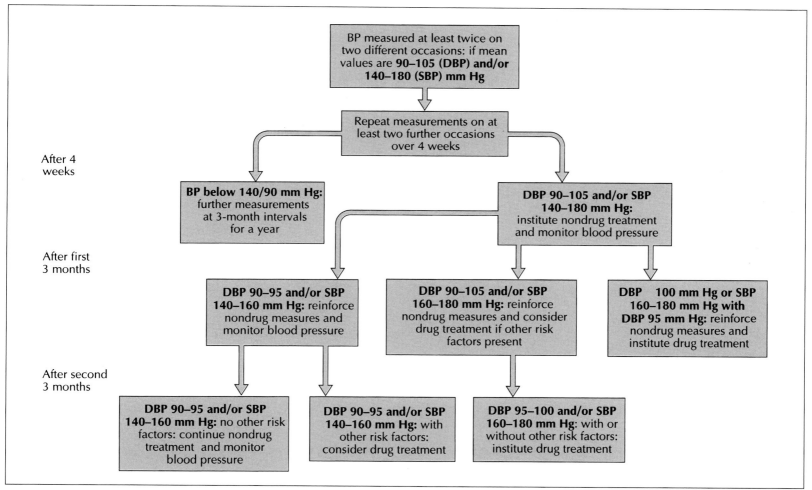

FIGURE 13-20. Management of mild hypertension. *Mild hypertension* is defined as diastolic blood pressure (DBP) of 90 to 105 mm Hg and/or systolic blood pressure (SBP) of 140 to 180 mm Hg. Drug treatment should be instituted more promptly in patients with evidence of substantial risk of cardiovascular disease or in patients with blood pressure above the mild hypertension range. Although the World Health Organization and Joint National Committee disagree on the definition of "mild" hypertension, both groups recommend nondrug treatment for 3 months before initiating drug treatment in this group. Many experts are sanguine about patient compliance with nondrug treatment, however, and would disagree with this recommendation. Although weight loss will correct hypertension in many who are overweight, and reduction in salt or alcohol intake will help if these are used to excess, the ability of physicians to persuade patients to change their behavior—unless they have a strong support group and show evidence of being prepared to change their behavior—remains ambiguous.

CLASSIFICATION OF HYPERTENSION BY BLOOD PRESSURE LEVEL

	SYSTOLIC BP, *mm Hg*		DIASTOLIC BP, *mm Hg*
Normotension	<140	and	<90
Mild hypertension	140–180	and/or	90–105
Borderline hypertension	140–160	and/or	90–95
Moderate and severe hypertension	≥180	and/or	≥105
ISH	≥140	and	<90
Borderline ISH	140–160	and	<90

FIGURE 13-21. Classification of hypertension by blood pressure (BP) level. In moderate and severe hypertension, risk is indicated by reporting the actual systolic and diastolic blood pressures. ISH—isolated systolic hypertension.

CLASSIFICATION OF HYPERTENSION BY EXTENT OF ORGAN DAMAGE

Stage I   No objective signs of organic changes

Stage II   At least one of the following signs of organ involvement:
Left ventricular hypertrophy (radiography electrocardiography, echocardiography)
Generalized and focal narrowing of the retinal arteries
Proteinuria and/or slight elevation of plasma creatinine concentration (1.2–2.0 mg/dL)
Ultrasound or radiologic evidence of atherosclerotic plaque (carotid arteries, aorta, iliac and femoral arteries)

Stage III   Both symptoms and signs have appeared as a result of organ damage, including:
Heart: angina pectoris, myocardial infarction, heart failure
Brain: TIA, stroke, hypertensive encephalopathy
Optic fundi: retinal hemorrhages and exudates with or without papilledema
Kidney: plasma creatinine concentration above 2.0 mg/dL, renal failure
Vessels: dissecting aneurysm, symptomatic arterial occlusive disease

FIGURE 13-22. Classification of hypertension by extent of organ damage. TIA—transient ischemic attack.

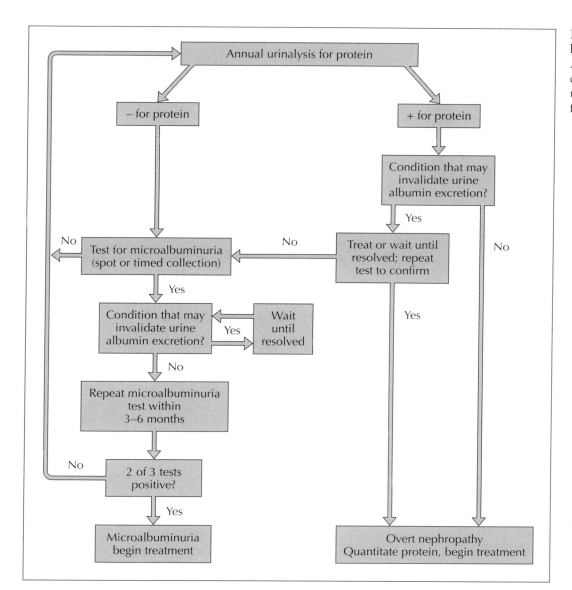

FIGURE 13-23. Screening for microalbuminuria. The American Diabetes Association flow diagram outlines the crucial role played by assessment of urine for protein excretion in planning for therapeutics.

1999 AMERICAN DIABETES ASSOCIATION RECOMMENDATIONS FOR HYPERTENSION CONTROL

Goal blood pressure is < 135/85 mm Hg

ACE inhibitors should be instituted in patients with type 1 diabetes when microalbuminuria is identified, even in the normotensive patient

Progression from microalbuminuria is less well substantiated in patients with type 2 diabetes, and should such a patient show progression or develop hypertension ACE inhibitors are indicated

---

FIGURE 13-24. American Diabetes Association recommendations for hypertension control. Current evidence strongly favors the aggressive approach to blood pressure control in patients with diabetes mellitus. The findings from the Hypertension Optimal Treatment Study and the UK Prospective Diabetes Study both favor a goal systolic blood pressure of less than 130 mm Hg, and a goal diastolic blood pressure of less than 85 mm Hg. Note also that the angiotensin-converting enzyme (ACE) inhibitor has become the first step when treatment is indicated. In most patients, two or three drugs will be required to achieve goal blood pressure.

BLOOD PRESSURE GOALS FOR PATIENTS WITH HYPERTENSION AND TYPE 2 DIABETES

JNC VI: < 130/85 mm Hg *or*
        125/75 mm Hg, if proteinuria is > 1.0 g/24 h
ADA/NKF: 130/80 mm Hg

FIGURE 13-25. Blood pressure goals for patients with hypertension and type 2 diabetes as recommended by the Joint National Committee on Hypertension-VI (JNC-VI), and both the American Diabetes Association (ADA) and National Kidney Foundation (NKF). (*Data from* the Sixth Report of the JNC on Prevention, Detection, Evaluation, and Treatment of High Blood Pressure [14], the ADA [15], and the NKF [16].)

REFERENCES

1. Joint National Committee on Detection, Evaluation, and Treatment of High Blood Pressure: The Fifth Report of the Joint National Committee on Detection, Evaluation, and Treatment of High Blood Pressure (JNCV). *Arch Intern Med* 1993, 153:153–183.

2. World Health Organization/International Society of Hypertension: Guidelines for the Management of Mild Hypertension: memorandum from a World Health Organization–ISH Meeting. *Hypertens Res* 1993, 16:149–161.

3. Roberts J: Blood pressure of persons 18–74 years, United States, 1971–72. Data from the National Health Survey, Washington, DC: National Center for Health Statistics, 1975; DHEW publication no. 75-1632. (Vital and Health Statistics; series 11, no.150).

4. Rowland M, Roberts J: Blood pressure levels and hypertension in persons ages 6–74 years: United States, 1971–72. Hyattsville, MD: National Center for Health Statistics, October 1982; DHHS publication no 82-1250. (Advance data from Vital and Health Statistics; no. 84).

5. Task Force on Blood Pressure Control in Children: Report of the Second Task Force on Blood Pressure Control in Children–1987. *Pediatrics* 1987:79:1–25.

6. Management Committee: Treatment of mild hypertension in the elderly. *Med J Aust* 1981, 2:398–402.

7. Amery A, Birkenhöger W, Brixko P, *et al.*: Mortality and morbidity results from the European Working Party on High Blood Pressure in the Elderly trial. *Lancet* 1985, 1:1349–1151.

8. Coope J, Warrender TS: Randomised trial of treatment of hypertension in elderly patients in primary care. *BMJ* 1986, 293:1145–1151.

9. Dahlof B, Lindholm L, Hansson L, *et al.*: Morbidity and mortality in the Swedish Trial in Old Patients with Hypertension (STOP-Hypertension). *Lancet* 1991, 338:1281–1284.

10. MRC Working Party: Medical Research Council trial of treatment of hypertension in older adults: principal results. *BMJ* 1992, 304:405–412.

11. SHEP Cooperative Research Group: Prevention of stroke by anti-hypertensive drug treatment in older persons with isolated systolic hypertension. *JAMA* 1991, 265:3255–3264.

12. Hypertension Detection and Follow-up Program Cooperative Group: The effect of treatment on mortality in "mild" hypertension: results of the Hypertension Detection and Follow-up Program. *N Engl J Med* 1982, 307:976–980.

13. American Diabetes Association: Clinical Practice Recommendations, 1999. Diabetic nephropathy. *Diabetes Care* Suppl 1 1999, 22:S66–S69.

14. *The Sixth Report of the Joint National Committee on Prevention, Detection, Evaluation, and Treatment of High Blood Pressure.* Bethesda: National Institutes of Health; 1997:41–52. NIH Publication no. 98-4080.

15. American Diabetes Association: Treatment of hypertension in adults with diabetes: clinical practice recommendations. *Diabetes Care* 2002, S71–S73.

16. National Kidney Foundation: Important facts about proteinuria and kidney disease. http//www.kidney.org/general/news/proteinuria.cfm. Accessed June 6, 2002.

NEWER ANTIHYPERTENSIVE AGENTS

Domenic A. Sica

The therapies available for the effective treatment of hypertension or end-organ complications of hypertension continue to experience almost a geometric growth in their numbers. Such a proliferation of therapies creates a conundrum of sorts for the treating physician. The physician is called upon to position a new drug class in comparison to traditional therapies, oftentimes without adequate information to reach such therapeutic distinctions. In addition, as new members of a drug class inevitably become available, it is incumbent upon the physician to determine the relevance of supposed pharmacokinetic and pharmacodynamic differences. This is the case with the angiotensin-receptor antagonists (AT_1-RAs). Seven such compounds are currently marketed in the United States and considerable controversy exists as to the significance of differences—both pharmacokinetic and pharmacodynamic—among individual class members. This is very much analogous to the present situation with angiotensin-converting enzyme (ACE) inhibitors, among which compounds 10 are available in the United States.

Angiotensin-receptor antagonists have been available since 1995, when the first such compound, losartan, was released. Since that time, six other AT_1-RAs have been released. These compounds block the AT_1-receptor in a very selective fashion, thereby eliminating virtually all of the harmful effects of angiotensin II. Because These compounds interrupt the short feedback loop of the renin-angiotensin axis; thus, their use can be accompanied by a reactive increase in angiotensin II concentrations. The degree to which angiotensin II levels rise is a primary determinant of AT_2-receptor stimulation. The significance of AT_2-receptor stimulation is unresolved in humans, although it is suggested that vasodilatation accompanies stimulation of this receptor. AT_1-RAs do not interfere with the activity of ACE, and thus they do not increase bradykinin levels, which distinguishes these drugs from ACE inhibitors. Individual AT_1-RAs have differing affinities for their target receptor, which may, in part, explain some of the observed treatment differences when head-to-head studies have been conducted with class members. For the most part, AT_1-RAs reduce blood pressure comparably to diuretics, β-blockers, calcium-channel blockers, and ACE inhibitors. Angiotensin-receptor antagonist monotherapy may be less effective in blacks; however, this relative resistance to an AT_1-RA can be overcome by its being administered together with a diuretic.

It was originally proposed that one of the major benefits of this drug class would be an ability to temper the negative effects of angiotensin II at a tissue level and thereby to provide benefits beyond what might be expected with blood pressure reduction alone. This promise has been realized, with positive outcomes data now available for angiotensin-receptor antagonists in congestive heart failure, diabetic nephropathy in type 2 diabetes, and stroke protection. These findings relative to end-organ protection are not dissimilar to what has been observed with ACE inhibitors. Angiotensin-receptor antagonists are unique among all drug classes in that their side effect profile is comparable to that observed with placebo. This is an important factor in the expanding use of this drug class. This drug class holds increasing promise and should see expanded use in the coming years.

A promising drug class is that of the vasopeptidase inhibitors. These compounds both inhibit ACE and simultaneously (in a dose-dependent fashion) retard the breakdown of atrial natriuretic peptide. Omapatrilat is the most clinically developed member of this class. The reduction in blood pressure with omapatrilat can be quite dramatic, particularly regarding systolic blood pressure, and far superior to what is observed with ACE inhibitor treatment. Omapatrilat has proved effective in heart failure management. In addition, it has been shown to modify the progression of renal failure in experimental models in a manner that positively distinguishes it from ACE inhibitors. Unfortunately, the potent blood pressure–reducing ability of this compound is counterbalanced by a high incidence rate of angioedema associated with its use. This potentially life-threatening side effect will likely stall development or preclude regulatory approval of omapatrilat and other similar compounds in this class.

ANGIOTENSIN-RECEPTOR ANTAGONISTS

PHYSIOLOGIC FUNCTIONS OF AT$_1$ RECEPTORS ACCORDING TO THEIR LOCATION

LOCATION	FUNCTION
Kidney	
Glomerulus	Mesangial cell contraction
Proximal tubule	Increased reabsorption of sodium
Juxtaglomerular apparatus	Decreased renin secretion
Heart	Inotropic effect and release of growth factors with ensuing stimulation of cardiac myocyte hypertrophy and increased extracellular matrix production
Blood vessels	Vasoconstriction with an increase in afterload as well as local release of growth factors
Adrenal gland	Aldosterone and catecholamine release
Brain	Vasopressin release, stimulation of thirst; autonomic activity and cardiovascular reflexes
Sympathetic nervous system	Increased sympathetic outflow

Figure 14-1. Physiologic functions of AT$_1$-receptors according to their location. Angiotensin receptors are ubiquitous in the body, although the physiologic significance of receptors in sites such as the gonads, peripheral blood cells, and many regions of the brain are still uncertain. AT$_1$ is the subtype that mediates the best-known actions of angiotensin. AT$_2$ is the subtype that predominates in fetal tissues; its role there and in some adult tissue is incompletely understood. A number of pathophysiologic events occur—some good and some bad—when angiotensin II stimulates an AT$_1$-receptor. The response to AT$_1$-receptor stimulation is relevant on a cellular, vascular, and whole-organ level. Conversely, blockade of the AT$_1$-receptor interrupts an assortment of maladaptive processes with both short- and long-term favorable consequences.

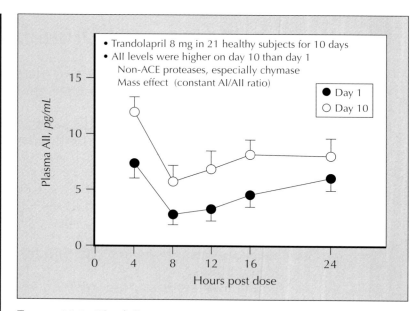

FIGURE 14-2. The failure to suppress angiotensin II concentrations completely with continuous administration of the angiotensin-converting enzyme (ACE) inhibitor trandolapril. This process has been termed *angiotensin II escape* and is linked to the production of angiotensin II by non–ACE-dependent enzymatic pathways found in the heart, kidney, and vascular wall, among other locations. The phenomenon of angiotensin II escape has been observed in normal volunteers, hypertensives, and patients with congestive heart failure. An alternative explanation for angiotensin II escape may simply be that of a return of angiotensin II levels to baseline during the latter portion of a dosing interval as pharmacologic suppression of ACE fades. (*Adapted from* Mooser *et al.* [1] and van den Meiracker [2].)

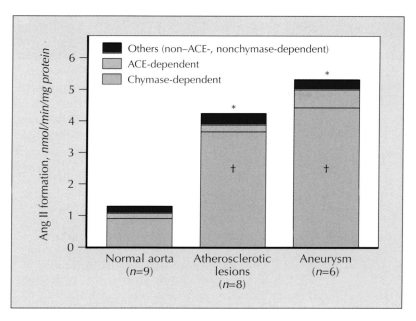

FIGURE 14-3. Angiotensin II formation in normal and dysfunctional vessels. Chymase, which originates from mast cells, is the major in vitro angiotensin II–forming enzyme in the human heart and aorta. In dysfunctional vessels, *total* angiotensin II production increases whether it is generated from angiotensin-converting enzyme (ACE), chymase, or other non–ACE-dependent pathways. The predominant site of angiotensin II production by each of these pathways differs. Chymase-positive mast cells were located predominantly in the tunica adventitia of normal and atheromatous aortas, whereas ACE-positive cells were localized in endothelial cells of normal aorta and in macrophages of atheromatous neointima. The chymase and non–ACE-dependent pathways for production of angiotensin II are not interfered with by ACE inhibition, leading to so-called "angiotensin-II escape" with long-term ACE inhibitor therapy. Angiotensin II escape has been suggested as a detrimental property of ACE inhibition, in which case angiotensin-receptor antagonist therapy might prove a more effective means of eliminating activity in the renin-angiotensin axis. (*Adapted from* Ihara *et al.* [3].)

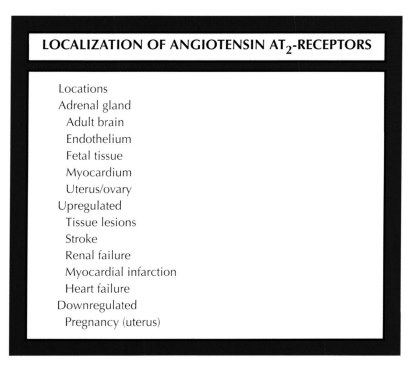

FIGURE 14-4. Localization of AT_2-receptors. There is now a great deal of evidence that the AT_2-receptor is an important physiologic regulator of blood pressure and kidney function. The AT_2-receptor appears to act as a modulator of complex biologic programs involved in embryonic development, cell differentiation, and tissue protection and regeneration, as well as in programmed cell death. The evidence indicates that the AT_2-receptor subserves a counter-regulatory protective role to the AT_2-receptor and that at least some of the beneficial effects of AT_1-receptor blockade are attributable to increased angiotensin II stimulation of the unblocked AT_2-receptor. It is now clear that the AT_2-receptor mediates a vasodilator cascade of signaling molecules, including bradykinin, nitric oxide, and cyclic GMP. There also is strong evidence that the AT_2-receptor, at least in part, mediates pressure natriuresis. It has yet to be determined whether the level of AT_2-receptor stimulation with angiotensin-receptor antagonists separates individual compounds in a relevant fashion. (*Adapted from* Unger [4].)

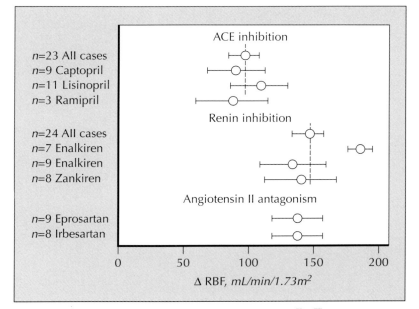

FIGURE 14-5. Meta-analysis of the renovascular response to pharmacologic interruption of the renin system in healthy young men who were in balance on a 10-mEq daily sodium intake. Each agent was studied at the top of its dose–renovascular response relationship. The similarity of the responses to renin inhibition and angiotensin-receptor antagonists makes it highly likely that this represents the contribution of endogenous renin-dependent angiotensin II formation triggered by the low-salt diet. From the ratio of the flow increase induced by angiotensin-converting enzyme (ACE) inhibition and the alternative blockers of the renin-angiotensin axis, one can calculate that approximately two thirds of angiotensin II formation under these conditions is ACE dependent and alternative, non-ACE pathways generate one third. This observation is further supported by infusion studies with a small molecular weight peptide ([Pro[11], D-Ala[12]] angiotensin I), which can only be converted to angiotensin II by chymase. Infusion of this peptide into the renal artery results in a decrease in renal blood flow and a reduction in afferent and efferent arteriolar diameter consistent with an angiotensin II effect. (*Adapted from* Hollenberg *et al.* [5] and Murakami [6].)

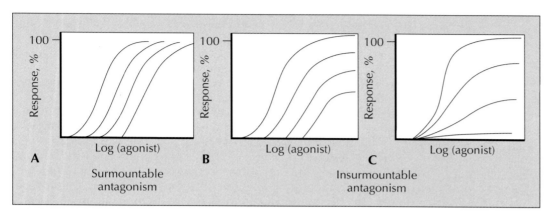

FIGURE 14-6. Surmountable and insurmountable binding characteristics. **A,** Losartan, a type of surmountable antagonist, produces parallel rightward shifts of the agonist concentration-response curves with no alteration in the agonist maximal response. **B,** Valsartan, irbesartan, and the active metabolite of losartan (EXP-3174), all types of insurmountable antagonists, can also elicit relatively parallel shifts of the agonist concentration-response curves but also show a depression of the maximal response to the agonist that cannot be overcome with increasing concentrations of the agonist. **C,** Candesartan represents an insurmountable antagonist that can elicit nonparallel shifts of the agonist concentration-response curves, again depressing the maximal response to the agonist that cannot be overcome with increasing concentrations of the agonist. The noncompetitive, insurmountable antagonism shown in **B** and **C** is thought by many to reflect very tight binding of the blocker to the receptor, which results in nonequilibrium kinetics and a very prolonged sojourn on the receptor. (*Adapted from* McConnaughey *et al.* [7].)

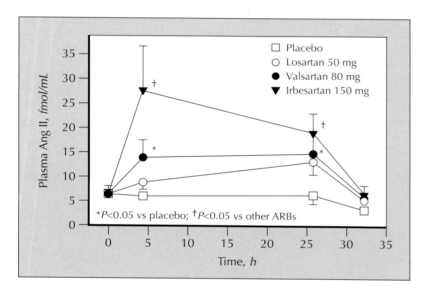

FIGURE 14-7. Plasma angiotensin II levels. Time course of the reactive rise in plasma angiotensin II levels induced by the administration of a single dose of placebo, losartan, valsartan, and irbesartan in normotensive subjects. Values are mean ± SEM. The extent to which angiotensin II levels rise following administration of an AT_1-receptor antagonist reflects both the degree and the duration of drug binding to this receptor. It has been suggested but not proved that the level of change in angiotensin II concentrations will define the extent of AT_2-receptor stimulation. Study-specific conditions such as single versus multiple dosing and/or the dose of medications being compared can importantly influence this finding. (*Adapted from* Mazzolai *et al.* [8] and Maillard *et al.* [9].)

PHARMACOLOGIC EFFECTS OF ACE INHIBITORS AND ANGIOTENSIN-RECEPTOR ANTAGONISTS

	ANGIOTENSIN-RECEPTOR ANTAGONISTS	ACE INHIBITORS
Plasma renin activity	↑	↑
Plasma angiotensin II	↑	↓ short-term but ↔ to ↑ in the long term
Bradykinin levels	↔	↑
AT_1-receptor stimulation	↓	↓
AT_2-receptor stimulation	↑	Indeterminate

FIGURE 14-8. Neurohumoral effects of angiotensin-receptor antagonists contrasted with those of angiotensin-converting enzyme (ACE) inhibitors. ACE inhibitor therapy is accompanied by an increase in plasma renin activity as a consequence of interrupting the short feedback loop, which controls activity in the renin-angiotensin axis. Because angiotensin-receptor antagonists interfere with this same pathway, but further downstream, their use is also accompanied by a rise in the concentration of upstream components, including angiotensin II. The increase in angiotensin II levels with angiotensin-receptor antagonist therapy is of limited pathophysiologic significance because the AT_1-receptor is effectively blocked and may be useful if AT_2-receptor stimulation ultimately proves relevant. Alternatively, the rise in angiotensin II levels with an ACE inhibitor reflects so-called "angiotensin-II escape" and may be clinically relevant because the AT_1-receptor can, at least in theory, be stimulated [10,11].

Losartan	Hepatic P_{450} 3A4, 2C9/10	E3174
x	Potency	10–40x
Competitive	AT_1 antagonism	Noncompetitive
1.5–2.5	Half-life (h)	6–9
34	V_D (L)	12

FIGURE 14-9. The chemical structures of losartan and its E-3174 metabolite. Losartan, released in 1995, was the first angiotensin-receptor antagonist. It is active in its parent form, although its predominant effect relates to its E-3174 metabolite. The P-450 isozymes 3A4 and 2C9/10 are responsible for the conversion of losartan to E-3174. The metabolism of losartan to its active carboxylic acid metabolite E-3174 is a two-step oxidative reaction with an aldehyde intermediate, E-3179. Reduced concentrations of E-3174 have been observed in fewer than 1% of healthy subjects and patients with hypertension given losartan in pharmacokinetic studies, and likely relate to a mutation in the *CYP2C9* gene. The other angiotensin-receptor antagonists requiring metabolic conversion from a prodrug form are candesartan cilexetil and olmesartan medoxomil [12,13].

EFFECT OF INDUCTION AND SUPPRESSION OF CYTOCHROME P$_{450}$ ON THE METABOLISM OF LOSARTAN

DRUG	ISOZYME	LOSARTAN	E-3174
Fluconazole [15]	2C9	↑	↓
Itraconazole [15,21]	3A4	No effect	No effect
Erythromycin [19]	3A4	No effect	No effect
Cimetidine [20]	Nonspecific	↑18%	No effect
Rifampin [19]	1A, 2C, 3A4	↓35%	↓ 40%
Phenytoin [22]	2C9	↑17%	↓ 63%
Phenobarbital [18]	Nonspecific	↓ 20%	↓ 20%
Grapefruit juice [23]	3A4	↑	↓

FIGURE 14-10. Effect of induction and suppression of cytochrome P-450 on the metabolism of losartan. A number of drugs are known to influence the activity of the cytochrome P-450 system, either stimulating or suppressing its activity. In theory, enzyme inhibitors or suppressors could either increase or decrease the concentration of the E-3174 metabolite. Of the studies conducted to date, inconsequential changes in the concentration of E-3174 occur when either enzyme inhibitors (fluconazole) or enzyme inducers (phenobarbital) are administered. Grapefruit juice, an inhibitor of cytochrome P-450 and activator of P-glycoprotein, slows the absorption of losartan and decreases conversion to E-3174. These findings are indicative of simultaneous CYP 3A4 inhibition and P-glycoprotein activation by coadministered grapefruit juice. To date, drug–drug interactions involving the P-450 system do not appear to influence the blood pressure–reducing ability of losartan [14–23].

BIOAVAILABILITY OF THE ANGIOTENSIN-RECEPTOR ANTAGONISTS

DRUG	BIOAVAILABILITY, %	FOOD EFFECT
Candesartan cilexetil [24]	15	No
Eprosartan [25–27]	6–29	AUC ↓≈25%
Irbesartan [28,29]	60-80	No
Losartan [30]	33	AUC ↓≈10%
Olmesartan [31]	26	No
Telmisartan [32]	42–58	AUC ↓ 6%–24%
Valsartan [33]	25	AUC ↓≈50%

FIGURE 14-11. The bioavailability of the individual angiotensin-receptor antagonists is variable. Some of these compounds can have a significant food effect, but it has yet to be established that this is relevant to the blood pressure–lowering capacity of an individual compound. These compounds have not been studied relative to day-to-day variability in absorption. If day-to-day absorptive differences exist for a compound, it would likely only be relevant to the poorly absorbed compounds. The data in this table refer to extent of absorption and not how quickly absorption begins or the subsequent rate at which it proceeds. The latter is relevant to the onset of action of these compounds. For example, although eprosartan has a low absolute bioavailability, its absorption begins shortly after it is ingested, thereby effecting prompt receptor blockade [24–33].

MODE OF ELIMINATION FOR AT$_1$-RAs

DRUG	RENAL	HEPATIC
Candesartan [34]	60	40
Eprosartan [35]	30	70 (unchanged)
Irbesartan [36]	1	99 (2C9)
Losartan [37]	10	90 (2C9/3A4)
Olmesartan [38]	35–50	50–65 (unchanged)
E-3174 [37]	50	50
Telmisartan [39]	1	99 (unchanged)
Valsartan [40]	30	70 (unchanged)

FIGURE 14-12. Mode of elimination of angiotensin-receptor antagonists. These compounds are cleared by a combination of renal and hepatic mechanisms, with the latter typically predominating. This is in contradistinction to angiotensin-converting enzyme (ACE) inhibitors, which undergo a predominantly renal mode of elimination. Angiotensin-receptor antagonists do not accumulate when dosed to steady state in patients with renal failure. This pharmacologic distinction may prove useful in treating the congestive heart failure patient prone to blood pressure and glomerular filtration rate drops with ACE inhibitors.

AT$_1$-RA PROPERTIES AND DIALYSANCE IN ESRD PATIENTS

COMPOUND	PROTEIN BINDING, %	MOLECULAR WEIGHT, D	HEMODIALYSANCE, cc/min
Losartan [41]	98.7	461	0
Eprosartan [42]	98.0	521	11
Irbesartan [36]	90.0	429	0
Losartan [43]	98.7	461	0
E-3174 [43]	99.8	437	0
Olmesartan	99.0	559	NA
Telmisartan [39]	99.5	515	0
Valsartan [44]	95.0	436	NA

FIGURE 14-13. Molecular weight, protein binding, and dialysance for the angiotensin-receptor antagonists. These compounds have a low molecular weight and typically are very highly protein bound. The latter typically limits their dialysance. Efficacy data for the angiotensin-receptor antagonists in end-stage renal disease are limited. Of the available data, there appears to be little difference between these compounds and angiotensin-converting enzyme inhibitors in the end-stage renal disease population.

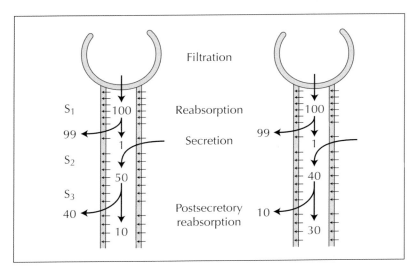

FIGURE 14-14. Depiction of fractional uric acid handling in a previously described four-component model of renal urate handling, including filtration, reabsorption, secretion, and post-secretory reabsorption (*left*). Uric acid handling in the presence of losartan is depicted on the *right*. In the presence of losartan, filtration and reabsorption of uric acid are likely to be unchanged. Secretion and postsecretory reabsorption are likely both blocked. The sum of these processes typically results in a time-dependent rise in fractional uric acid excretion to 30%. This is marked by a reduction in serum uric acid of between 0.5 and 1.0 mg/dL, which is sufficient to lessen the risk of diuretic-related hyperuricemia. Losartan-related uricosuria is unique to the parent molecule and is not seen with either its E-3174 metabolite or other angiotensin-receptor antagonists. It is not associated with adverse renal consequences because losartan also increases urine pH, which, in turn, increases uric acid solubility and diminishes the risk of stone formation. The significance of losartan-induced uricosuria (and hypouricemia) is unclear. (*Adapted from* Sica *et al.* [45].)

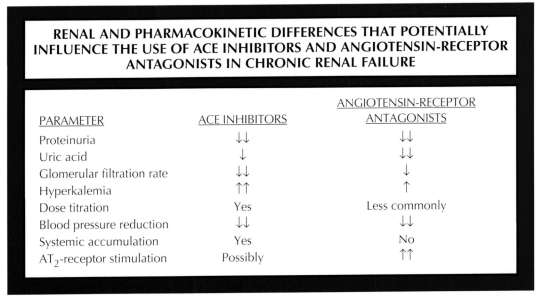

RENAL AND PHARMACOKINETIC DIFFERENCES THAT POTENTIALLY INFLUENCE THE USE OF ACE INHIBITORS AND ANGIOTENSIN-RECEPTOR ANTAGONISTS IN CHRONIC RENAL FAILURE

PARAMETER	ACE INHIBITORS	ANGIOTENSIN-RECEPTOR ANTAGONISTS
Proteinuria	↓↓	↓↓
Uric acid	↓	↓↓
Glomerular filtration rate	↓↓	↓
Hyperkalemia	↑↑	↑
Dose titration	Yes	Less commonly
Blood pressure reduction	↓↓	↓↓
Systemic accumulation	Yes	No
AT$_2$-receptor stimulation	Possibly	↑↑

FIGURE 14-15. The antiproteinuric effects of these compounds are comparable. The angiotensin-receptor antagonist losartan is the only one of the drugs in this class that lowers uric acid, a process accomplished by a direct tubular effect of losartan—and not the E-3174 metabolite—on tubular handling of uric acid. This process is recognized to occur in renal failure as well as in the presence of normal renal function. The fall in glomerular filtration rate, in a kidney functionally dependent on angiotensin II, is theorized to be greater with angiotensin-converting enzyme (ACE) inhibitors than with angiotensin-receptor antagonists. This is proposed to be secondary to the effect of bradykinin on efferent arteriolar tone, a phenomenon not observed with angiotensin-receptor antagonists. Hyperkalemia has been observed to occur somewhat less frequently with angiotensin-receptor antagonists, although the reason for this is still not clearly established. A final consideration in contrasting ACE inhibitors and angiotensin-receptor antagonists is the pharmacokinetic profile of the drugs in these classes. The active forms of ACE inhibitors are almost entirely cleared renally with the exception of fosinoprilat and trandolaprilat. Angiotensin-receptor antagonists are predominantly hepatically cleared or renally/hepatically cleared; as such, these drugs do not systemically accumulate when dosed to steady state in renal failure patients [46–49].

RENAL AND PHARMACOKINETIC DIFFERENCES THAT POTENTIALLY INFLUENCE THE USE OF ACE INHIBITORS AND ANGIOTENSIN-RECEPTOR ANTAGONISTS IN END-STAGE RENAL DISEASE

PARAMETER	ACE INHIBITORS	ANGIOTENSIN-RECEPTOR ANTAGONISTS
Angioneurotic edema	Yes	Yes, but less so
Dialyzer reactions	Yes	No
Residual renal function	↓↓	↓
Dialyzability	Yes	No
Hyperkalemia	↑↑	↑
Dose titration	Yes	Less commonly
Blood pressure reduction	↓↓	↓↓
Systemic accumulation	Yes	No
AT_2-receptor stimulation	Possibly	↑↑

FIGURE 14-16. Renal and pharmokinetic differences that potentially influence the use of angiotensin-converting enzyme (ACE) inhibitors and angiotensin-receptor antagonists in end-stage renal disease (ESRD). The angiotensin-receptor antagonists and ACE inhibitors are pharmacokinetically, pharmacodynamically, and toxicologically distinctive in the ESRD patient. ACE inhibitors are associated with angioneurotic edema, a phenomenon that occurs with angiotensin-receptor antagonists but much less frequently. ACE inhibitors can also trigger anaphylactoid dialyzer reactions, particularly when polysulfone dialyzers are in use. These types of membranes carry a significant negative charge load and therein promote activation of Hageman factor (with the resultant generation of bradykinin) when surface contact with blood occurs. Anaphylactoid dialyzer reactions have not been observed with angiotensin-receptor antagonists. Residual renal function is postulated to change less with angiotensin-receptor antagonists, although this has not been formally studied. A major difference between ACE inhibitors and angiotensin-receptor antagonists is that of dialyzability. Several of the ACE inhibitors—*eg*, captopril, enalapril, and lisinopril—are dialyzable, whereas all of the angiotensin-receptor antagonists are not dialyzable. In dosing an ACE inhibitor in renal failure and ESRD, dose titration is still used, whereas dose titration is uncommon with angiotensin-receptor antagonists. In non–dialysis-dependent chronic renal failure, hyperkalemia has been observed to occur somewhat less with angiotensin-receptor antagonists, although the reason for this is still not clearly established. The occurrence of hyperkalemia in ESRD with either ACE inhibitor or angiotensin-receptor antagonist therapy has not been systematically examined [43,50–56].

RENAL AND PHARMACOKINETIC DIFFERENCES THAT POTENTIALLY INFLUENCE THE EFFECT OF ACE INHIBITORS AND ANGIOTENSIN-RECEPTOR ANTAGONISTS ON RENAL FUNCTION IN CHF

PARAMETER	ACE INHIBITORS	ANGIOTENSIN-RECEPTOR ANTAGONISTS
Afferent arteriolar resistance	Minimal change	Minimal change
Efferent arteriolar resistance	↓↓	↓
Glomerular filtration rate	↓	↓
Hyperkalemia	↑↑	↑
Dose titration	Yes	Less commonly
Blood pressure reduction	↓↓	↓
Systemic accumulation	Yes	No
AT_2-receptor stimulation	Possibly	↑↑

FIGURE 14-17. Renal and pharmacokinetic differences that potentially influence the effect of angiotensin-converting enzyme (ACE) inhibitors and angiotensin-receptor antagonists on renal function in congestive heart failure (CHF). Both ACE inhibitors and angiotensin-receptor antagonists minimally change afferent arteriolar resistance. Alternatively, ACE inhibitors decrease efferent arteriolar resistance more so than do angiotensin-receptor antagonists. This may be linked to the change in bradykinin, which occurs with an ACE inhibitor. Bradykinin can dilate the efferent arteriole. This has been the basis of the hypothesis that angiotensin-receptor antagonists reduce glomerular filtration rate in heart failure patients less so than ACE inhibitors. In the only available study to date (Losartan in Heart Failure [ELITE]), in which an ACE inhibitor (captopril) was compared with an angiotensin-receptor antagonist (losartan), each compound was associated with a similar number of episodes of glomerular filtration rate decline throughout the 48 weeks of the study. The subjects in this study were mainly class II and III congestive heart failure patients; therefore, any difference in how ACE inhibitors or angiotensin-receptor antagonists affected renal function would be less likely to emerge. A factor that clearly distinguishes ACE inhibitors from angiotensin-receptor antagonists is the nonaccumulating nature of the angiotensin-receptor antagonists in congestive heart failure or renal failure. Both blood pressure and glomerular filtration are closely related to the blood levels of these drugs in the congestive heart failure patient—unlike what is seen in the hypertensive patient. This phenomenon would be expected to translate into less protracted changes in renal function in the congestive heart failure patient, who might experience a transient decline in renal function. It may also explain the observation that serum potassium increases less with angiotensin-receptor antagonists than with ACE inhibitors. The pertinence of AT_2-receptor stimulation remains to be determined [57–60].

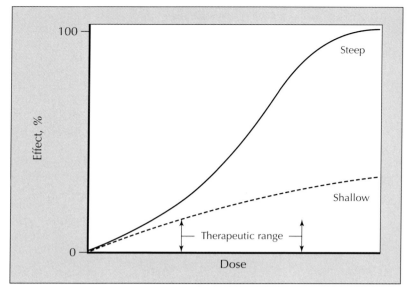

FIGURE 14-18. Dose–response relationship for antihypertensive medications. This relationship can be shallow, with small blood pressure decrements occurring with dose titration, as might be the case with diuretic therapy. Alternatively, the slope of the line describing this relationship can be steep. In the case of angiotensin-receptor antagonists, doses in the low end of the dosing range typically elicit the greatest response; thereafter, dose escalation produces a fall in blood pressure, which is proportionally less than the amount by which the dose is increased [61].

BLOOD PRESSURE–LOWERING EFFECTS AND TISSUE PROTECTIVE PROPERTIES OF ANGIOTENSIN-RECEPTOR ANTAGONISTS

Angiotensin-receptor antagonists reduce systolic and diastolic blood pressure comparable to what is seen with ACE inhibitors, β-blockers, diuretics, and calcium channel blockers.

Angiotensin-receptor antagonists exhibit a moderately steep dose-response slope at beginning doses and a lesser response as doses are increased.

The addition of a diuretic, such as hydrochlorothiazide, to an angiotensin-receptor antagonist results in an additive reduction in blood pressure. This occurs in a dose-dependent fashion for the diuretic.

The maximal blood pressure reduction with an angiotensin-receptor antagonist is usually achieved only after several weeks of therapy. This probably relates to a long-term effect attributable to the resetting of hemodynamics and/or vascular remodeling.

Angiotensin-receptor antagonists are now formally indicated in congestive heart failure and type 2 diabetic nephropathy on the basis of randomized, controlled clinical trials, which evaluated these drugs relative to hard outcomes.

Angiotensin-receptor antagonists have a side-effect profile that is indistinguishable from placebo and in some cases is better than placebo, particularly related to headache.

FIGURE 14-19. Blood pressure–lowering effects of angiotensin-receptor antagonists.

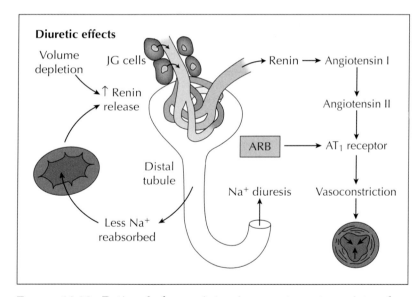

FIGURE 14-20. Rationale for angiotensin-receptor antagonist and diuretic combination in the treatment of hypertension. Diuretic-related volume contraction stimulates the renin-angiotensin-aldosterone system. In this setting, angiotensin-receptor antagonists exhibit a greater vasodepressor effect. The dose of diuretic used—to the extent that volume contraction occurs—may be important to the final response.

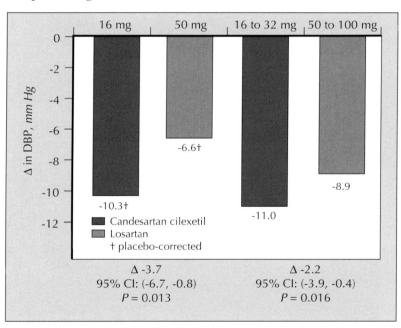

FIGURE 14-21. Change in trough diastolic blood pressure comparing monotherapy with candesartan to losartan. The greater blood pressure reduction observed with candesartan in these trials served as the basis for additional studies designed to more carefully assess differences between these two members of the angiotensin-receptor antagonist class. These additional studies have shown candesartan to be superior to losartan at the maximum recommended doses administered once daily. Candesartan cilexetil, 32 mg once daily, consistently lowered trough, peak, and 48-hour postdose diastolic blood pressure more effectively than losartan 100 mg once daily. The US Food and Drug Administration has recently granted candesartan a superiority label over losartan based on these studies [62–64].

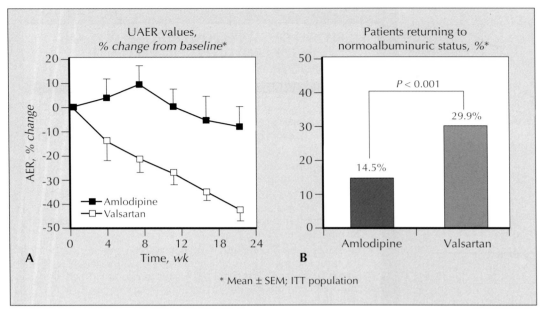

randomly assigned to 80 mg/d valsartan or 5 mg/d amlodipine for 24 weeks. A target BP of 135/85 mm Hg was sought by dose-doubling followed by addition of bendrofluazide and doxazosin as needed. Over the study period, BP reductions were similar between the two treatments (systolic/diastolic 11.2/6.6 mm Hg for valsartan; 11.6/6.5 mm Hg for amlodipine). The primary endpoint was the percent change in UAER from baseline to 24 weeks. The UAER at 24 weeks was 56% of baseline with valsartan and 92% of baseline with amlodipine ($P < 0.001$). Valsartan lowered UAER similarly in both the hypertensive and the normotensive subgroups. **B,** More patients reverted to normoalbuminuria with valsartan (29.9% vs 14.5%; $P = 0.001$). For the same level of attained BP and the same degree of BP reduction, valsartan lowered UAER more effectively than amlodipine in patients with type 2 diabetes and microalbuminuria, including the subgroup with baseline normotension. This indicates a BP-independent antiproteinuric effect of valsartan [65].

FIGURE 14-22. Change in urine albumin excretion rate (UAER) in microalbuminuric type 2 diabetes patients comparing valsartan to amlodipine. The Microalbuminuria Reduction with Valsartan (MARVAL) study evaluated the blood pressure (BP)–independent effect of valsartan on UAER in type 2 diabetes patients with microalbuminuria. **A,** A total of 332 patients with type 2 diabetes and microalbuminuria, with or without hypertension, were

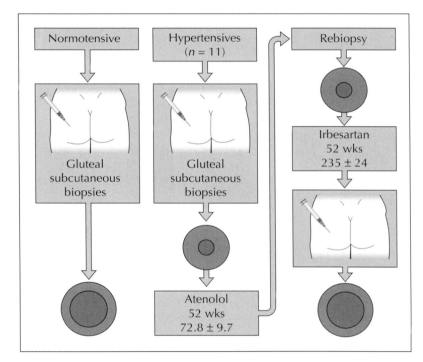

FIGURE 14-23. Structural changes in small arteries following treatment with the β-blocker atenolol and thereafter the angiotensin-receptor antagonist irbesartan. Eleven essential hypertensive patients (51 ± 2 years [range 38– 65]; 75% male) previously randomly assigned to treatment with atenolol for 1 year with good blood pressure control were crossed over to treatment with irbesartan for an additional year. Small resistance arteries were dissected from gluteal subcutaneous biopsy specimens that were performed before and after 1 year of atenolol and then 1 year of irbesartan treatment. Blood pressure control with irbesartan (129 ± 3.3/85 ± 1.8 mm Hg) was identical to that achieved previously with atenolol (131 ± 3.3/84 ± 1.1 mm Hg). Following 1 year of treatment, the arterial media width-to-lumen ratio (M/L) of resistance arteries (lumen diameter, 150–350 microns), which had remained unchanged under atenolol treatment, decreased from 8.44 ± 0.45% when patients were on atenolol, to 6.46 ± 0.30% ($P < 0.01$), when patients received irbesartan. Maximal acetylcholine-induced endothelium-dependent relaxation was 81.1% ± 4.1% when patients were on atenolol, unchanged from before starting treatment with the β-blocker, and was normalized by irbesartan (to 94.8 ± 2.0%, $P < 0.01$) (data not shown). Crossing over essential hypertensive patients with well-controlled blood pressure from the β-blocker atenolol to the angiotensin-receptor antagonist irbesartan corrected persistently altered vascular structure and endothelial function, suggesting a structural and endothelial vascular protective effect of antihypertensive treatment with the angiotensin-receptor antagonist [66].

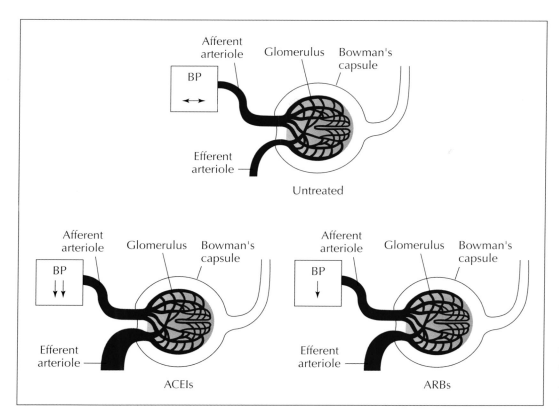

FIGURE 14-24. The importance of drug accumulation determines the duration of effect of angiotensin-converting enzyme (ACE) inhibitors in either congestive heart failure or renal insufficiency. Both of these are conditions wherein reduced renal function slows renal elimination of an ACE inhibitor, the majority of which is exclusively renally cleared (with the exception of fosinoprilat and trandolaprilat). This is less an issue with angiotensin-receptor antagonists in that they are predominantly hepatically cleared. The *double down arrows* for blood pressure change with ACE inhibitors, as contrasted with a *single down arrow* for blood pressure change with angiotensin-receptor blockers (ARBs), represent a greater effect attributable to accumulation, and not a specific difference in effect between these two drug classes. In addition, efferent arteriolar diameter is greater with ACE inhibitors than with ARBs, reflecting the influence of bradykinin on this postglomerular vessel. This is manifested in lower glomerular capillary pressures and a propensity for a greater fall in glomerular filtration rate. Although this relationship has been demonstrated experimentally, these findings have, as of yet, not been replicated in humans.

SIDE EFFECTS

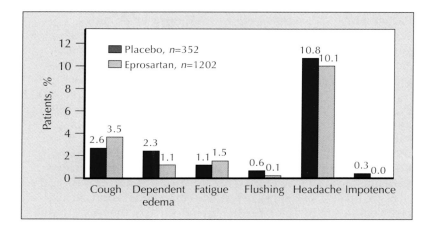

FIGURE 14-25. Selected adverse events reported among patients taking eprosartan in placebo-controlled trials. The numbers of adverse events would suggest a side-effect profile indistinguishable from placebo. This is particularly the case for headache. In fact, headache appears to occur less frequently with eprosartan. This is likely a class effect. The basis of the reduction in headaches with angiotensin-receptor antagonists is likely the well-established association between blood pressure reduction and improvement in quality of life indices [67].

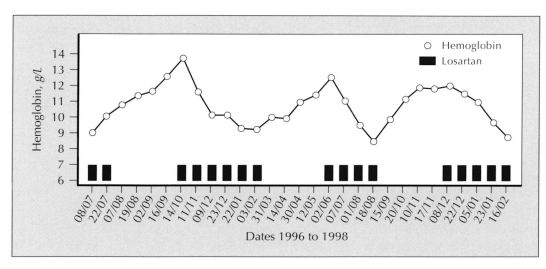

FIGURE 14-26. ACE inhibitors and angiotensin-receptor antagonists both cause certain similar side effects. This is the case for reduction in red blood cell production. Erythropoietin production and possibly its marrow effect are reduced with both drug classes. The relationship between losartan and hemoglobin concentration in a dialysis patient is shown. As losartan is started and stopped, there is as much as a 4-g change in hemoglobin concentration. Subsequent observations have shown this to be a class effect for angiotensin-receptor antagonists as has been previously shown to be the case with ACE inhibitors. On occasion, this angiotensin-receptor antagonist property has proved useful in the management of posttransplant erythrocytosis [68].

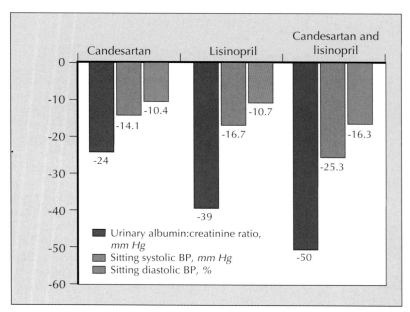

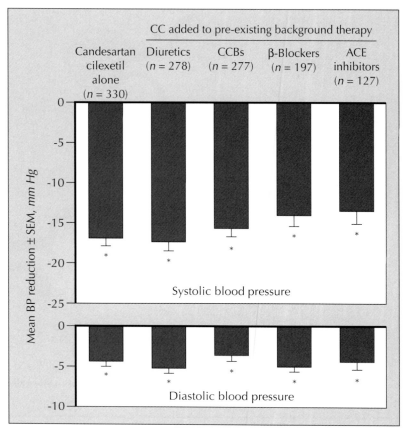

FIGURE 14-27. Comparison of the effects of candesartan or lisinopril, or both, on blood pressure (BP) and urinary albumin excretion in patients with microalbuminuria, hypertension, and type 2 diabetes. This trial was a prospective, randomized, parallel group, double-blind study with a 4-week placebo run-in period and 12-weeks' monotherapy with candesartan (16 mg/d) or lisinopril (20 mg/d) followed by 12-weeks' monotherapy or combination treatment. BP and urinary albumin:creatinine ratio were determined throughout the study. At 24 weeks, the mean reduction in diastolic BP with combination treatment (16.3 mm Hg; *P* < 0. 001) was significantly greater than that with candesartan (10.4 mm Hg; *P* < 0.001) or lisinopril (10.7 mm Hg; *P* < 0.001). The reduction in urinary albumin:creatinine ratio with combination treatment (50%; *P* < 0.001) was greater than with candesartan (24%; *P* = 0.05) and lisinopril (39%; *P* < 0.001). In this trial, candesartan 16 mg/d was as effective as lisinopril 20 mg/d in reducing BP and microalbuminuria in hypertensive patients with type 2 diabetes. Combination treatment was well tolerated and more effective in reducing BP. The difference in albumin excretion in the combination therapy group in this study was at least, in part, attributable to the observed BP differences. Other studies examining the effect of combination ACE inhibitor and angiotensin-receptor antagonist therapy on urine protein excretion have observed quite variable reductions in urine protein excretion [69–70].

FIGURE 14-28. This large-scale, 8-week, open-label, clinical experience trial evaluated the efficacy of the angiotensin receptor antagonist candesartan cilexetil (16 to 32 mg once daily) either alone or as add-on therapy in 6465 hypertensive patients. These patients had either untreated or uncontrolled hypertension (systolic blood pressure [SBP] 140 to 179 mm Hg or diastolic blood pressure [DBP] 90 to 109 mm Hg inclusive at baseline) despite a variety of antihypertensive medications, including diuretics, calcium antagonists, angiotensin-converting enzyme (ACE) inhibitors, and α- or β-blockers, either singly or in combination. Candesartan cilexetil as monotherapy (in 51% of hypertensive patients) reduced mean SBP/DBP by 18.7/13.1 mm Hg. As add-on therapy (in 49% of hypertensive patients), candesartan cilexetil reduced mean SBP/DBP further, irrespective of the background therapy: diuretics (17.8/11.3 mm Hg), calcium antagonists (16.6/11.2 mm Hg), β-blockers (16.5/10.4 mm Hg), ACE inhibitors (15.3/10.0 mm Hg), α-blockers (16.4/10.4 mm Hg). The further BP-lowering effect of candesartan cilexetil as add-on therapy was independent of age, sex, and race [71].

COMPARISON OF RECENT ANGIOTENSIN-RECEPTOR ANTAGONIST TRIALS IN TYPE 2 DIABETIC NEPHROPATHY PATIENTS

STUDY DESIGN	IDNT	IRMA 2	RENAAL	MARVAL
	IRB 300 mg vs AML 10 mg vs PLA	IRB 150 mg vs 300 mg vs PLA	LOS 50–100 mg vs PLA	VAL 80 mg vs AML
Patients, n	1715	590	1513	332
Patient type	HTN/type 2 diabetes/nephropathy	HTN/type 2 diabetes/microalbuminuria	Type 2 diabetes/nephropathy	Type 2 diabetes/microalbuminuria/SBP < 180 and/or DBP < 105 mm Hg
Duration	Mean 2.6 y	2 y	Mean 3.4 y	24 wk
Endpoints	Primary composite: doubling of serum creatinine/ESR/death	Time to onset of nephropathy with UAER > 200 µg/min/30% greater than baseline	Primary composite: doubling of serum creatinine/ESRD/death	Δ UAER
Results	Risk of primary endpoint 20% lower with IRB vs PLA; 23% lower vs AML; lower doubling of serum creatinine; ESRD with IRB; no difference in deaths	IRB was renoprotective (5.2% reached endpoint in 300-mg group; 9.7% reached endpoint in 150-mg group vs 14.9% in PLA ($P = 0.08$)	Risk of primary endpoint lower by 16% ($P = 0.02$) with LOS; lower doubling of serum creatinine, ESRD with LOS; no difference in deaths	VAL significantly lowered UAER (44%) vs AML (17%) ($P < 0.001$)

FIGURE 14-29. The Reduction in End-Points in NIDDM with the Angiotensin-II Antagonist Losartan Study (RENAAL) and the Irbesartan Diabetic Nephropathy Trial (IDNT) are two recently reported hard endpoint trials conducted in patients with advanced stages of diabetic nephropathy. Two other studies—the Irbesartan Microalbuminuria Study (IRMA-2) and the Microalbuminuria Reduction with Valsartan (MARVAL)—were trials conducted in patients with type 2 diabetes with microalbuminuria; a cardio-vascular risk factor associated with early-stage diabetic nephropathy. Both the MARVAL and the IRMA-2 trial demonstrated a significant reduction in urine albumin excretion independent of blood pressure reduction. Likewise, in the IDNT and RENAAL, a positive effect on the composite endpoint of doubling of serum creatinine/dialysis/death, was seen with the drugs irbesartan and losartan [65,72–74].

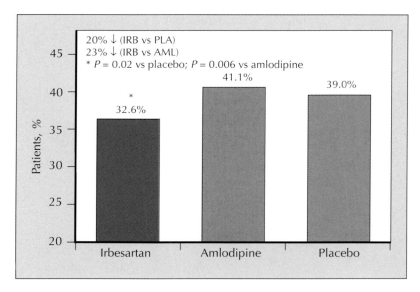

FIGURE 14-30. The Irbesartan Diabetic Nephropathy Trial (IDNT) had three treatment limbs, including placebo, amlodipine, and irbesartan, and involved 1715 patients. Patients randomly assigned to the placebo group were treated with antihypertensive agents as needed (primarily diuretics, β-blockers, and centrally-acting agents) with CCBs disallowed in all treatment limbs. The irbesartan dose in the IDNT was titrated from 75 to 300 mg/d. The dose of amlodipine was titrated from 2.5 to 10 mg in the IDNT. The goal systolic BP was 135 mm Hg or lower (or 10 mm Hg lower than the value at screening if it was more than 145 mm Hg) and a diastolic BP of 85 or lower. These goal BP values were somewhat lower than those in the RENAAL trial. Although patients in the IDNT who were randomly assigned to receive amlodipine as initial therapy achieved reductions in BP comparable with those in the irbesartan and placebo groups, the percentage of patients reaching the primary endpoint in this arm (41%) was slightly greater than the percentage of patients in the placebo arm (39%) and significantly greater than irbesartan. These data provide the basis for the labeled indication for irbesartan in the treatment of diabetic nephropathy in type 2 diabetic patients [74].

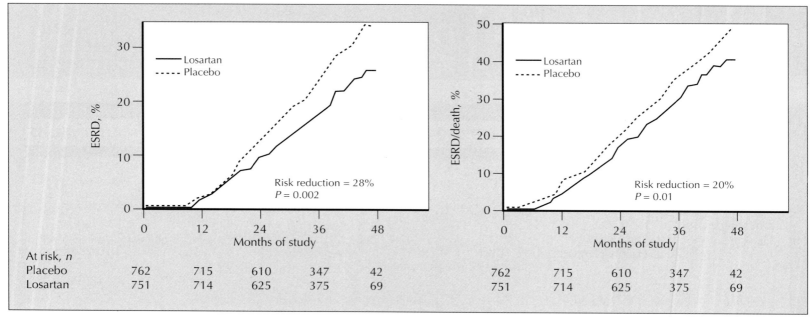

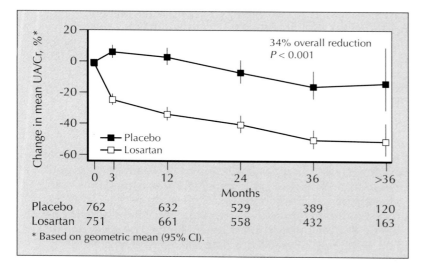

FIGURE 14-31. The Reduction in End-Points in NIDDM with the Angiotensin-II Antagonist Losartan Study (RENAAL) studied 1513 patients. It had a placebo treatment limb, which, in fact, was a conventional therapy treatment limb with placebo added. RENAAL patients randomized to the placebo group were treated with antihypertensive agents as needed (primarily diuretics, CCBs, β-blockers, and peripheral α-antagonists) to a goal BP of under 140 systolic/90 diastolic. In both the losartan-treated and placebo groups, approximately 80% of patients required a CCB to achieve BP control, which in most cases was a dihydropyridine CCB. In the RENAAL trial, losartan was given in a dose of either 50 or 100 mg/d. There was a 16% reduction in the number of patients who reached the primary endpoint (doubling of serum creatinine, ESRD, or death) in losartan-treated patients in RENAAL versus those randomly assigned to the placebo group. The single endpoint of ESRD and the double endpoint of ESRD/death were reduced by 28% and 20%, respectively, with losartan therapy [73].

FIGURE 14-32. The effect on urine albumin/creatinine was studied in the Reduction in End-Points in NIDDM with the Angiotensin-II Antagonist Losartan Study (RENAAL). In this study there was a significant reduction in the urinary protein excretion rate favoring losartan, which occurred independent of blood pressure changes. This reduction in urinary protein excretion likely contributed to the observed favorable effect on outcomes with losartan [73].

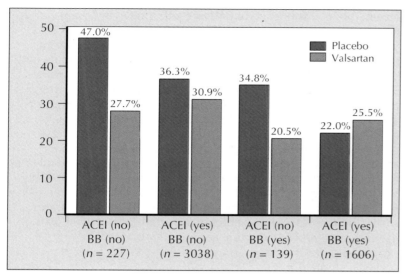

FIGURE 14-33. Treatment outcomes for valsartan versus placebo were studied in the Valsartan Heart Failure Trial (Val-HeFT). A total of 5010 patients with heart failure of New York Heart

Association (NYHA) class II, III, or IV were randomly assigned to receive 160 mg of valsartan or placebo twice daily. The primary outcomes were mortality and the combined endpoint of mortality and morbidity, defined as the incidence of cardiac arrest with resuscitation, hospitalization for heart failure, or receipt of intravenous inotropic or vasodilator therapy for at least 4 hours. Overall mortality was similar in the two groups. The incidence of the combined endpoint, however, was 13.2% lower with valsartan than with placebo ($P = 0.009$), predominantly because of a lower number of patients hospitalized for heart failure: 455 (18.2%) in the placebo group and 346 (13.8%) in the valsartan group ($P < 0.001$). The findings in treatment groups based on concomitant medications offered two additional relevant observations: first, there was a 44% risk reduction in the primary endpoint if patients not being treated with ACE inhibitors were given valsartan, rather than placebo. Second, patients receiving an ACE inhibitor, β-blocker, and valsartan had a somewhat worse outcome although the reason for this could not be determined. This latter observation was obtained in a post-hoc analysis; similar findings have not been found in other studies to date [75].

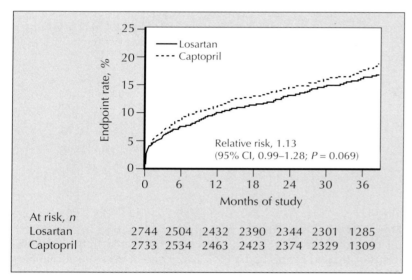

FIGURE 14-34. Kaplan-Meier curves for primary endpoint of all-cause mortality in the Optimal Trial in Myocardial Infarction with the Angiotensin-II Antagonist Losartan (OPTIMAAL). A total of

5477 patients with confirmed acute myocardial infarction and heart failure during the acute phase, or a new Q-wave anterior infarction or reinfarction, were randomly assigned and titrated to a target dose of losartan (50 mg once daily) or captopril (50 mg three times daily) as tolerated. The primary endpoint was all-cause mortality. There were 946 deaths during a mean follow-up of 2.7 years: 499 (18%) in the losartan group and 447 (16%) in the captopril group (relative risk, 1.13; $P = 0.07$). Losartan was significantly better tolerated than captopril, with fewer patients discontinuing study medication (458 [17%] vs 624 [23%]; $P < 0.0001$). The fact that there was a nonsignificant difference in total mortality in favor of captopril would suggest that ACE inhibitors should remain first-choice treatment in patients after complicated acute myocardial infarction. The 50-mg dose of losartan used in this trial may have contributed to some of these findings. Additional information concerning angiotensin-receptor antagonist therapy in the postmyocardial infarction patient will be forthcoming in 2003 with the results of the Valsartan in Acute Myocardial Infarction Trial (VALIANT). Although the role of losartan in patients intolerant of ACE inhibition is not clearly defined, it can be considered in such patients [76,77].

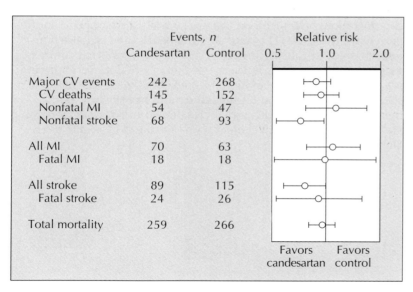

FIGURE 14-35. Cardiovascular events and total mortality in the Study on Cognition and Prognosis in the Elderly (SCOPE) in elderly patients with mild hypertension. SCOPE enrolled 4937 patients aged 70 or older with systolic blood pressures between 160 and 179 and diastolic pressures between 90 and 99 mm Hg, and normal cognitive function. The trial was a comparison of two treatment strategies: candesartan 8 to 16 mg/d versus diuretic, calcium channel blocker, or β-blocker therapy. The primary endpoint of SCOPE was a composite of death/myocardial infarction/stroke, which was not significantly different between the two groups. However, candesartan was associated with a 28% relative reduction in nonfatal stroke ($P = 0.041$). This was despite the fact that there was only a small difference in blood pressure reduction between the two groups (-3.2 mm Hg systolic and -1.6 mm Hg diastolic). These findings relative to stroke are similar to those of the Losartan Intervention for Endpoints trial (LIFE) [78].

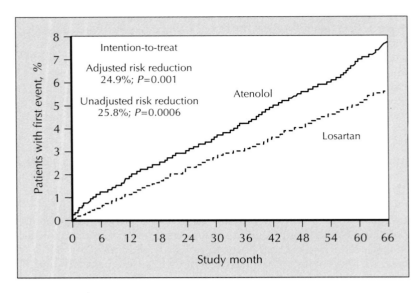

FIGURE 14-36. Proportion of patients with first event as fatal and nonfatal stroke in the Losartan Intervention for Endpoints trial (LIFE). This was a double-masked, randomized, parallel-group trial of losartan versus atenolol in 9193 hypertensive patients with left ventricular hypertrophy [79,80]. In both randomized groups, 50 mg of losartan or atenolol was the starting dose. Thereafter, hydrochlorothiazide (HCTZ) (12.5–25.0 mg/d), as well as other agents, was permitted with the exception of β-blockers, ACE inhibitors, or ARBs if BP remained persistently high during follow-up. There was no significant difference between the losartan and the atenolol treatment groups in adjusted relative risk for the primary endpoint component of cardiovascular mortality. For the primary endpoint, there was a 13.0% overall relative risk reduction on losartan. The curves for stroke, though, separated early, and the outcome was highly in favor of losartan, showing a 24.9% relative risk reduction compared with atenolol (*P* = 0.001) [79,80].

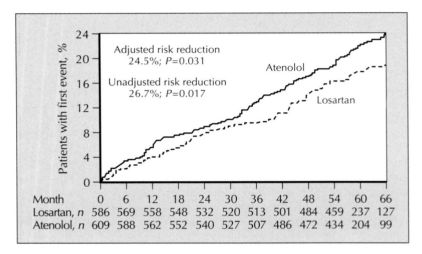

FIGURE 14-37. Diabetes substudy of the Losartan Intervention for Endpoints trial (LIFE). In the diabetic subset, the findings were somewhat different from those in the total study population. Losartan-treated patients demonstrated a 39% reduction in total mortality (*P* = 0.002), a 37% reduction in cardiovascular mortality (*P* = 0.028), and a 24% reduction in reaching the primary composite endpoint [79].

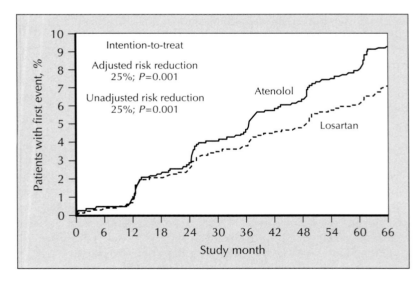

FIGURE 14-38. Proportion of patients in the Losartan Intervention for Endpoints trial (LIFE) with new-onset diabetes. In this trial, the losartan-treated group had a 25% lower rate of new-onset diabetes development. New-onset diabetes mellitus occurred in 242 patients receiving losartan (13.0 per 1000 person-years) and 320 receiving atenolol (17.5 per 1000 person-years). In this trial, new-onset diabetes could be strongly predicted by a specific risk score incorporating baseline serum glucose concentration (nonfasting), body mass index, serum high-density lipoprotein cholesterol concentration, systolic blood pressure, and history of prior antihypertensive drug use. The unusual nonlinear shape of these lines reflects point-in-time diagnosis of diabetes at clinic visits, rather than a continuous occurrence as with other pre-defined endpoints. It is likely that one explanation for these findings is that atenolol treatment worsened insulin sensitivity and losartan did not; therefore, the greater rate of diabetes development with atenolol and not a specific positive effect with losartan. (*Adapted from* Dahlof *et al*. [80–82]).

STRUCTURE AND PHARMACOLOGY

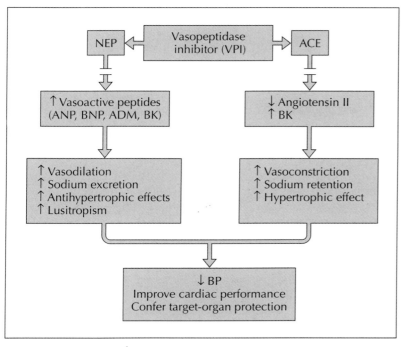

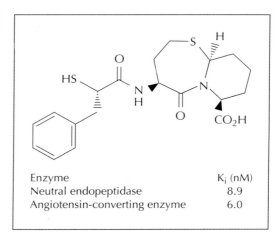

Enzyme	K_i (nM)
Neutral endopeptidase	8.9
Angiotensin-converting enzyme	6.0

FIGURE 14-40. Chemical structure of omapatrilat, a vasopeptidase inhibitor. Omapatrilat is a mercaptoacyl derivative of a bicyclic thiazepinone dipeptide surrogate and has a molecular weight of 408.5. Omapatrilat displays equipotent, highly selective competitive activity against neutral endopeptidase (NEP) and ACE. Kinetic analyses have shown that omapatrilat inhibits NEP and ACE in a linear and competitive manner in a single nmol/L range for both enzymes. (*Adapted from* Burnett [84].)

FIGURE 14-39. Mechanism of action of vasopeptidase inhibitors. Several of these agents have been synthesized and a few have been evaluated in clinical trials. Omapatrilat is the most clinically developed vasopeptidase inhibitor. ACE—angiotensin-converting enzyme; ANP—atrial natriuretic peptide; NEP—neutral endopeptidase. (*Adapted from* Weber [83].)

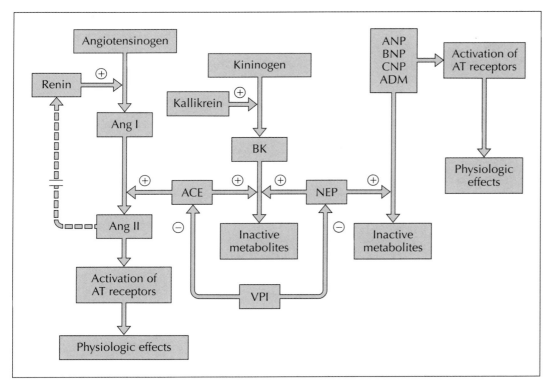

FIGURE 14-41. Vasopeptidase inhibitors (VPIs) are single molecules that simultaneously inhibit neutral endopeptidase (NEP) and angiotensin converting enzyme. Vasopeptide inhibitors elevate levels of vasodilator peptides and inhibit the production of the vasoconstrictor substance angiotensin-II (Ang II). By inhibiting both enzymes, VPIs target multiple pathways of cardiovascular regulation at both the systemic and the tissue level. Vasopeptide inhibitors have a potentiating effect on the half-life of bradykinin, which may vary according to tissue-type being sampled. AT–angiotensin; BK—bradykinin; ANP—atrial natriuretic peptide; BNP—brain natriuretic peptide; CNP—C-type natriuretic peptide.

THE PHARMACOKINETICS OF OMAPATRILAT

Omapatrilat has a long half-life (14–19 h) over the expected dosing range.

Omapatrilat is rapidly absorbed as indicated by a short T_{max} (0.5–2.0 h). It has an absolute oral bioavailability of 31%.

Omapatrilat undergoes minimal accumulation with repeated dosing with an accumulation index well below 2.

C_{max} and AUC of omapatrilat are independent of renal, cardiac, and hepatic function, and no dosage adjustment is required for omapatrilat when it is administered to patients with renal, cardiac, or hepatic disease.

Omapatrilat metabolites do not accumulate in a clinically significant fashion when it is administered to renal failure patients.

Omapatrilat is not dialyzable.

FIGURE 14-42. The pharmacokinetic profile of omapatrilat [85–88].

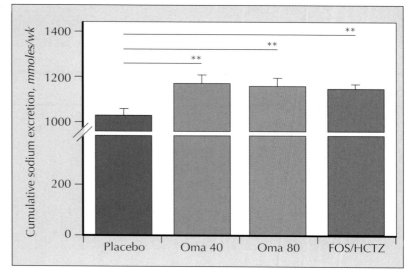

FIGURE 14-43. Effect of omapatrilat (40 or 80 mg/d) and fosinopril/hydrochlorothiazide (20/12.5 mg/d) (FOS/HCTZ) on cumulative 1-week sodium excretion in normotensive subjects. (ANOVA, $P = 0.01$.) Baseline sodium excretion was comparable in all four groups. Although the acute natriuretic response to FOS/HCTZ was significantly greater than that observed with omapatrilat over the ensuing week, the cumulative sodium excretion induced by both doses of omapatrilat was at least as great as that induced by the dose of FOS/HCTZ. *Asterisks* indicate $P < 0.01$ vs placebo. (*Adapted from* Regamey *et al.* [89]).

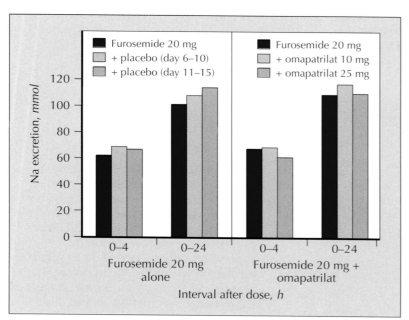

FIGURE 14-44. Single doses of omapatrilat of up to 500 mg in normal subjects does not produce an acute natriuretic response. Pharmacodynamic effects of combination therapy with omapatrilat and furosemide have also been evaluated. In a randomized, parallel-design study of two groups of 13 healthy subjects, both groups received furosemide 20 mg daily for 15 days with concomitant daily treatment of either placebo for days 6 to 15 or omapatrilat 10 mg on days 6 to 10, escalated to omapatrilat 25 mg on days 11 to 15. Furosemide alone produced the expected natriuresis 0 to 4 hours after dosing: coadministration of omapatrilat produced no additional natriuresis or diuresis. Effective renal plasma flow and glomerular filtration rate also did not change in either treatment group. These studies would suggest that the coadministration of either 10 or 25 mg of omapatrilat with 20 mg of furosemide does not affect the pharmacodynamics of furosemide at steady state. (*Adapted from* Uderman *et al.* [90]).

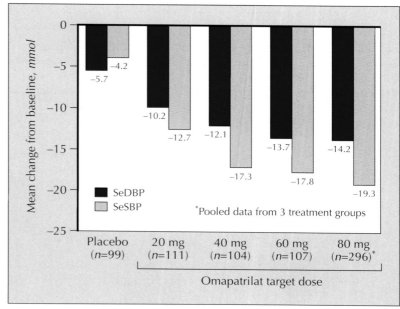

FIGURE 14-45. Mean change from baseline in trough seated diastolic blood pressure and seated systolic blood pressure after 9 weeks of treatment. The change in systolic blood pressure and diastolic blood pressure after omapatrilat 80 mg at peak was -25.8/16/9 mm Hg. With the 80-mg dose, diastolic blood pressure was normalized (<90 mm Hg at trough) in 69% of subjects overall and in 83% of subjects with Stage I hypertension at baseline. Trough-to-peak ratios of 61% to 78% for seated diastolic blood pressure indicated efficacy with once-daily administration of omapatrilat. (*Adapted from Zusman et al.* [91].)

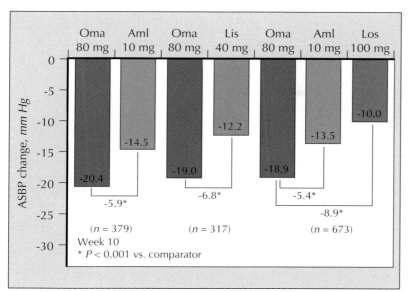

FIGURE 14-46. Changes in 24-hour average ambulatory systolic blood pressure (SBP) with omapatrilat versus amlodipine, lisinopril, or losartan at maximally recommended doses. In the comparison trial with lisinopril, the doses of omapatrilat and lisinopril were forced dose-titrated to 80 and 40 mg, respectively. After 6 weeks at the maximum dose, the 24-hour average SBP was 6.8 mm Hg lower with omapatrilat. In a similar study, omapatrilat was compared with the calcium-channel blocker amlodipine. The differences in the whole-day SBP values were 5.9 mm Hg, favoring omapatrilat. Likewise, at maximal doses, omapatrilat reduced whole-day SBP values by 8.9 mm Hg compared with losartan. (*Adapted from* Asmar *et al.* [92] and Ruilope *et al.* [93].)

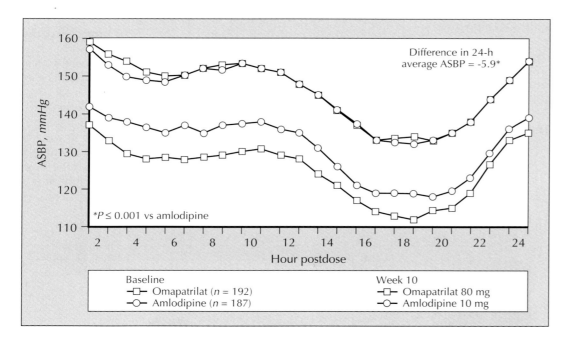

FIGURE 14-47. Twenty-four-hour systolic blood pressure profile for omapatrilat versus amlodipine. The differences in the whole-day SBP values were 5.9 mm Hg favoring omapatrilat. Throughout the 24 hours of study the change in blood pressure for omapatrilat consistently exceeded that for amlodipine. (*Adapted from* Ruilope *et al.* [93].)

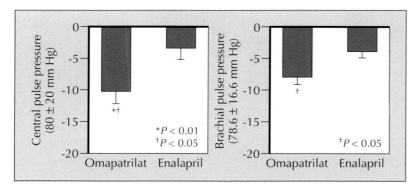

FIGURE 14-48. Central and brachial pulse pressure changes following treatment with omapatrilat and enalapril. Pulse pressure and conduit vessel stiffness was assessed in a 12-week, double-blind, randomized comparison of monotherapy with enalapril (40 mg/d) versus omapatrilat (80 mg/d) in patients with systolic hypertension. Omapatrilat compared with enalapril produced greater reductions in peripheral (-8.2 ± 12.2 vs 4.0 ± 12.2 mm Hg; *P* < 0.05) and central (-10.2 ± 16.2 vs -3.2 ± 16.9 mm Hg; *P* < 0.01) pulse pressures. These data suggest that aortic stiffness is maintained by partially reversible mechanisms and underscore a potential role for pharmacologic modulation of natriuretic peptides in the treatment of hypertension. (*Adapted from* Mitchell *et al.* [94].)

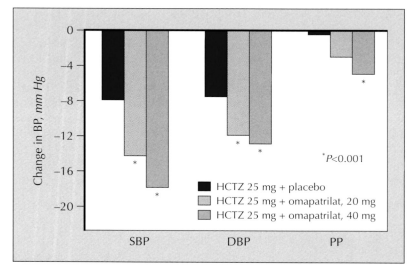

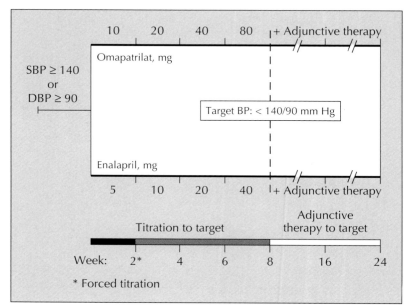

FIGURE 14-49. Study evaluating the safety and efficacy of omapatrilat given in conjunction with hydrochlorothiazide (HCTZ) to subjects unresponsive to HCTZ alone. Subjects with seated diastolic blood pressure between 93 and 110 mm Hg while on diuretic therapy were randomly assigned to omapatrilat 10 mg or 20 mg titrated to 20 and 40 mg/d at week 4. At week 8, additional reductions in systolic, diastolic, and pulse pressures were significant with omapatrilat. Because the antihypertensive effects of omapatrilat and HCTZ appear to be additive, it is unlikely that the effects of omapatrilat on blood pressure are entirely due to diuretic or natriuretic effects. (*Adapted from* Ferdinand *et al.* [95]).

FIGURE 14-50. Study design for the Omapatrilat Cardiovascular Treatment Assessment Versus Enalapril (OCTAVE) trial. This was a randomized, double-blind comparison of omapatrilat and enalapril in 25,267 hypertensive subjects aged over 18 years with a blood pressure equal to or greater than 140 mm Hg systolic and/or 90 mm Hg diastolic either on treatment or not.

The purpose of this trial was twofold; first, to establish whether omapatrilat would be superior to enalapril in clinical use conditions; therein systolic blood pressure from baseline to week 8 was assessed per study group and the use of new adjunct antihypertensives was evaluated from week 8 to 24; second, to determine the frequency of angioedema in comparison to the ACE inhibitor drug class particularly as relates to supposed high-risk patient subsets, such as the black patient.

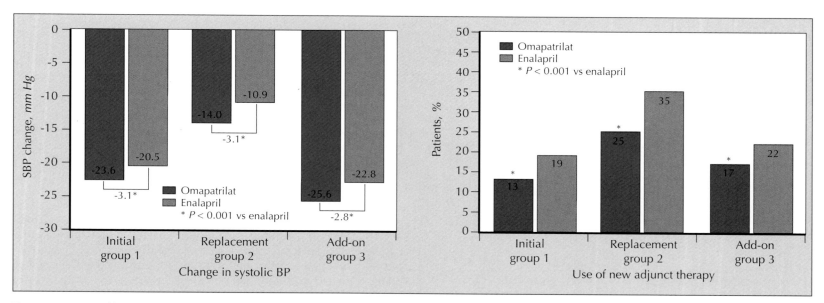

FIGURE 14-51. Efficacy results in the Omapatrilat Cardiovascular Treatment Assessment Versus Enalapril (OCTAVE) trial at week 24. Initial (group 1) were untreated hypertensives (*n* = 9292) randomly assigned to enalapril or omapatrilat (baseline blood pressure 156/96); replacement (group 2) were patients with persistent (JNC stage I) hypertension despite treatment (*n* = 11,224) also randomized to either enalapril or omapatrilat

(baseline blood pressure 150/91); add-on (group 3) were patients with persistent (JNC stage II) hypertension despite treatment (*n* = 4751) randomized to enalapril or omapatrilat (baseline blood pressure 166/97). There was a greater reduction in blood pressure in all case with omapatrilat, despite more frequent use of maximal doses and adjunctive therapy with enalapril [96].

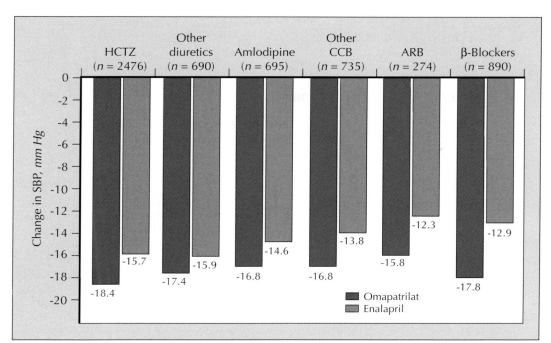

FIGURE 14-52. Change in systolic blood pressure at week 24 in the Omapatrilat Cardiovascular Treatment Assessment Versus Enalapril (OCTAVE) trial for patients receiving adjuncts after week 8. There was clearly a greater blood pressure reduction with omapatrilat, despite more frequent use of maximal doses and adjunctive therapy with enalapril irrespective of what was given as adjunctive therapy. These more favorable results were found irrespective of age, race, or the presence of a comorbid condition [96].

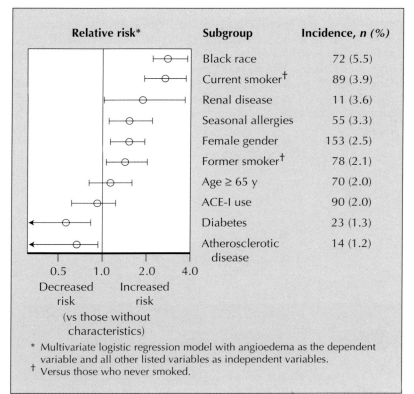

FIGURE 14-53. Summary of angioedema risk with omapatrilat in subgroups. The overall angioedema risk with omapatrilat was considerably higher in black hypertensives, current smokers, and individuals with renal disease and less so in those with diabetes. This risk of angioedema has proved to be a limiting factor in the regulatory approval of omapatrilat and has slowed the experimental development of other compounds in this class [96].

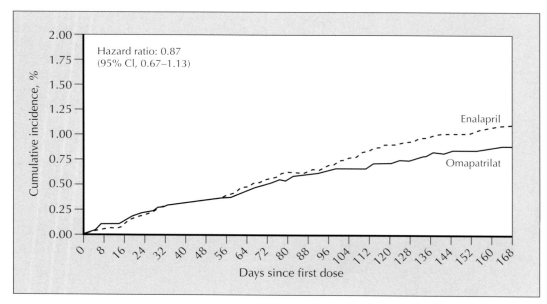

FIGURE 14-54. Cumulative incidence of cardiovascular events in the Omapatrilat Versus Enalapril Randomized Trial of Utility in Reducing Events (OVERTURE). A total of 5770 patients with New York Heart Association class II to IV heart failure were randomly assigned to double-blind treatment with either enalapril (10-mg BID [n = 2884]) or omapatrilat (40 mg once daily [n = 2886]) for a mean of 14.5 months. The primary endpoint (the combined risk of death or hospitalization for heart failure requiring intravenous treatment) was used prospectively to test both a superiority and noninferiority hypothesis. A primary endpoint was achieved in 973 patients in the enalapril group and in 914 patients in the omapatrilat group (hazard ratio, 0.94; 95% CI 0.86–1.03; P = 0.187])—a result that fulfilled prespecified criteria for noninferiority but not for superiority. The omapatrilat group also had a 9% lower risk of cardiovascular death or hospitalization (P = 0.024) and a 6% lower risk of death (P = 0.339). Omapatrilat reduces the risk of death and hospitalization in chronic heart failure but was not more effective than ACE inhibition alone in reducing the risk of a primary clinical event. (*Adapted from* Packer *et al.* [97].)

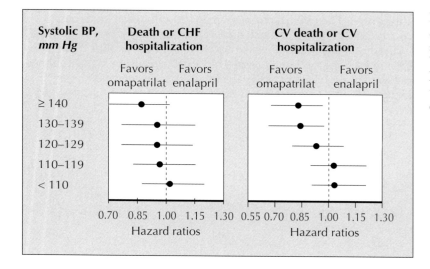

FIGURE 14-55. Omapatrilat and enalapril hazard ratios reported according to the systolic blood pressure value at the onset of the study in the Omapatrilat Versus Enalapril Randomized Trial of Utility in Reducing Events (OVERTURE). Those patients with the highest systolic blood pressure (> 140 mm Hg) at the beginning of the study showed the greatest difference between omapatrilat and enalapril for the primary endpoint. (*Adapted from* Packer *et al.* [97].)

REFERENCES

1. Mooser V, Nussberger J, Juillerat L, *et al.*: Reactive hyperreninemia is a major determinant of plasma angiotensin II during ACE inhibition. *J Cardiovasc Pharmacol* 1990, 15:276–282.

2. van den Meiracker AH, Man in 't Veld AJ, Admiraal PJ, *et al.*: Partial escape of angiotensin converting enzyme (ACE) inhibition during prolonged ACE inhibitor treatment: does it exist and does it affect the antihypertensive response? *J Hypertens* 1992, 10:803–812.

3. Ihara M, Urata H, Kinoshita A, *et al.*: Increased chymase-dependent angiotensin II formation in human atherosclerotic aorta. *Hypertension* 1999, 33:1399–1405.

4. Unger T: The angiotensin type 2 receptor: variations on an enigmatic theme. *J Hypertens* 1999, 17:1775–1786.

5. Hollenberg NK, Fisher ND, Price DA: Pathways for angiotensin II generation in intact human tissue. Evidence from comparative pharmacological interruption of the renin system. *Hypertension* 1998, 32:387–392.

6. Murakami M, Matsuda H, Kubota E, *et al.*: Role of angiotensin-II generated by angiotensin converting enzyme-independent pathways in canine kidney. *Kidney International* 1997, 63:S132–S135.

7. McConnaughey MM, McConnaughey JS, Ingenito AJ: Practical considerations of the pharmacology of angiotensin receptor blockers. *J Clin Pharmacol* 1999, 39:547–559.

8. Mazzolai L, Maillard M, Rossat J, *et al.*: Angiotensin II receptor blockade in normotensive subjects: A direct comparison of three AT1 receptor antagonists. *Hypertension* 1999, 33:850–855.

9. Maillard MP, Wurzner G, Nussberger J, *et al.*: Comparative angiotensin II receptor blockade in healthy volunteers: the importance of dosing. *Clin Pharmacol Ther* 2002, 71:68–76.

10. Ribstein J, Picard A, Armagnac C, *et al.*: Inhibition of the acute effects of angiotensin II by the receptor antagonist irbesartan in normotensive men. *J Cardiovasc Pharmacol* 2001, 37:449–460.

11. Cooper ME, Webb RL, de Gasparo M: Angiotensin receptor blockers and the kidney: possible advantages over ACE inhibition? *Cardiovasc Drug Rev* 2001, 19:75–86.

12. Yasar U, Forslund-Bergengren C, Tybring G, *et al.*: Pharmacokinetics of losartan and its metabolite E-3174 in relation to the CYP2C9 genotype. *Clin Pharmacol Ther* 2002, 71:89–98.

13. McCrea JB, Cribb A, Rushmore T, et al.: Phenotypic and genotypic investigations of a healthy volunteer deficient in the conversion of losartan to its active metabolite E-3174. Clin Pharmacol Ther 1999, 65:348–352.

14. McCrea JB, Cribb A, Rushmore T, et al.: Phenotypic and genotypic investigations of a healthy volunteer deficient in the conversion of losartan to its active metabolite E-3174. Clin Pharmacol Ther 1999, 65:348–352.

15. Kazierad DJ, Martin DE, Blum RA, et al.: Effect of fluconazole on the pharmacokinetics of eprosartan and losartan in healthy male volunteers. Clin Pharmacol Ther 1997, 62:417–425.

16. Meadowcroft AM, Williamson KM, Patterson JH, et al.: The effects of fluvastatin, a CYP2C9 inhibitor, on losartan pharmacokinetics in healthy volunteers. J Clin Pharmacol 1999, 39:418–424.

17. McCrea JB, Low MW, Furtek CI, et al.: Ketoconazole does not affect the systemic conversion of losartan to E-3174. Clin Pharmacol Ther 1996, 59:A169.

18. Goldberg MR, Lo MW, Deutsch PJ, et al.: Phenobarbital minimally alters plasma concentrations of losartan and its active metabolite E-3174. Clin Pharmacol Ther 1996, 59:268–274.

19. Williamson KM, Patterson JH, McQueen RH, et al.: Effects of erythromycin or rifampin on losartan pharmacokinetics in healthy volunteers. Clin Pharmacol Ther 1998, 63:316–323.

20. Goldberg MR, Lo MW, Bradstreet TE, et al.: Effects of cimetidine on pharmacokinetics and pharmacodynamics of losartan, an AT1-selective non-peptide angiotensin II receptor antagonist. Eur J Clin Pharmacol 1995, 49:115–119.

21. Kaukonen KM, Olkkola KT, Neuvonen PJ: Fluconazole but not itra-conazole decreases the metabolism of losartan to E-3174. Eur J Clin Pharmacol 1998, 53:445–449.

22. Fischer TL, Pieper JA, Graff DW, et al.: Evaluation of potential losartan-phenytoin drug interactions in healthy volunteers. Clin Pharmacol Ther 2002, 72:238–246.

23. Zaidenstein R, Soback S, Gips M, et al.: Effect of grapefruit juice on the pharmacokinetics of losartan and its active metabolite E3174 in healthy volunteers. Ther Drug Monit 2001, 23:369–373.

24. Riddell JG: Bioavailability of candesartan is unaffected by food in healthy volunteers administered candesartan cilexetil. J Hum Hypertens 1997, 11(Suppl 2):S29–S30.

25. Tenero D, Martin D, Ilson B, et al.: Pharmacokinetics of intravenously and orally administered eprosartan in healthy males: absolute bioavailability and effect of food. Biopharm Drug Disp 1998, 19:351–356.

26. Bottorff MB, Tenero DM: Pharmacokinetics of eprosartan in healthy subjects, patients with hypertension, and special populations. Pharmacotherapy 1999, 19:73S–78S.

27. Chapelsky MC, Martin DE, Tenero DM, et al.: A dose proportionality study of eprosartan in healthy male volunteers. J Clin Pharmacol 1998, 38:34–39.

28. Vachharajani NN, Shyu WC, Chando TJ, et al.: Oral bioavailability and disposition characteristics of irbesartan, an angiotensin antagonist, in healthy volunteers. J Clin Pharmacol 1998, 38:702.

29. Vachharajani NN, Shyu WC, Mantha S, et al.: Lack of effect of food on the oral bioavailability of irbesartan in healthy male volunteers. J Clin Pharmacol 1998, 38:433–436.

30. Lo MW, Goldberg MR, McCrea JB, et al.: Pharmacokinetics of losartan, an angiotensin II receptor antagonist, and its active metabolite, EXP3174 in humans. Clin Pharmacol Ther 1995, 58:641–649.

31. Laeis P, Puchler K, Kirch W: The pharmacokinetic and metabolic profile of olmesartan medoxomil limits the risk of clinically relevant drug interaction. J Hypertens 2001, 19(Suppl 1):S21–S32.

32. Stangier J, Schmid J, Turck D, et al.: Absorption, metabolism, and excretion of intravenously and orally administered [14C] telmisartan in healthy volunteers. J Clin Pharmacol 2000, 40:1312–1322.

33. Flesch G, Muller P, Lloyd P: Absolute bioavailability and pharmaco-kinetics of valsartan, an angiotensin II receptor antagonist, in man. Eur J Clin Pharmacol 1997, 52:115–120.

34. de Zeeuw D, Remuzzi G, Kirch W: The pharmacokinetics of candesartan cilexetil in patients with renal or hepatic impairment. J Human Hypertens 1997, 11(Suppl 2):S37–S42.

35. Martin DE, Chapelsky MC, Ilson B, et al.: Pharmacokinetics and protein binding of eprosartan in healthy volunteers and in patients with varying degrees of renal impairment. J Clin Pharmacol 1998, 38:129–137.

36. Sica DA, Marino MR, Hammett JL, et al.: The pharmacokinetics of irbesartan in renal failure and maintenance hemodialysis. Clin Pharmacol Ther 1997, 62:610–618.

37. Sica DA, Shaw WC, Lo MW, et al.: The pharmacokinetics of losartan in renal insufficiency. J Hypertens 1995, 13(Suppl 1):S49–S52.

38. von Bergmann K, Laeis P, Puchler K, et al.: Olmesartan medoxomil: influence of age, renal and hepatic function on the pharmacokinetics of olmesartan medoxomil. J Hypertens 2001, 19(Suppl 1):S33–S40.

39. Stangier J, Su CA, Brickl R, Franke H: Pharmacokinetics of single-dose telmisartan 120 mg given during and between hemodialysis in subjects with severe renal insufficiency: comparison with healthy volunteers. J Clin Pharmacol 2000, 40:1365–1372.

40. Prasad P, Mangat S, Choi L, et al.: Effect of renal function on the phar-macokinetics of valsartan. Clin Drug Invest 1997, 13:207–214.

41. Pfister M, Schaedeli F, Frey FJ, Uehlinger DE: Pharmacokinetics and haemodynamics of candesartan cilexetil in hypertensive patients on regular haemodialysis. Br J Clin Pharmacol 1999, 47:645–651.

42. Kovacs SJ, Tenero DM, Martin DE, et al.: Pharmacokinetics and protein binding of eprosartan in hemodialysis-dependent patients with end-stage renal disease. Pharmacotherapy 1999, 19:612–619.

43. Sica DA, Halstenson C, Gehr TWB, Keane W: Pharmacokinetics and blood pressure response of losartan in end-stage renal disease. Clin Pharmacokinet 2000, 38:519–526.

44. Leidig MF, Delles C, Kuchenbecker C, et al.: Pharmacokinetics of valsartan in hypertensive patients on long-term hemodialysis. Clin Drug Invest 2001, 21:59–66.

45. Sica DA, Schoolwerth A: Losartan and uric acid. Curr Opin Nephrol Hypertens 2002, 11:475–482.

46. Sica DA, Cutler RE, O'Connor DT, Ford NF: Comparison of the steady-state pharmacokinetics of fosinopril, lisinopril and enalapril in patients with chronic renal insufficiency. Clin Pharmacokinetics 1991, 20:420–427.

47. Sica DA: Pharmacology and clinical efficacy of angiotensin receptor blockers. Am J Hypertens 2001, 14:242S–247S.

48. Laverman GD, Navis G, Henning RH, et al.: Dual renin-angiotensin system blockade at optimal doses for proteinuria. Kidney Int 2002, 62:1020–1025.

49. Toto R: Angiotensin II subtype 1-receptor blockers and renal function. Arch Intern Med 2001, 161:1492–1499.

50. Vleeming W, van Amsterdam JGC, Stricker BH, et al.: ACE inhibitor-induced angioedema. Incidence, prevention, and management. Drug Safety 1998, 18:171–188.

51. van Rijnsoever EW, Kwee-Zuiderwijk WJM, Feenstra J: Angioneurotic edema attributed to the use of losartan. Arch Intern Med 1998, 158:2063–2065.

52. Sica DA, Black HR: ACE inhibitor-related angioedema: can angiotensin-receptor blockers be safely used? Journal of Clinical Hypertension 2002, 4:375–380.

53. Verresen L, Fink E, Lemke HD, Vanrenterghem Y: Bradykinin is a mediator of anaphylactoid reactions during hemodialysis with AN69 membranes. Kidney International 1994, 45:1497–1503.

54. Saracho R, Martin-Malo A, Martinez I, et al.: Evaluation of the Losartan in Hemodialysis (ELHE) study. Kidney Int 1998, 54(Suppl 68):S125–S129.

55. Sica DA, Gehr TWB: The pharmacokinetics of angiotensin converting enzyme inhibitors in end-stage renal disease. Semin Dialysis 1994, 7:205–213.

56. Sica DA, Gehr TWB: Risk-benefit ratio of angiotensin-receptor blockers vs. angiotensin-converting enzyme inhibitors in end-stage renal disease. Drug Safety 2000, 22:350–359.

57. Pitt B, Segal R, Martinez FA, et al.: Randomised trial of losartan versus captopril in patients over 65 with heart failure) (Evaluation of Losartan in the Elderly Study, ELITE). Lancet 1997, 349:747–752.

58. Kon V, Fogo A, Ichikawa I: Bradykinin causes selective efferent arteriolar dilation during angiotensin I converting enzyme inhibition. Kidney International 1993, 44:545–550.

59. Schoolwerth A, Sica DA, Ballermann BJ, Wilcox CS: Renal consid-erations in angiotensin converting enzyme inhibitor therapy. A statement for healthcare professionals from the Council on the Kidney in Cardiovascular Disease and the Council for High Blood Pressure Research of the American Heart Association. Circulation 2001, 104:1985–1991.

60. Bakris GL, Siomos M, Richardson D, *et al.*: ACE inhibition or angiotensin receptor blockade: impact on potassium in renal failure. VAL-K Study Group. *Kidney Int* 2000, 58:2084–2092.

61. Sica DA: Rationale for fixed-dose combinations in the treatment of hypertension: the cycle repeats. *Drugs* 2002, 62:443–462.

62. Andersson OK, Neldam S: The antihypertensive effect and tolerability of candesartan cilexetil, a new generation angiotensin II antagonist in comparison with losartan. *Blood Pressure* 1998, 7:53–59.

63. Gradman AH, Lewin A, Bowling BT, *et al.*: Comparative effects of candesartan cilexetil and losartan in patients with systemic hypertension. *Heart Disease* 1999, 1:52–57.

64. Easthope SE, Jarvis B: Candesartan cilexetil: an update of its use in essential hypertension. *Drugs* 2002, 62:1253–1287.

65. Viberti G, Wheeldon NM: Microalbuminuria reduction with valsartan in patients with type 2 diabetes mellitus: a blood pressure-independent effect. *Circulation* 2002, 106:672–678.

66. Schiffrin EL, Park JB, Pu Q: Effect of crossing over hypertensive patients from a beta-blocker to an angiotensin receptor antagonist on resistance artery structure and on endothelial function. *J Hypertens* 2002, 20:71–78.

67. Hedner T: Management of hypertension: the advent of a new angiotensin II receptor antagonist. *J Hypertens* 1999, 17(suppl):S21–S25.

68. Schwarzbeck A, Wittenmeier KW, Hallfritzsch U: Anaemia in dialysis patients as a side-effect of sartanes. *Lancet* 1998, 352:286.

69. Mogensen CE, Neldam S, Tikkanen I, *et al.*: Randomised controlled trial of dual blockade of renin-angiotensin system in patients with hypertension, microalbuminuria, and non-insulin dependent diabetes: the Candesartan and Lisinopril Microalbuminuria (CALM) study. *BMJ* 2000, 321:1440–1444.

70. Sica DA: The practical aspects of combination therapy with angiotensin receptor blockers and angiotensin-converting enzyme inhibitors. *J Renin Angiotensin Aldosterone Syst* 2002, 3:66–71.

71. Weir MR, Weber MA, Neutel JM, *et al.*: Efficacy of candesartan cilexetil as add-on therapy in hypertensive patients uncontrolled on background therapy: a clinical experience trial. ACTION Study Investigators. *Am J Hypertens* 2001, 14:567–572.

72. Parving H-H, Lehnert H, Bröchner-Mortensen J, *et al.*: The effect of irbesartan on the development of diabetic nephropathy in patients with type 2 diabetes. *N Engl J Med* 2001, 345:870–878.

73. Brenner BM, Cooper ME, de Zeeuw D, *et al.*: Effects of losartan on renal and cardiovascular outcomes in patients with type 2 diabetes and nephropathy. *N Engl J Med* 2001, 345:861–869.

74. Lewis EJ, Hunsicker LG, Clarke WR, *et al.*: Renoprotective effect of the angiotensin-receptor antagonist irbesartan in patients with nephropathy due to type 2 diabetes. *N Engl J Med* 2001, 345:851–860.

75. Cohn JN, Tognoni G: A randomized trial of the angiotensin-receptor blocker valsartan in chronic heart failure. *N Engl J Med* 2001, 345:1667–1675.

76. Dickstein K, Kjekshus J: Effects of losartan and captopril on mortality and morbidity in high-risk patients after acute myocardial infarction: the OPTIMAAL randomised trial. Optimal Trial in Myocardial Infarction with Angiotensin II Antagonist Losartan. *Lancet* 2002, 360:752–760.

77. Pfeffer MA, McMurray J, Leizorovicz A, *et al.*: Valsartan in acute Myocardial Infarction Trial (VALIANT): rationale and design. *Am Heart J* 2000, 140:727–750.

78. Hansson L, Lithell H, on behalf of the SCOPE Study Investigators: The Study on Cognition and Prognosis in Elderly Hypertensives (SCOPE). Abstracts of Hypertension Prague 2002 Joint 19th Scientific Meeting of the International Society of Hypertension and 12th European Meeting on Hypertension, June 23–27, 2002, Prague, Czech Republic; abstract 0162.

79. Lindholm LH, Ibsen H, Dahlof B, *et al.*: Cardiovascular morbidity and mortality in patients with diabetes in the Losartan Intervention For Endpoint reduction in hypertension study (LIFE): a randomised trial against atenolol. *Lancet* 2002, 359:1004–1010.

80. Dahlof B, Devereux RB, Kjeldsen SE, *et al.*: Cardiovascular morbidity and mortality in the Losartan Intervention For Endpoint reduction in hypertension study (LIFE): a randomised trial against atenolol. *Lancet* 2002, 359:995–1003.

81. Lindholm LH, Ibsen H, Borch-Johnsen K, *et al.*: Risk of new-onset diabetes in the Losartan Intervention For Endpoint reduction in hypertension study. *J Hypertens* 2002, 20:1879–1886.

82. Sica DA, Weber M: The Losartan Intervention for Endpoint Reduction (LIFE) trial-have angiotensin-receptor blockers come of age? *J Clin Hypertens (Greenwich)* 2002, 4:301–305.

83. Weber MA: Vasopeptidase inhibitors. *Lancet* 2001, 358:1525–1532.

84. Burnett JC Jr.: Vasopeptidase inhibition: a new concept in blood pressure management. *J Hypertens* 1999, 17(suppl 1): S37–S43.

85. Kostis JB, Klapholz M, Delaney C, *et al.*: Pharmacodynamics and phar-macokinetics of omapatrilat in heart failure. *J Clin Pharmacol* 2001, 41:1280–1290.

86. Malhotra BK, Iyer RA, Sauce KM, *et al.*: Oral bioavailability and disposition of [^{14}C] omapatrilat in healthy subjects. *J Clin Pharmacol* 2001, 41:833–841.

87. Sica DA, Liao W, Gehr TW, *et al.*: Disposition and safety of omapatrilat in subjects with renal impairment. *Clin Pharmacol Ther* 2000, 68:261–269.

88. O'Grady P, Vesterqvist O, Malhotra B, *et al.* Omapatrilat in patients with hepatic cirrhosis. Pharmacodynamics and pharmacokinetics. *Eur J Clin Pharmacol* 2001, 57:249–257.

89. Regamey F, Maillard M, Nussberger J, *et al.*: Renal hemodynamic and natriuretic effects of concomitant angiotensin-converting enzyme and neutral endopeptidase inhibition in men. *Hypertension* 2002, 40:266–272.

90. Uderman H, Vesterqvist O, Manning J Jr, *et al.*: Omapatrilat: neuro-hormonal and pharmacodynamic profile when administered with furosemide. *J Clin Pharmacol* 2001, 41:1291–1300.

91. Zusman R, Atlas S, Kochar M, *et al.*: Efficacy and safety of omapatrilat, a vasopeptidase inhibitor. *Am J Hypertens* 1999, 12:125A.

92. Asmar R, Fredebohm W, Senftleber I, *et al.*: Omapatrilat compared with lisinopril in treatment of hypertension as assessed by ambulatory blood pressure. *Am J Hypertens* 2000, 13:143A.

93. Ruilope LM, Plantini P, Grossman E, *et al.*: Randomized, double-blind comparison of omapatrilat with amlodipine in mild-to-moderate hypertension. *Am J Hypertens* 2000, 13:134A.

94. Mitchell GF, Izzo JL, Lacourciere Y, *et al.*: Omapatrilat reduces pulse pressure and proximal aortic stiffness in patients with systemic hypertension. Results of the Conduit Hemodynamics of Omapatrilat International Research Study. *Circulation* 2002, 105:2955–2961.

95. Ferdinand K, Saini R, Lewin A, *et al.*: Efficacy and safety of omapatrilat with hydrochlorothiazide for the treatment of hypertension in subjects nonresponsive to hydrochlorothiazide alone. *Am J Hypertens* 2001, 14:788–793.

96. Cardiorenal Advisory Panel, Food and Drug Administration; July 18–19, 2002. http://www.fda.gov/ohrms/dockets/ac/02/slides/3877S2_02_ Bristol-Myers-Efficacy-Safety.ppt. Accessed October 9, 2002.

97. Packer M, Califf RM, Konstam MA, *et al.*: Comparison of omapatrilat and enalapril in patients with chronic heart failure: the Omapatrilat Versus Enalapril Randomized Trial of Utility in Reducing Events (OVERTURE). *Circulation* 2002, 106:920–926.

Accurate and Reliable Blood Pressure Measurement in the Clinic and Home

Clarence E. Grim
Carlene Minks Grim

This chapter reviews the guidelines for accurate and reliable blood pressure (BP) measurement and quality assurance methods that must be implemented in the day-to-day practice of medicine if the proven benefits of detecting and treating high BP are to be translated to the population.

Mastering BP measurement accuracy is the first step toward long-term control. The fact that most practitioners (or persons measuring BP for them today) did not learn or rarely practice or insist on good BP measurement technique may harm more patients than all other medical mistakes combined. Research suggests that poor measurement may be one of the weakest links in the community chain of BP control [1,2]. Problems with observer variations in BP readings, even in trained observers, have also been well documented.

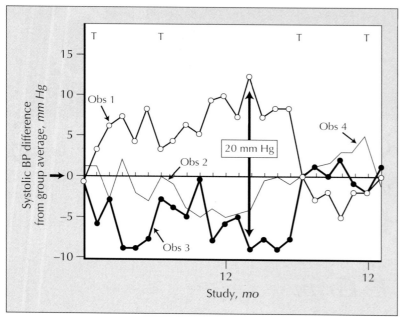

FIGURE 15-1. The effect of training on blood pressure (BP) observer errors. One large research study has indicated that even those who have been retrained benefit from repeated reminders of performance standards. The data in this figure were collected from trained research nurses during the British Heart Study [3]. At the end of the study the investigators were interested in the quality of the BPs taken during the 2 years of the survey. They pooled all BPs taken by all trained observers and then subtracted this number from the pressure taken by each observer. The plot is of the difference (and sign) of the BPs recorded by each nurse by each month of the study. The observers were trained and standardized at the beginning of the study, and the procedure was to be repeated every 6 months as shown at the top of the figure by a "T." Note that at the first T, the BPs recorded were all very close together. However, over time the BPs recorded by observer 1 became consistently higher than the other two observers and observer 2 became progressively lower. With the second training the observer differences narrowed again. However, the training was considered to be tedious and unnecessary by the nurses. It was not repeated for 18 months. Note that at 14 months into the study the BPs recorded by observer 1 and 2 differed by an average of 20 mm Hg systolic. After retraining at 18 months the BPs finally became much closer together. The authors suggest that for research studies, repeated training and testing should be done every few months, but that this would not be practical in routine practice. We disagree. Because major health decisions and treatments are based on readings taken in the clinic, the most rigid quality control should be in place in the day-to-day measurement of BP in the clinic. (*Adapted from* Bruce *et al.* [3].)

HISTORY OF INDIRECT MEASUREMENT OF ARTERIAL BLOOD PRESSURE

1733: Stephen Hales first estimated arterial pressure in the horse.

1828: Nearly 100 years later, Poiseuille introduced the mercury manometer indirect method to reliably measure arterial pressure.

1847: Permanent blood pressure recordings, using a mercury manometer and a rotating smoked drum, were developed by Ludwig.

1876: von Basch developed a clinically useful way to measure the systolic pressure by recording the direct pressure necessary to occlude the pulse at the wrist.

1896: Riva-Rocci connected the manometer to an inflatable cuff that encircled the arm. Indeed, Riva-Rocci's report of the steps and pitfalls necessary for accurate and reliable blood pressures includes nearly all of the steps that we know and teach today. This article has recently been reprinted [4].

1901: von Recklinghausen documented the importance of cuff width, and the standard 12-cm-wide cuff was adopted for "normal" arms.

1905: Korotkoff described the sounds heard over a partially occluded artery that even today remain the simplest and most accurate way to measure blood pressure noninvasively in human and animals.

FIGURE 15-2. The history of indirect measurement of arterial blood pressure (BP). With the advent of standard methods, it became apparent that elevated BP was an important predictor of premature death and disability in patients who reported feeling ill. The term "hypertensive cardiovascular disease" was coined by Janeway [5] after following 458 symptomatic patients with a systolic pressure greater than 160 mm Hg (by palpation) from 1903 to 1912. He noted that 53% of men and 32% of the women had died in this 9-year period, and 50% of those deaths occurred in the first 5 years after being seen. Cardiac insufficiency and stoke accounted for 50% of the deaths and uremia for 30%. By 1914 the life insurance industry had learned that even in asymptomatic men, the measurement of BP was the best way to predict premature death and disability; all insurance examiners were urged to learn to use this most valuable of medical instruments. As stated by Fisher [6] in 1914, "No practitioner of medicine should be without a sphygmomanometer. This is a most valuable aid in diagnosis."

Standardized BP readings predict premature death and disability and cause of death and disability in asymptomatic persons. Population-wide studies of BP in men and women began in 1948 with the Framingham Heart study. The standardized measurement of BP using the guidelines developed by the American Heart Association [7] demonstrated that cardiovascular risk increased continuously from the lowest to the highest levels of pressure and that the systolic pressure was the most predictive measure. At least 91% of those who developed heart failure had high BP before they developed overt congestive heart failure (CHF) [8]. The impact of BP was found to be even more devastating in American blacks in Evans County, GA [9] where 60% of all deaths in black women were attributed to high BP.

These results and the discovery of drugs that lowered BP led to the implementation of large-scale trials in the 1960s, to determine at what level of pressure the risks of lowering high BP outweighed the risks of not lowering it. The design and implementation of these trials required ways to assure that BP would be measured with the same accurate and reliable method by all personnel across several study centers over at least 5 years. Methods of training during these trials and the National Health and Nutrition Examination Survey evolved into a standardized training, certification, and quality assurance program [10] that needs to be translated to the day-to-day practice of medicine if the impressive benefits of these trials are to be translated to the population. We have modeled our videotutored training and certification program on their experiences [2]. This chapter is based on this training program. It should be remembered that in most of the large-scale trials, the difference in BP between the treated and untreated groups over 5 years was less than 10/5 mm Hg. Thus errors of this magnitude, if too low, will deny the proven benefits of treatment to millions of person who truly have high BP but who will be falsely told their BP is normal. (*Adapted from* Janeway [11] and O'Brien *et al.* [12].

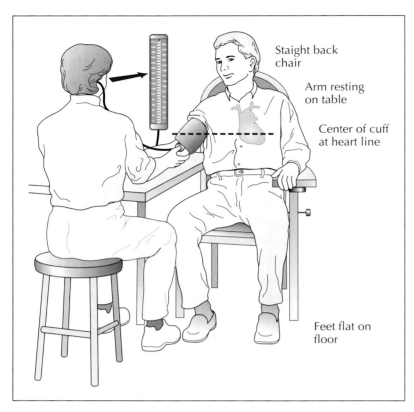

Staight back chair

Arm resting on table

Center of cuff at heart line

Feet flat on floor

FIGURE 15-3. The measurement of blood pressure (BP) in the clinic. If patients are to benefit from the impressive advances made in the treatment of high BP, the office team must have a system that guarantees that BPs taken in your facility are done following the steps needed to get an accurate and reliable BP. This requires that the personnel who measure BP not only have the knowledge and skills required for accurate BP measurement but also that they actually perform every measurement using correct techniques. In the ideal office for BP measurement the patient must be seated in a chair with arm support on both sides and a stand to support the arm when standing BP is being measured. The setting should be quiet and relaxed with a straight back chair for seated readings and an adjustable stand to support the arm for standing readings. Do not measure BP on the examining table, as sitting without back support increases the BP about 5 mm Hg [13]. The chair should be moveable and a table or desk placed so that BP can be easily measured in either arm. It must be easy to adjust the height of the arm so that the middle of the cuff is at heart level (at the 4th intercostal space). The manometer should be placed so the scale is visible at eye level when the observer is seated. We recommend that the observer also be seated, as this decreases extraneous sounds generated by not being able to rest the observer's arms on the table to minimize muscle noise. You should listen to the room to be certain that the heating or air conditioning fans are quiet so that you can hear the soft diastolic sounds. Other sources of noise should also be minimized.

Preparing the patient should be a part of the measurement process. The purpose of preparation is to inquire about, note, and control for factors that cause changes in BP in order to get the best standardized estimate of the pressure at the time. When possible, apply the cuff and discuss the procedure prior to the rest period, then leave the patient alone for 5 minutes. If the patient is not wearing a short-sleeved shirt, provide a gown or have them remove their arm from their sleeve, and remind them to wear a loose, short sleeve garment for future readings. Explanation should include how the measurement is performed and that there should be no talking by the patient or the observer during this time. Also tell the patient that at least two readings will be taken. Some patients worry that something is wrong if more that one pressure measurement is done. The patient is to sit straight against the back of the chair with the feet resting flat on the floor and legs uncrossed. The observer should also inquire about factors that might affect BP now: pain, tobacco use or caffeine ingestion during the last 30 minutes, over-the-counter medications, full bladder, or strenuous exercise.

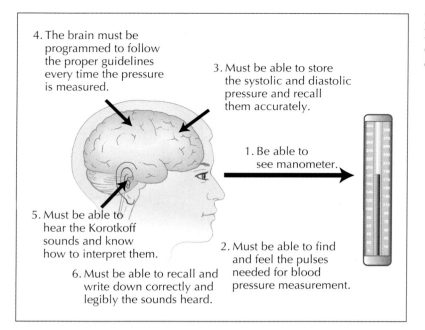

4. The brain must be programmed to follow the proper guidelines every time the pressure is measured.

3. Must be able to store the systolic and diastolic pressure and recall them accurately.

1. Be able to see manometer.

5. Must be able to hear the Korotkoff sounds and know how to interpret them.

2. Must be able to find and feel the pulses needed for blood pressure measurement.

6. Must be able to recall and write down correctly and legibly the sounds heard.

FIGURE 15-4. The skills a good blood pressure observer must have. Skills 1, 3, 5, and 6 can be tested by standardized video tests or multistethoscope testing [2]. Skills 2 and 4 are evaluated by observing as blood pressure measurement is performed.

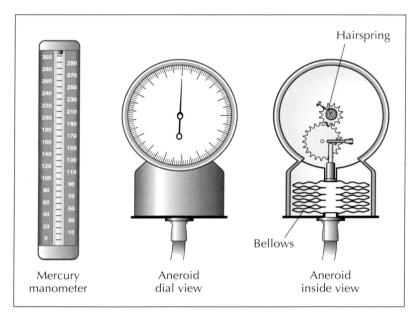

Hairspring

Bellows

Mercury manometer

Aneroid dial view

Aneroid inside view

FIGURE 15-5. The equipment. A mercury manometer and an aneroid gauge (one intact and one with the face removed). The mercury manometer is the primary standard for all pressure measurements. All who measure blood pressure with non-mercury devices should have at least one reference mercury device available to check other devices regularly. The tube containing the mercury needs to be large enough to allow rapid increases and decreases in pressure. The 2-mm graduated markings should be on the tube. The standard glass tube, which can break, should be replaced with either a Mylar-wrapped glass tube or a plastic tube.

The aneroid device, as seen on the inside view, is made up of a delicate system of gears and bellows that can be easily damaged by rough handling and "fatigues" with use and time, leading to inaccuracy. Current research suggests that at least 30% of these devices in use are out of calibration and the error is almost always too low [14,15].

To detect an inaccurate aneroid device, inspect the face for cracks and the needle should be in the zero range. If it is out of this range, it is almost always inaccurate and should be removed from use until recalibrated. How often these devices should be checked has not been determined. The practitioner should realize that once an aneroid device is out of calibration it is difficult to detect the problem without calibrating it against a mercury device. Measurements with an inaccurate device will only be recognized *after* it has been found to be faulty. In a busy office this will lead to dangerous mismeasurement until the next inspection is carried out.

A. CALIBRATING THE MANOMETER

READING	YOUR READING	ELECTRONIC DEVICE	DEVICE ERROR DIFFERENCE (+ OR -)
Systolic 1	122	127	+5
Diatolic 1	78	66	-12
Systolic 2	118	119	+1
Diastolic 2	70	64	-6
Systolic 3	116	110	-6
Diastolic 3	68	65	-3
		Avg systolic error	5+1-6/3=0
		Avg diastolic error	(-12-6-3)/3=7
		Comment	Device reads 7 mm Hg too low diastolic

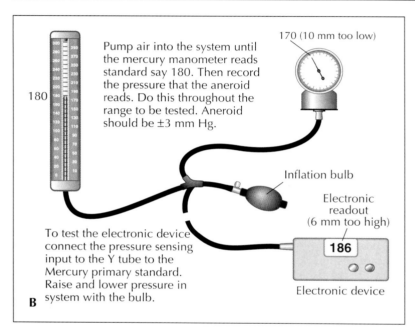

Pump air into the system until the mercury manometer reads standard say 180. Then record the pressure that the aneroid reads. Do this throughout the range to be tested. Aneroid should be ±3 mm Hg.

180

170 (10 mm too low)

Inflation bulb

Electronic readout (6 mm too high)

186

Electronic device

To test the electronic device connect the pressure sensing input to the Y tube to the Mercury primary standard. Raise and lower pressure in system with the bulb.

B

FIGURE 15-6. Calibrating the manometer. **A,** If you have another observer record the pressure with you with a double stethoscope, you will have a more accurate estimate of agreement. Do this at least three times. Compare the average of your readings to those of the electronic device. If this differs by more that 4 mm Hg, the electronic device should be returned to the manufacturer. **B,** Mercury, aneroid, and electronic devices connected by a Y tube. If a mercury device is at zero and the column rises and falls rapidly with inflation-deflation, the manometer is accurate.

The aneroid device must be checked by connecting it to a mercury device with a "Y" tube. Wrap the cuff around a book or can and inflate to 200 mm Hg. Wait 1 minute. Record the pressure. If it is lower than 170, there is a leak that must be found and corrected. This can be done by inflating to 200 mm Hg and then pinching off the tubing to locate the leak. If pinching just before the inflation bulb stops the leak, the leak is in the valve, which can be taken apart and cleaned or replaced. If the leak continues when the tubing is pinched just before the manometer, the leak is in the manometer, and in this case 1) note whether Hg rises and falls smoothly; 2) locate and correct any leaks by replacing the appropriate part, although a leak of less than 2 mm/s can be tolerated in a pinch, as this is the correct deflation rate; and 3) date the device to indicate when it was last

inspected or repaired. Now reinflate again to 200. Deflate the level in the system and check the aneroid readings against the mercury set at the critical decision points for BP: 180, 160, 140, 130, 120, 110, 100, 90, 80, and 70 mm Hg. If the reading differs more than 3 mm Hg at any reading, the aneroid device must be recalibrated by trained personnel or discarded.

To calibrate an electronic device, replace the aneroid device with the electronic instrument in the Y system and check the pressure levels registered on the electronic manometer as noted previously. Activate the inflation mechanism and compare the pressure on the digital display with the mercury as above. In some cases you must squeeze the rolled up bladder to simulate a pulsating arm.

Does the electronic device work on this particular patient? Because electronic devices are not accurate in up to 30% of people, verify reading accuracy in every patient using the following protocol: Choose the correct cuff size and center it over the brachial artery. Palpate the pulse in antecubital fussa and place the bell over the point of strongest pulsation. Trigger the automatic device and listen as it records the pressure. Immediately record your pressure readings at K1 and K5, then record and compare the device pressures.

The British Medical Society regularly reviews the state of the market for devices for blood pressure measurement for hospital, clinic, home, and ambulatory measurements. The last review, done in December 2001, shows the dismal state of the market for accurate and reliable devices [16]. It is interesting that no aneroid device has passed the standards set up by the US American Association for Medical Instrumentation (AAMI) and the British Hypertension Society. Unfortunately, in the United States these devices are not required to meet these standards. We discuss here only the devices for home use. Of the 21 devices that have been formally tested, only five have passed both standards: HEM-737, HEM-713C, HEM-735C, HEM-72C, and the HEM-705CP, all manufactured by Omron Corporation (Tokyo, Japan). Of the five devices for office use that have been tested, only two have passed the standards: Datascope Accutor Plus (Datascope, Montvale, NJ) and the CAS model 9010 (CAS Medical Systems, Inc., Branford, CT). It is interesting that some of the most widely used devices in hospitals and clinics have failed this objective evaluation. All who are involved in using automated devices should keep up to date on the testing results and ensure that devices that are used on their patients should be only those that have passed the standards. One must also validate as accurate at least every 6 months any device that is used on one's patients.

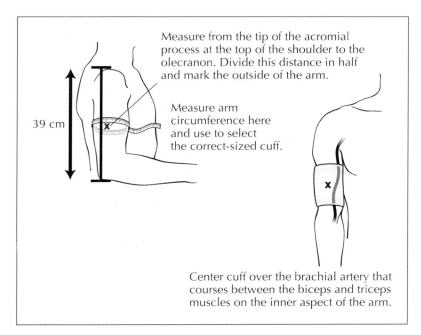

Measure from the tip of the acromial process at the top of the shoulder to the olecranon. Divide this distance in half and mark the outside of the arm.

39 cm

Measure arm circumference here and use to select the correct-sized cuff.

Center cuff over the brachial artery that courses between the biceps and triceps muscles on the inner aspect of the arm.

FIGURE 15-7. Selecting the most accurate cuff. Measure the arm circumference at the midbiceps area. Have the subject stand and hold the arm along the side with the forearm flexed at 90°. Place the 0 end of the tape measure at the acromial process at the top shoulder and measure to the tip of the elbow (olecranon). Divide this length in half and place a small mark on the lateral biceps area. This mark is used later to speed up location of the brachial artery pulse and to position the cuff. Now let the forearm hang down and measure the circumference of the upper arm in a plane parallel to the floor. The tape should lie against the skin without indenting the skin. This circumference is used to select the correct cuff from those recommended by the American Heart Association. The width of the cuff bladder should encircle at least 40% of the arm, and the length of the bladder must encircle at least 80% of the arm. Most cuffs in use are not marked correctly. The correct way to mark the cuff is shown in Figure 15-8.

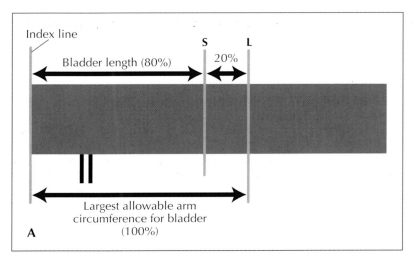

Index line

Bladder length (80%)

20%

S   L

Largest allowable arm circumference for bladder (100%)

A

FIGURE 15-8. The cuff and arm circumference. **A,** It is important to mark the blood pressure cuff so that it is used on arms of acceptable size for the bladder cuff width. **B,** Blood pressure cuff sizes, arm circumference ranges, and bladder widths and lengths.

Many cuffs are not marked at all or are not marked correctly. We recommend doing this measurement yourself and marking the cuff correctly. The observer is where the index line falls when the cuff is placed around the arm. If the index line falls to the right of the "L" line when placed on the arm, use a larger cuff. If the index line falls to the left of the "S" line, use a smaller cuff.

B. BLOOD PRESSURE CUFF SIZES, ARM CIRCUMFERENCE RANGES, AND BLADDER WIDTHS AND LENGTHS

CUFF SIZES	ARM CIRCUMFERENCE RANGE AT MIDPOINT, cm	BLADDER WIDTH, cm	BLADDER LENGTH, cm
Newborn	≤6	3	6
Infant	6-15	5	15
Child	16–21	8	21
Small adult	22–26	10	24
Adult	27–34	13	30
Large adult	35–44	16	38
Adult thigh	45–52	20	42

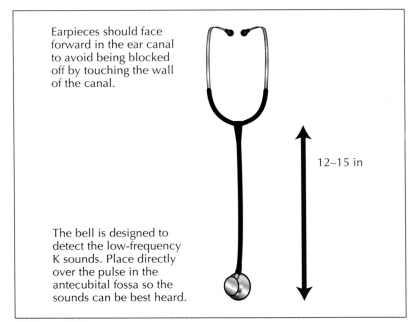

Earpieces should face forward in the ear canal to avoid being blocked off by touching the wall of the canal.

12–15 in

The bell is designed to detect the low-frequency K sounds. Place directly over the pulse in the antecubital fossa so the sounds can be best heard.

FIGURE 15-9. The stethoscope. The bell or low-frequency detector of the stethoscope chest piece is designed for the low-frequency Korotkoff (K) sounds and can be placed more precisely over the source of the K sounds. The tubing should be thick and 12 to 15 inches in length. For sound transmission, earpieces should be worn in the direction of the ear canal, *ie,* toward the patient.

Sometimes the K sounds will be hard to hear. There are two methods to make these sounds louder. The first uses the increased flow of blood into an arm that has been rendered transiently ischemic by exercise. To do this maneuver, inflate the cuff to the maximum inflation level (MIL) (*see* Fig. 15-11) and have the patient forcefully open and close their fist 10 times. Then have them relax the hand and measure the pressure in the standard fashion. If this does not work, the next method combines the first with "draining" the blood out of the arm by holding it straight up over the head for 1 minute, then inflating the cuff another 30 mm Hg above the MIL. The arm is then lowered and the fist squeezed 10 times.

CUFF PLACEMENT AND PULSE DETECTION

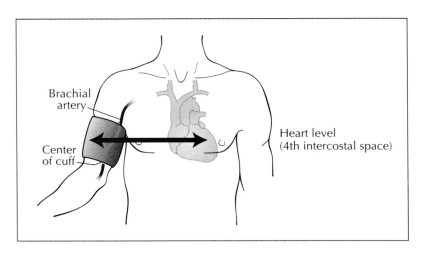

Brachial artery

Center of cuff

Heart level (4th intercostal space)

FIGURE 15-10. Palpate the brachial artery to place the cuff so it exerts pressure evenly and directly over the artery along the inner surface of the arm. Adjust the arm height so that the center of cuff on the arm is at heart level (4th intercostal space). If the center of the cuff is above the this line the pressure measured will be falsely low. If the center is below this line it will be falsely high. Each 1.3 cm displacement from this point will change pressure plus or minus 1 mm Hg.

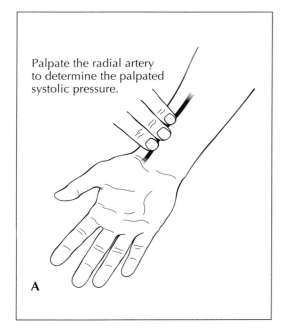

Palpate the radial artery to determine the palpated systolic pressure.

A

B. STEPS TO DETERMINING THE MAXIMUM INFLATION LEVEL

1. Inflate the cuff to 60 mm Hg, then inflate by 10- to 15-mm increments until the pulse can no longer be felt. Inflate another 10 to 15 mm Hg and then deflate at 2 mm/s. Note where the pulse reappears as you deflate the cuff. This is the palpated systolic pressure, which is very close to the true intra-arterial systolic pressure.

2. Release the pressure completely

3. Add 30 mm Hg to the pressure; this is the MIL

4. Place the bell of the stethoscope over the palpated brachial pulse in the antecubital fossa, inflate to at least the MIL, release the pressure at a steady 2 mm Hg/s, and record the readings

FIGURE 15-11. Determining the palpated systolic pressure and the maximum inflation level (MIL). The reason for estimating the palpated systolic pressure and the MIL is to assure that an auscultatory gap does not give the observer a wrong reading. After a rest period of at least 5 minutes, find the MIL. Palpate the radial artery at the wrist (**A**). Use this pulse to determine when the pressure in the cuff has exceeded the systolic pressure. Then determine the MIL as described in **B**.

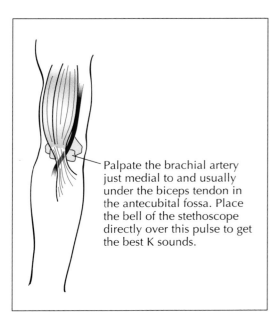

Palpate the brachial artery just medial to and usually under the biceps tendon in the antecubital fossa. Place the bell of the stethoscope directly over this pulse to get the best K sounds.

FIGURE 15-12. Where to listen for the blood pressure sounds. Palpate the brachial artery just medial to and usually under the biceps tendon in the antecubital fossa. Place the bell of the stethoscope directly over this pulse to get the best Korotkoff (K) sounds. If you do not feel this pulse, do not use this arm. Extending the arm as straight as possible makes the brachial artery easier to feel in the antecubital area.

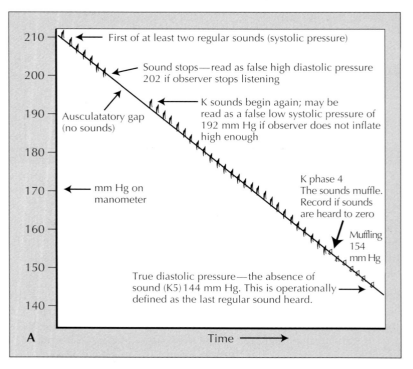

A

210 — First of at least two regular sounds (systolic pressure)

200 — Sound stops—read as false high diastolic pressure 202 if observer stops listening

190 — K sounds begin again; may be read as a false low systolic pressure of 192 mm Hg if observer does not inflate high enough

Auscultatatory gap (no sounds)

180 —

170 — mm Hg on manometer

K phase 4
The sounds muffle.
Record if sounds are heard to zero

160 —
Muffling
154
mm Hg

150 —
True diastolic pressure—the absence of sound (K5)144 mm Hg. This is operationally defined as the last regular sound heard.

140 —

Time ⟶

B. STEPS TO RECORD THE BLOOD PRESSURE READING

1. Inflate the cuff quickly to the MIL
2. Immediately begin to deflate at 2 mm/s
3. Remember the systolic pressure at the point where you hear the first of at least two regular sounds
4. Repeat this number silently to yourself with each heart beat until you detect the diastolic pressure at the point where the last regular sound is heard
5. If K sounds are heard to 0, repeat the reading and note the K4 or muffling and record all three sounds (eg, 142/66/0)
6. Record the arm, position, cuff used, and the systolic and diastolic pressure
7. Wait 1 min

Repeat the reading two more times. Experts recommend discarding the first two readings and averaging the last two.

FIGURE 15-13. Recording the pressure and the auscultatory gap. **A,** Range of Korotkoff (K) sounds. **B,** Steps to recording the reading. The palpated systolic pressure can be used in envi-

ronments that are too noisy to hear sounds. This may be used in an ambulance or in a large crowd or at a health fair where there is loud music. MIL—maximum inflation level.

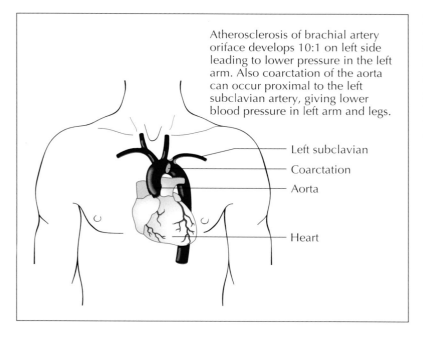

Atherosclerosis of brachial artery oriface develops 10:1 on left side leading to lower pressure in the left arm. Also coarctation of the aorta can occur proximal to the left subclavian artery, giving lower blood pressure in left arm and legs.

Left subclavian

Coarctation

Aorta

Heart

FIGURE 15-14. Which arm should be used? At the first visit blood pressure should be recorded in both arms. This is the only way to avoid missing a large difference between the two arms. This error can be as much as 100 mm Hg. The most common cause of a difference is hemodynamically significant atherosclerotic stenosis of the left subclavian artery. In the screening situation where only one side is to be used, the subject should be asked if they know if one arm is higher and then use that one. Otherwise use the right arm.

OBSERVER

BP Measurement

GRADING BP ACCURACY AND RELIABILITY

Name _____ Date _____

View the videotape and record your answers in the spaces below.

Example Number		Your answer			T	Correct answer	Difference (record sign [±] of diff.)
Example 1	Sys	1	2	8	-	126	+2
	Dias		5	8	-	62	–4
Example 2	Sys	2	2	0	-	220	0
	Dias	1	1	0	-	118	–8
Video 1	Sys				-		
	Dias				-		
Video 2	Sys				-		
	Dias				-		
Video 3	Sys				-		
	Dias				-		
Video 4	Sys				-		
	Dias				-		
Video 5	Sys				-		
	Dias				-		
Video 6	Sys				-		
	Dias				-		
Video 7	Sys				-		
	Dias				-		
Video 8	Sys				-		
	Dias				-		
Video 9	Sys				-		
	Dias				-		
Video 10	Sys				-		
	Dias				-		
Video 11	Sys				-		
	Dias				-		
Video 12	Sys				-		
	Dias				-		

A

BP Measurement – Quality Assessment

GRADING BP ACCURACY AND RELIABILITY ACCURACY:

Subtract the correct answer from your answer and place this difference (with sign) in the "Difference" column. Count and record the differences you have from the correct answers in the table below.

Accuracy Table

Range	0	±2	±4	±6	≥±8
Count					

To be graded as accurate you should have at least 22 answers that are ±2 and only 2 can be ±4 mm Hg.

ARE YOU ACCURATE?   YES   NO

If you have answers that are ±8 or greater it is likely that you misread the manometer by about 10 mm Hg.

RELIABILITY:

Each of the examples you saw in the standardized video-test was repeated in the sequence. You should be ±2 mm Hg in all of the repeat pairs. Complete the table below to assess your reliabilty.

Pair	1 and 11	2 and 8	3 and 10	4 and 7	5 and 9	6 and 12
±2?						

ARE YOU RELIABLE?   YES   NO

If you are not reliable it is likely you need to read the manometer more carefully or you have a memory problem.

DIRECTION BIAS:

If you read above or below the correct answer, you have direction bias. Record the number of times your answers are above the correct answer (number of +'s) and the number of times you were below the correct answer (number of –'s) in the table below.

+'s =	Least freq. sign	1	2	3	4	5	6	7
–'s =	Sum of +'s, –'s	8–10	11–12	13–15	16–17	18–20	21–22	23–24

You should have about 50% +'s and –'s. Enter the sum of +'s and –'s here = _____. If this is ≤ 7, you do not have direction bias. If ≥8, match your sum of +'s and –'s with the cell in the bottom row of the table above. If your least frequent sign is ≤ the value in the cell above it (in the top row) you have direction bias ($P < 0.05$). If you tend to read the systolic too low and the diastolic too high you may have a hearing problem.

TERMINAL DIGIT BIAS:

The last digit of a BP reading should end in an even number if you follow AHA guidelines. Count the number of times your answers ended in 0 and enter it into the "n" row in the table below under the 0's column. Repeat for 2's, 4's, 6's, and 8's. Any answer ending in an odd number is wrong.

End digit =	0's	2's	4's	6's	8's	odd#?
n =						
n^2 =						

Now square each "n" and enter it in the n^2= row. Now add the n^2 in this row and enter here Σn^2 = _____. If $\Sigma n^2 \geq 161$ you have terminal digit bias ($P < 0.05$). You need to be more careful.

DO YOU HAVE TERMINAL DIGIT BIAS?   YES   NO

BETWEEN OBSERVER BIAS can be assessed by comparing your answers with others who watched the same video.

B

FIGURE 15-15. Testing observer accuracy with the standardized videotest (**A**) or triple stethoscope (**B**). We have developed this form to standardize the evaluation of observer accuracy under two circumstances. For videotape testing, the observers being tested view a test tape of 12 examples and then the correct answers are provided. This same form can be used with a double stethoscope testing method, in which the instructor listens with the student. The results are graded in the same way. The form can also be used to assess terminal digit bias on 12 random blood pressure (BP) readings.

At least yearly all staff who take BP should 1) be observed while taking seated/standing BP and have their technique corrected if needed; 2) be tested with a multistethoscope for their ability to hear and record the BPs accurately; 3) be tested with a standardized video test for accuracy, reliability, terminal digit bias, and direction bias. Those who have these errors should be counseled and retested every month until there is no bias; and 4) be assessed for terminal digit bias in readings taken on 12 previous patients.

Although the American Heart Association standards for BP measurement have been published since 1939, these standards are rarely taught to those who today are being trained to take BP.

If the observer is inaccurate, we suggest reviewing the teaching videotapes and then one-on-one teaching of the actual technique. Then the observer should be retested with the videotape and by return demonstration testing. Those who cannot master the technique and are not accurate and reliable should not be measuring BPs. (*Adapted from* Grim and Grim [2].)

EQUIPMENT INSPECTION FOR QUALITY ASSURANCE

TESTING THE MERCURY MANOMETER

Check the "0". Top of meniscus should rest at the zero mark. Add/remove Hg.

Inflate to 200 mm Hg. Wait 1 minute. Record pressure. If lower than 170 there is a leak. Release pressure.

Note whether Hg rises and falls smoothly

Locate and correct any leaks by replacing appropriate part

Date device to indicate that it was inspected/repaired today

FIGURE 15-16. Testing the mercury manometer. At least once a year, a staff member should inspect each device, document the results, and initiate maintenance if needed.

TESTING THE ANEROID MANOMETER

Does the needle rest at zero? (Discard devices with stop pins.)

Inflate to 200 and check pressure release as for mercury above

Using a Y connector, connect to a mercury device and record the readings at the critical decision points

If any reading is off by ≥4 mm Hg, remove it from service

Place a date on the device that indicates that it was inspected today

FIGURE 15-17. Testing the aneroid manometer. At least twice a year, a staff member should inspect each device, document the results, and initiate maintenance if needed.

FIGURE 15-18. Testing the stethoscope. The stethoscope should be checked periodically for wear and damage.

CHECKING THE STETHOSCOPE

Check ear pieces for obstruction

Check/replace/shorten tubing as needed

Check for a low-frequency detector

REFERENCES

1. McKay DW, Campbell NR, Parab A, *et al.*: Clinical assessment of blood pressure. *J Hum Hypertens* 1990, 4:639–645.

2. Grim CM, Grim CE: A curriculum for the training and certification of blood pressure measurement for health care providers. *Can J Cardiol* 1995, 11(suppl H): 38H–42H.

3. Bruce NG, Shaper AG, Walker M, Wannamethee G: Observer bias in blood pressure studies. *J Hypertens* 1988, 6:375–380.

4. Zanchetti A, Mancia G: The centenary of blood pressure measurement: a tribute to Scipione Riva-Rocci. *J Hypertens* 1996, 14:1–12.

5. Janeway TC: A clinical study of hypertensive cardiovascular disease. *Arch Intern Med* 1913, 12:755–798.

6. Fisher JW: The diagnostic value of the sphygmomanometer in examinations for life insurance. *JAMA* 1914, 63:1752–1754.

7. Perloff D, Grim CM, Flack J, *et al.*: Recommendations for human blood pressure determination by sphygmomanometry. *Circulation* 1993, 88:2460–2470.

8. Levy D, Larson MG, Vasan RS, *et al.*: The progression from hypertension to congestive heart failure. *JAMA* 1996, 275:1557–1562.

9. Deubner DC, Tyroler HA, Cassel JC, *et al.*: Attributable risk, population risk and population attributable risk fraction of death associated with hypertension in a biracial community. *Circulation* 1975, 52:901–908.

10. Curb JD, Labarthe DR, Cooper SP, *et al.*: Training and certification of blood pressure observers. *Hypertension* 1983, 5:610–614.

11. Janeway TC: *The Clinical Study of Blood Pressure: A Guide to the Use of the Sphygmomanometer.* New York and London: Appleton & Co.; 1904.

12. O'Brien ET, Semple PF, Brown WCB: Riva-Rocci centenary exhibition: On the Occasion of the 16th Scientific Meeting of the International Society of Hypertension in Glasgow, 23–27 June 1996. *J Human Hyperten* 1996, 10:705–721.

13. Cushman WC, Cooper KM, Horne RA, Meydrech EF: Effect of back support and stethoscope head on seated blood pressure. *Am J Hypertens* 1990, 3:240–241.

14. Bailey RH, Knaus VL, Bauer JH: Aneroid sphygmomanometers: an assessment of accuracy at a university hospital land clinics. *Arch Intern Med* 1991, 151:1409–1412.

15. Meert RM, Grim CE: Inaccurate blood pressure measurement in the clinical setting: causes and control. Am J Hypertens 2000, 13:A24.

16. O'Brien E: State of the market for devices for blood pressure management. *Blood Press Monit* 2001, 6:281–286.

Felodipine
  pharmacologic properties of, 165
Fibroelastic hyperplasia
  vascular morphology in, 87
Fibromuscular hyperplasia
  renal artery stenosis in, 78, 81
Flux gene
  in hypothetical hypertension model, 10
Framingham Study
  blood pressure measurement in, 327
  in cardiovascular risk assessment, 109–124
  on weight-blood pressure relation, 30

G

G protein
  adrenoceptors and, 43
  angiotensin receptors and, 71–72
Gender
  hypertension and
    cardiovascular risk in, 112, 121–123
    in old age, 264
  isolated systolic and diastolic blood pressure and, 110
  mortality trends and, 284
Genes. See also Genetics
  angiotensin-converting enzyme, 68
  angiotensinogen, 67
  candidate, 8
  hypothetical hypertension-promoting, 10
  renin, 65
Genetic linkage
  principles of, 11
  in rat hypertension model, 7
Genetics
  diet and, 32
  drug effects and, 31
    racial factors in, 204
  expression array in, 33
  of glucocorticoid-remediable aldosteronism, 1–2, 11, 145
  in pathogenesis of hypertension, 1–17
    adducin in, 14
    angiotensinogen gene in, 13–14
    in brachydactyly, 12
    environmental interactions and, 1–2, 23–33
    familial dyslipidemic hypertension in, 16–17
    in hyperaldosteronism, 11
    hypothetical model of, 10
    in Liddle's syndrome, 12
    linkage study in, 11
    parent-child studies in, 3
    population studies in, 3
    rat models of, 1, 4–9
    sodium transport in, 15–16
    twin studies in, 4
    vascular mechanisms in, 85–86
Gestational hypertension
  criteria for, 260
Glomerular filtration rate
  in renal disease, 216–221
Glucagon stimulation test
  in pheochromocytoma, 149
Glucocorticoid-remediable hyperaldosteronism, 1–2, 11, 145
Glucose intolerance
  hypertension associated with, 109–110
Glucose tolerance
  antihypertensive agents and, 171
Growth factors
  in hypertension, 99

H

Handgrip testing
  blood pressure and, 44
Headache
  from eprosartan, 311
Health perception
  as quality of life component, 245–246
  treatment compliance and, 243
Heart failure. See also Congestive heart failure

hypertension-related risk of, 117
Heart Outcomes Prevention Evaluation study, 181, 236–237
Heart rate
  in borderline hypertension, 56
  cardiovascular disease risk and, 121
  circadian pattern of, 45
  as hypertension predictor, 51–52
  spectral analysis of, 46, 50
  sympathetic tone and, 60
Hemodialysance
  angiotensin-receptor antagonists and, 307
Hemodynamics
  of hypertension, 58–60
  of renin-angiotensin-aldosterone system, 214–215
High-density lipoprotein cholesterol
  antihypertensive agents and, 172
  cardiovascular disease risk and, 115–116, 118, 122–123
Home blood pressure monitoring, 258, 276–280
Hydralazine
  guidelines for use of, 289
  in hypertensive emergency, 268, 295
  in pregnancy, 261
  side effects of, 294
Hydrochlorothiazide
  in diabetic renal disease, 231
  in obese patients, 206
  omapatrilat and, 320
  in primary aldosteronism, 141
  race and age and, 197–204
  side effects of, 171
18-Hydroxycorticosterone
  in primary aldosteronism, 138
11β-Hydroxylase deficiency syndrome
  characteristics of, 130
  mineralocorticoid receptors in, 135
17α-Hydroxylase deficiency syndrome
  characteristics of, 131
Hyperaldosteronism
  glucocorticoid-remediable, 1–2, 11, 145
Hypercortisolism, 132–134
Hyperinsulinemia
  as possible factor in hypertension, 30
Hyperkinetic borderline hypertension, 37, 51–52
  β-adrenergic responsiveness and, 55
Hyperlipidemia
  familial combined, 2, 16–17
Hyperplasia
  primary aldosteronism from, 138
Hypertension
  borderline. See Borderline hypertension
  cardiovascular risk in, 185–187
    assessment of, 109–124
  classification of
    by age, 296
    by blood pressure, 298
    by organ damage, 298
  as complex syndrome component, 16
  defined, 285
  diagnostic algorithm for, 280
  essential. See Essential hypertension
  familial dyslipidemic, 2, 16–17
  family history of, 56
  first-line, 156
  heart rate as predictor of, 51
  hemodynamics of, 58–60
  heterogeneity of, 156
  isolated systolic, 269–271
  mild
    defined, 297
    treatment study of, 179, 194–196
  pathogenesis of
    genetics and environment in, 1–33
    nervous system in, 37–60
    renin-angiotensin system in, 63–82
    vascular mechanisms in, 85–106
  prevention of, 188
  public awareness of, 176, 243, 285
  pulmonary, 88
  renal causes of, 81–82
  renovascular, 76–82

risk factors for, 16
secondary, 127–153. See also Secondary hypertension; specific disorders
treatment of. See also Antihypertensive agents; specific drugs
  ADA guidelines for, 299–300
  benefits of, 187
  compliance and quality of life and, 241–255
  extreme, 258, 267–271
  failures in, 294
  Joint National Committee guidelines for, 285–296
  mechanisms of drug action in, 155–173
  mild, 297
  new agents in, 301–322
  nonpharmacologic, 188–196
  patient selection in, 185–207
  renal injury and, 209–238
  special situations in, 257–280
  trials of, 175–183
  WHO guidelines in, 297
  vascular characteristics of, 106
Hypertension Detection and Follow-up Program, 178, 242
Hypertensive crisis
  guidelines for, 295–296
Hypertensive emergency, 295–296
  defined, 267
  survival rates in, 268
  treatment of, 268
Hypertensive urgency
  defined, 267
Hypokalemia
  in mineralocorticoid-induced hypertension, 129
  in primary aldosteronism, 136, 138, 140

I

Indapamide
  mechanism and site of action of, 158
Inferior petrosal sinus catheterization
  in Cushing's syndrome, 134
Insulin sensitivity
  antihypertensive agents and, 171
INTERSALT study, 18–19, 24–25, 193
Intrinsic sympathomimetic activity
  of β-blockers, 160–161
Ion transport
  in pathogenesis of hypertension, 99–100
Irbesartan
  in diabetic renal disease, 234–235
  pharmacologic effects of, 304
    arterial, 310
  trials of, 313
Irbesartan Diabetic Nephropathy Trial, 313
Irbesartan Microalbuminuria Study-2, 313
Isolated systolic hypertension
  borderline, 272
  cardiovascular risk in, 269, 271
  defined, 285
  treatment of, 270
  trials of, 269–271
Isometric exercise
  blood pressure and, 44, 55

J

Janeway
  on blood pressure measurement, 327
Japanese population
  angiotensinogen gene and, 14
Joint National Committee
  blood pressure classification of, 285
  guidelines of, 283, 285–296
    adverse drug effects noted in, 292–294
    antihypertensive agents in, 287–292
    for hypertensive crisis, 295–296
    for lifestyle modification, 287
    for treatment failures, 294
    treatment principles in, 285–286
  mortality statistics of, 284
Juxtaglomerular apparatus
  anatomy of, 64

Omapatrilat
  angioedema from, 321
  development of, 302
  pharmacology of, 318–322
  structure of, 317
  trials of, 318–321
    hydrochlorothiazide and, 320
Omapatrilat Cardiovascular Treatment Assessment
    Versus Enalapril trial, 320–321
OPTIMAAL trial, 315
Organ responsiveness testing, 45–48
Organ transplantation
  cyclosporine-induced hypertension in, 274
OVERTURE trial, 322
Owsjannikow
  rabbit studies of, 38
Oxidative stress
  endothelial dysfunction and, 93–95

P

Paleolithic diet
  modern *versus*, 23
Panic attacks
  hypertension in, 206
Papua New Guinea
  lack of hypertension in, 24
Parasympathetic nervous system
  organization of, 39
Parasympathetic tone
  in blood pressure regulation, 42
  in hypertension, 57
  integrating factors in, 57
  sympathetic *versus*, 40
Parent-child studies
  of blood pressure, 3
Pathogenesis of hypertension
  genetics and environment in, 1–33
  nervous system in, 37–60
  renin-angiotensin system in, 63–82
  vascular mechanisms in, 85–106
Patient positioning
  for blood pressure measurement, 328, 331–332
Patient selection
  for antihypertensive therapy, 185–207
Perindopril
  in rat hypertension models, 6
Perindopril Protection Against Recurrent Stroke Study, 182
Peripheral artery disease
  hypertension-related risk of diabetic, 119
Peripheral-acting adrenergic antagonists
  guidelines for use of, 289
  side effects of, 294
Personality traits
  in borderline hypertension, 58
Pharmacogenomics
  principles of, 31
Phenoxybenzamine
  in pheochromocytoma, 153
Phentolamine
  in hypertensive emergency, 268, 295
Phenylalkylamines
  pharmacologic properties of, 165
Pheochromocytoma
  catecholamines in, 147–150, 152
  conditions associated with, 146
  diagnosis of
    accuracy of tests for, 150
    differential, 146
    imaging in, 151
    strategies in, 152
  medical treatment of, 152
  normetanephrine in, 150
  overview of, 145
  pathologic features of, 146
  perioperative hemodynamics in, 153
  secondary hypertension in, 145–153
Physician visits
  blood pressure and, 44
Physician-patient perception differences
  treatment compliance and, 243

Pickering
  on hypertension genetics, 2
Placental weight
  adult blood pressure and, 28
Plasma aldosterone-plasma renin activity ratio
  in primary aldosteronism, 136
Plasma renin activity
  β-blockers and, 161
  in primary aldosteronism, 137, 140
  in renovascular hypertension, 79–80
Platt
  on hypertension genetics, 2
Potassium
  in essential hypertension, 136
  in hypertension pathogenesis, 15, 20, 100
    in vascular smooth muscle, 99
  mineralocorticoid-induced hypertension and, 129
  in primary aldosteronism, 136, 141
Potassium restriction
  effects on blood pressure of, 27
Potassium supplementation
  blood pressure and, 192
Prazosin
  mechanism of action of, 167
  in pheochromocytoma, 153
  race and age and, 199–204
Preeclampsia
  criteria for, 260
  pathophysiology of, 259
  prevention of, 262
Pregnancy
  hypertension in, 258-262
    classification of, 260
    treatment of, 257, 261–262, 290
Pressor stimuli
  blood pressure and, 44–45
Pressure loading
  vascular luminal diameter and, 89
Preventive therapy, 188
Primary aldosteronism
  adenoma versus hyperplasia in, 138
  diagnosis of, 136, 139–140
  hemodynamics in, 140
  hypertension in, 135
    plasma volume and, 141
    response to surgery and, 142
  hypokalemia in, 136
  imaging accuracy in, 139
  screening tests for, 138
  treatment of, 141–144
Propranolol
  in autonomic function testing, 50, 56
  in borderline hypertension, 56
  compliance study of, 242
  quality of life assessment with, 246–248
  race and, 197
Prostacyclin
  endothelial derivation of, 97
Protein restriction
  in renal disease, 220
Proteinuria
  in renal disease, 219–220, 229–231, 234–235, 237–238
Psychologic well-being
  as quality of life component, 244–246
Public awareness of hypertension, 176, 243, 285
Pulmonary disease
  antihypertensives in, 290
Pulmonary hypertension
  vascular morphology in, 88
Pulse detection
  in blood pressure measurement, 332–333
Pulse pressure
  cardiovascular disease risk and, 114

Q

Quality assurance
  in blood pressure measurement, 335–336
Quality of life
  antihypertensives and, 207, 241–255
  assessment of, 244–246

errors and problems in, 241, 248–249
  future directions in, 255
  relevance and sensitivity of, 249–255
  therapeutic applications of, 246–249
components of, 244
Questionnaires
  in quality of life assessment, 244–245

R

Race
  hypertension and, 258, 272–273
    antihypertensive selection for, 197–204
    pathogenesis of, 23, 272
  kidney function and, 212–213
    in renal disease, 220–221
  mortality trends and, 284
Radial artery
  in blood pressure measurement, 333
Radiotherapy
  in Cushing's syndrome, 133
Ramipril
  in diabetic renal disease, 226, 236
  race and, 273
  trials of, 181, 226–227
RAMP method
  in baroreceptor function testing, 46
Rand Mental Health Index
  in quality of life assessment, 253–254
Rat models of hypertension, 1, 4–9, 91
  in renal disease, 217–218
Recording techniques
  in blood pressure measurement, 334
RENAAL trial, 313–314
Renal artery stenosis
  causes of, 78
Renal disease
  antihypertensives in
    ACE inhibitors as, 205, 209, 217–218, 221–229, 307–308, 311
    angiotensin-receptor antagonists in, 209, 225, 307–308, 311
    diabetes and, 205, 229–238
    Joint National Committee guidelines for, 290
    multiple, 237
    nondiabetic disease and, 221–229
  hypertension in, 87, 209–210
    in benign nephrosclerosis, 87
  ideal blood pressure in, 209, 237
  in Liddle's syndrome, 12
  nephron injury in, 216
  patients at risk of, 215
  proteinuria in, 219–220, 229–231, 234–235, 237–238
  race and ethnicity in, 220
  renin-angiotensin-aldosterone system in, 216
  trials in
    clinical, 218–221, 313–314
    experimental, 217–218
Renin
  immunohistochemistry studies of, 66–67
  in primary aldosteronism, 137
  in renin-angiotensin system, 63–70, 75
    biosynthetic pathway in, 65
    metabolism in, 70
    release mechanisms in, 66
    sodium excretion and, 67
  in renovascular hypertension, 79–80
  in VA antihypertensive study, 203
Renin gene, 65
Renin-angiotensin system, 63–82
  anatomy and physiology of, 64–75
    metabolism in, 70
    overview of, 68
    renin release in, 66
    sodium excretion and, 67
  angiotensin-converting enzyme inhibitors and, 163, 303
  angiotensin-receptor antagonists and, 170, 303
  circulating components of, 76
  defined, 63
  genetics of, 65, 67–68
  pathophysiology of, 76–77
  reactive oxygen species produced by, 86
  in renovascular hypertension, 78–82